Nursing Children and Young People with ADHD

ADHD is one of the most commonly diagnosed behavioural disorders in children and young people. It is a complex and contested condition, with potential causes and treatments in biological, psychological and social domains. This is the first comprehensive text for nurses and other health professionals in this field.

Nursing Children and Young People With ADHD explores the evidence, incorporating and expanding on the new NICE guidelines for practice in this area, to provide an essential knowledge base for practice. The text covers: causes, diagnosis, comorbidity, user and carer perspectives, assessment, treatment and interventions (including those suitable for use in schools), prescribing and the legal background.

An invaluable text for pre-registration student nurses on mental health and children branches, this will also be a useful reference work for post-registration nurses and health professionals seeking evidence-based recommendations for practice.

Noreen Ryan is Nurse Consultant within Child and Adolescent Mental Health Services for Bolton Hospitals Trust. She is part of the NICE practice guidelines development group for the assessment and treatment of ADHD in children, adolescents and adults.

Tim McDougall is Nurse Consultant within Child and Adolescent Mental Health Services in Cheshire and Merseyside and a project manager within the Cheshire and Merseyside Child Health Development Programme.

Nursing Children and Young People with ADHD

Noreen Ryan and
Tim McDougall

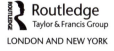

Routledge
Taylor & Francis Group

LONDON AND NEW YORK

2/09

First published 2009
by Routledge
2 Park Square, Milton Park, Abingdon, Oxon OX14 4RN

Simultaneously published in the USA and Canada
by Routledge
270 Madison Ave, New York, NY 10016

Routledge is an imprint of the Taylor & Francis Group, an informa business

Typeset in Garamond by
RefineCatch Limited, Bungay, Suffolk
Printed and bound in Great Britain by
CPI Antony Rowe, Chippenham, Wiltshire

British Library Cataloguing in Publication Data
A catalogue record for this book is available from the British Library

Library of Congress Cataloging-in-Publication Data
McDougall, Tim.
    Nursing children and young people with ADHD / Tim McDougall
and Noreen Ryan.
        p. ; cm.
    Includes bibliographical references.
    1. Attention-deficit hyperactivity disorder—Nursing.
2. Attention-deficit disorder in adolescence—Nursing.   I. Ryan,
Noreen, 1963–   II. Title.
    [DNLM: 1 Attention Deficit Disorder with Hyperactivity.
2. Adolescent.   3. Attention Deficit Disorder with Hyperactivity—
nursing.   4. Child. WS 350.8.A8 M137n 2009]
    RJ506.H9M42366 2009
    618.92'8589—dc22   2008028833

ISBN 10: 0–415–45410–7 (hbk)
ISBN 10: 0–415–45411–5 (pbk)
ISBN 10: 0–203–88423–X (ebk)

ISBN 13: 978–0–415–45410–0 (hbk)
ISBN 13: 978–0–415–45411–7 (pbk)
ISBN 13: 978–0–203–88423–2 (ebk)

Contents

10 Adults with ADHD   154

Introduction 155
How many adults have ADHD? 155
Service provision 155
How do symptoms of ADHD differ for adults? 156
ADHD and relationship difficulties 159
ADHD and parenting 160
Diagnosis 160
Assessment 162
Treatment 163
Summary 165

11 Nurse prescribing and ADHD   166

Introduction 166
Background to nurse prescribing 167
Clinical management plans 168
Training, skills and knowledge 168
Prescribing for children and young people 170
Medication trials 174
Monitoring response to treatment 177
Good practice in nurse prescribing 180
Summary 182

12 Good practice and the legal framework   183

Introduction 184
Policy 184
ADHD and the legal framework 187
Summary 190

Figures and tables

Figures

Tables

Authors

Noreen Ryan, RGN, RMN, ENB 603, ENB 998, BA (Hons), MSc, is Nurse Consultant and Clinical Lead at Bolton Hospitals NHS Trust. Whilst Noreen's key area of expertise is in relation to attention deficit hyperactivity disorder, she is also interested in neurodevelopmental disorders in general. As lead of the ADHD service in Bolton, Noreen is responsible for the strategic and clinical development of the service. As part of her consultation role Noreen provides expert opinions on ADHD, and helps other professionals develop skills and competencies to manage children and young people in a range of settings. After training as a general nurse, Noreen worked as a staff nurse on a neurosurgical unit. After completing post-registration Mental Health nurse training, Noreen worked on an older people's mental health ward before starting her career as a CAMHS nurse. Noreen has worked in both in-patient and community settings and has developed expertise in assessment, parenting interventions, groupwork, and nurse prescribing as well as providing liaison and consultation to colleagues in statutory and voluntary services in primary care, education and social services. Noreen is involved in the strategic development of ADHD services and helped develop the recently published National Institute for Health and Clinical Excellence guideline on ADHD.

Tim McDougall, RMN, BSc (Hons), PG Dip, Specialist Practitioner (Mental Health), ENB 603, is part-time Nurse Consultant (Tier 4 CAMHS) and Lead Nurse (CAMHS) at the Cheshire & Wirral NHS Foundation Trust. Tim is also part of the North West Care Services Improvement Partnership (CSIP) Children and Families Programme Team. Tim has worked in a range of CAMHS settings including community child mental health teams, adolescent in-patient services and secure adolescent forensic services. With a National profile in CAMHS and with over 80 book and journal publications, Tim has spoken at National and European conferences about the mental health of children and adolescents. Tim was formerly Nurse Advisor for CAMHS at the Department of Health in England and is primarily interested in the strategic development and leadership of CAMHS and nursing. Tim helped develop the National Institute for

Clinical Excellence (NICE) guideline for bipolar disorder and the Chief Nursing Officer review of mental health nursing, *From Values to Actions*. When Tim isn't working he enjoys reading, growing chillies and visiting Greek islands with his partner and three children.

Foreword

Nursing is already making an important contribution to the services for children with ADHD. The last decade has seen a rapid increase in service provision in the UK. In many areas there are now dedicated NHS clinics and different health disciplines are working well together; in most areas there has been better access for children to supervised medication. There are many different local styles of organisation and much remains to be done, but it is good to see how quickly services have advanced.

The involvement of nurses has been a highly valued development. ADHD is many things and can be seen in many ways – as this book makes clear – but it is certainly a condition that imposes persistent impairment of function on some children. The model of chronic disability works well, and the nursing disciplines have a grand tradition of helping people to cope with disabilities. Nurses have improved access, provided treatment more effectively and demonstrated a long-term commitment to care.

The increasing role of nurses has not, however, been supported by authoritative accounts of ADHD that are tailored to their context.

This book provides both theoretical bases and practical advice, and should prove a milestone in the development of community mental health nursing.

Better treatments and more precise assessments will emerge in time. The future development of services is likely to be multidisciplinary and based on practitioners' skills rather than their basic qualifications. One of the skills will be the ability to understand the perspectives of other workers. The tensions between education and health, for example, will call for willingness to learn from each other. The eclectic balance in this book should be helpful in communication between agencies.

Eric Taylor
Professor of Child and Adolescent Psychiatry
Kings College London, Institute of Psychiatry, UK
Chair, NICE Guidelines Development Group for ADHD

Preface

ADHD is one of the most commonly diagnosed behavioural disorders in children and young people. It is a complex and contested condition, with potential causes and treatments in the biological, the psychological and the social domains. This is the first comprehensive text for nurses and other health professionals in this field.

Nursing Children and Young People with ADHD explores the evidence, incorporating and expanding on the new NICE guidelines for practice in this area, to provide an essential knowledge base for practice. The text covers: causes, diagnosis, comorbidity, user and carer perspectives, assessment, treatment and interventions (including those suitable for use in schools), nurse prescribing and the legal background.

Covering topics such as basic descriptions of ADHD, context specific interventions in schools and more detailed information about pharmacology, it is hoped that this book will be of interest to the family of nursing professions and others. Appealing to a wide audience, it will be an invaluable text for pre-registration student nurses on mental health and children branches. This will also be a useful reference work for post-registration nurses and health professionals seeking evidence-based recommendations for practice.

Acknowledgements

The authors wish to thank the following people for their help and support in writing this book:

Noreen:

To my husband David for endless cups of tea, encouragement and a sympathetic ear when the going was tough. To my brothers John and James and their families, particularly my nieces Rebecca, Amy and Caitlin and nephews Matthew and Ewan for reminding us all about the joy of childhood. My friends Joanne and Denise for their incredible friendship and laughter, and ability to keep me knowing what is important. To Louise Brindle for her amazing ability to decipher my writing. To Tim without whom this book would not have happened.

Tim:

My children for providing me with something else to worry about; my partner Dr Gemma Wall for her tolerance, patience and support and lending me her frontal lobes for chapter 1; my colleague and friend Martin Bell for distracting me with scrabble when I should have been writing; and of course Noreen Ryan, my co-author, for her hard work, commitment and critical eye.

Abbreviations

AACAP	American Academy of Child and Adolescent Psychiatry
ADD	Attention deficit disorder
ADDISS	Attention Deficit Disorder Information and Support Service
ADHD	Attention deficit hyperactivity disorder
ADR	Adverse drug reaction
AKOS-R	ADHD Knowledge and Opinion Scale Revised
ASRS	Adult ADHD Self Report Scale
BADDS	Brown Attention Deficit Disorder Scale
BME	Black and minority ethnic
BNF	British National Formulary
CAARS	Conners Adult ADHD Rating Scale
CAMHS	Child and Adolescent Mental Health Services
CASR	Conners Adolescent Self Report
CBCL	Child Behaviour Checklist
CBT	Cognitive behavioural therapy
CD	Controlled drug
CGAS	Children's Global Assessment Scale
CMP	Clinical management plan
CNS	Central nervous system
CPRS	Conners Parent Rating Scale
CPT	Continuous Performance Test
CRS	Conners Rating Scale
CSIP	Care Services Improvement Partnership
CTRS	Conners Teacher Rating Scale
DAMP	Deficits in attention, motor control and perception
DBDC	Disruptive Behaviour Disorders Checklist
DCD	Developmental coordination disorder
DCSF	Department for Children, Schools and Families
DfES	Department for Education and Skills
DH	Department of Health
DSM	Diagnostic and Statistical Manual of Mental Disorders
EBD	Emotional and behavioural disorders

ECHR	European Convention on Human Rights
EEG	Electroencephalography
GHQ	General Health Questionnaire
HAS	Health Advisory Service
GP	General practitioner
HKD	Hyperkinetic disorder
HMSO	Her Majesty's Stationery Office
HSQ	Home Situations Questionnaire
ICD	International Classification of Diseases
IBP	Individual Behaviour Plan
IEP	Individual Education Plan
INCB	International Narcotics Control Board
IP	Independent prescriber
KSF	Knowledge Skills Framework
MDT	Multidisciplinary team
MFFT	Matching Familiar Figures Test
MHRA	Medicines and Healthcare Products Regulatory Agency
MRI	Magnetic resonance imaging
MTA	Multimodal Treatment Study of Children with ADHD
NANDA	North American Nursing Diagnosis Association
NCCMH	National Collaborating Centre for Mental Health
NHS	National Health Service
NICE	National Institute for Health and Clinical Excellence
NMC	Nursing and Midwifery Council
NPC	National Prescribing Centre
NSF	National Service Framework
OCC	Office of the Children's Commissioner for England
ODD	Oppositional defiant disorder
ONS	Office for National Statistics
PCT	Primary Care Trust
PE	Physical education
PET	Parent Effectiveness Training
PHSE	Personal, Health and Social Education
PMHW	Primary Mental Health Worker
RCP	Royal College of Psychiatrists
RCT	Randomised controlled trial
SDQ	Strengths and Difficulties Questionnaire
SEAL	Social and Emotional Aspects of Learning
SEN	Special Educational Needs
SENCO	Special Educational Needs Coordinator
SIGN	Scottish Intercollegiate Guidelines Network
SNRI	Serotonin noradrenaline reuptake inhibitor
SP	Supplementary prescriber
SPECT	Single photon emission computed tomography
SSRI	Selective serotonin reuptake inhibitor

UK	United Kingdom
US	United States of America
WASH-U-KSADS	Washington University Kiddie Schedule for Affective Disorders and Schizophrenia
WHO	World Health Organisation
WURS	Wender Utah Rating Scale

Introduction
Setting the scene

Nurses work with children and young people in a range of settings. This includes community and hospital-based health services, schools and colleges, social care settings and the youth justice system. Other primary care professionals including GPs, health visitors and social workers come into contact with children who have ADHD on a daily basis. ADHD is one of the most widely researched and written about disorders in child and adolescent mental health literature. It has been viewed through many different lenses and is as controversial as it is common. There is no single theory of ADHD and we will hear that it can be understood within biological, psychological and social domains.

Like any childhood disorder, understanding ADHD investigates the relationship between nature and nurture. The child's physical development, their early brain growth and neurological functioning represent the domain of nature. Life experiences, the social environment in which the child lives, early care giving and the opportunities that hinder and facilitate positive outcomes represent the domain of nurture. The interplay of nature and nurture is at the core of the assessment process. In recent years there has been an increase in our knowledge and understanding of the links between early childhood development and outcomes in adulthood. It is all too easy to blame the bad behaviour of children on poor parenting, bad diet, too much television and not enough discipline. However, this absolves us of the need to understand. This book will illustrate that there is no simple explanation for ADHD. Instead, it should be understood as a complex, multifaceted disorder where the unique combination of biological, psychological and environmental risk and protective factors combine to produce various outcomes in different children. Seeking to understand this complex interplay, assess how it impacts on the individual child or young person and their family, and planning effective treatment and management strategies requires much skill and patience and is at the heart of nursing interventions.

Much has been written and spoken about ADHD in the popular media and academic press. On the one hand this has enabled a process of normalisation, whilst on the other media coverage has served to fuel the controversy and perpetuate myths about ADHD. For some children and young people, a diagnosis enables an understanding and a framework within which to organise their day-to-day functioning. This can be a liberating and empowering experience. For others, being given a diagnosis of ADHD can generate powerful messages about not fitting in, and being different or less worthy than their peers. The diagnosis becomes stigmatising and an unhelpful barrier to getting along with life. Debate continues about what being diagnosed with ADHD means in a rapidly evolving world. This is in terms of family life and constitution, social expectations and changes in the ways children and young people are educated. The notion that preventative healthcare interventions can prevent all ills and provide a solution to the perceived problems of childhood behaviour problems is unfounded. However, what cannot be in doubt are the devastating difficulties encountered by children and young people and their families who are struggling to cope with and adjust to ADHD on a daily basis. Rarely does ADHD present as a discrete disorder, and we will hear that the problems associated with it are many and varied.

Nurses are encouraged to use 'evidence-based practice' in their day to day work with children and young people. Where it exists, the guidance and good practice recommended in this book is based on high-quality evidence, systematic reviews and the combined knowledge of experts in the field of ADHD. However, evidence about what works is lacking in some areas related to the care, treatment and management of children and young people with ADHD. Here, it is important for nurses and other professionals to articulate 'practice-based evidence' by sharing what children, young people and families want from ADHD service providers and by describing the lived experience of ADHD as it affects children and young people, families and the wider society in which they live. The nurse authors of this book have seen the evidence for themselves, and hope that the book will enable others to use the evidence of ADHD to inform their own nursing practice.

This book sets out the key theories of ADHD, the evidence regarding the aetiology, presentation, classification and prevalence of ADHD and key messages about the care, treatment and management of children and young people with ADHD. It is hoped that this will help the reader to navigate care pathways in health, education, social care and youth justice services, and define best practice for children and young people with ADHD in a range of settings. The National Institute for Health and Clinical Excellence (NICE) has published a major review of what works for children and young people with ADHD (NICE 2008). This highlights ADHD as a discrete disorder requiring specialist assessment and treatment and defines best practice in terms of care pathways, treatment modalities and outcomes. The guideline also reviews the evidence for the use of medication to ameliorate the core symptoms of hyperactivity, impulsivity and inattention. The guidance that emerges is based on the evidence from research, the expert opinions of professionals working in the field and the views of children and young people and their families. This guidance is referenced throughout this book.

It should be no surprise to readers that the authors of this book believe that

ADHD exists and is real. Noreen Ryan has ten years' experience of working specifically with children and young people who present with a cluster of symptoms that amount to a diagnosis of ADHD. Tim McDougall has worked with children and young people with ADHD in community settings, in-patient mental health wards and with young offenders in adolescent forensic services. Both authors have witnessed ADHD having a devastating effect and wide-ranging impact on the child or young person in terms of their place within a family, school, friendship circle and wider community network. They have seen the impact of incessant demands placed on good parents, the obstacles that hinder success and achievement in schools and the effects of social exclusion as children with ADHD and their families are demonised and ostracised. Both authors are optimistic that nurses have the individual and collective potential to make a difference to the lives of children and young people with ADHD and hope this book will be of use in enabling them to do so.

1 What is ADHD, and what is not?

Key points

- For many researchers and clinicians, ADHD is an international disorder with a strong genetic and neurological basis. However, for critics it is a powerful label of social control and a symbol of the medicalisation of childhood.
- ADHD has received much attention in research and in the media, and there exists much debate about causation, over- and underdiagnosis, the medications used to treat this condition and the long-term outcomes for children and young people. Debate continues about the usefulness of diagnosis, the rigidity of the psychiatric classification systems used to diagnose psychosocial difficulties and what are perceived to be the negative effects of labelling and stigmatisation of children and young people.
- Although our understanding of ADHD is becoming increasingly sophisticated, the exact causal pathways of ADHD remain unknown. International research suggests that a biological, psychological and social factors combine to produce ADHD. Cultural variations exist in relation to the degree to which ADHD is considered problematic.
- Determining prevalence rates for ADHD is far from straightforward and depends on a multitude of factors. These include the social and political attitudes of the day, the availability of service provision, and cultural beliefs about the nature and management of childhood behaviour problems (Sayal 2008).
- There is currently not enough evidence to support the restriction of diet as a cause or treatment for ADHD and no evidence for the benefits of adding vitamins, herbal remedies or metals.
- The process of understanding ADHD is complex and relies on skilled and experienced nurses and other practitioners to evaluate the broad range of information and make sense of it within the context of the child's individual development and wider family functioning.

What is ADHD?

A wide variety of terms are used to describe what will be referred to throughout this book as ADHD. This includes attention deficit disorder (ADD), attention deficit hyperactivity disorder (ADHD) and hyperkinetic disorder (HKD). The most widely used overarching term of ADHD refers to a neuro-developmental disorder characterised by a persistent pattern of hyperactivity, impulsivity and inattention that is more frequent and severe than is typically observed in individuals at a comparable level of development (American Psychiatric Association 1994). For the purposes of this book, ADHD is defined as a common behavioural disturbance of childhood, characterised by excessive hyperactivity, inattention and impulsiveness.

Whilst previously considered to be exclusively a disorder of childhood, it is now recognised that ADHD persists into adolescence, adulthood and older age. For children and young people to be diagnosed with ADHD, these symptoms should cause impairment in their psychological, social and educational development and functioning. For adults, impairment is also seen in their occupational and working lives. The degree to which young people are impaired varies, and depends on risk and resilience factors, the coexistence of other psychosocial difficulties and the support networks available to them.

Is ADHD new?

Contrary to popular belief, ADHD is not a new phenomenon. Reference to the hallmark features of inattention, hyperactivity and impulsivity has been made across the centuries (Dobson 2004). One of the first illustrations of ADHD was made in 1845 by Dr Heinrich Hoffman, a German physician and poet, who told the story of 'Fidgety Philip'. He described a child whose behaviour might today be recognised as ADHD (see Figure 1.1 below).

At the turn of the 20th century, two British paediatricians, Sir George Frederic Still and Alfred Tredgold, wrote of a group of children who were described as defiant, emotional, lawless and disinhibited (Tredgold 1908; Still 1902). Believing that these children had a 'morbid and abnormal defect of moral control', these paediatricians suggested that the behaviours of the children were biological and constitutional rather than a product of poor parenting or child rearing. Their findings fuelled public controversy, clinical uncertainty and scientific debate (Biederman and Faraone 2005), and to a large extent this debate continues today.

Another landmark in the history of ADHD was the worldwide epidemic of encephalitis which occurred between 1917 and 1928. Many children survived this outbreak, but were left with impaired attention, hyperactivity, lack of coordination and poor impulse control (Wender 1995). Historical records note that many children who had suffered encephalitis were later diagnosed with *'encephalitis lethargica'* or *'post-encephalitic behaviour disorder'*, the characteristics of which would today be referred to as ADHD (Adler and Chua 2002).

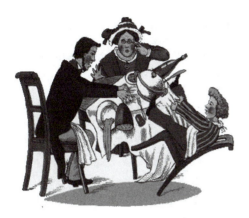

'Let me see if Philip can
Be a little gentleman;
Let me see if he is able
To sit still for once at table.'
Thus spoke, in earnest tone,
The father to his son;
And the mother looked very grave
To see Philip so misbehave.
But Philip he did not mind
His father who was so kind.
He wriggled
And giggled,
And then, I declare,
Swung backward and forward
And tilted his chair,
Just like any rocking horse;–
'Philip! I am getting cross!'

See the naughty, restless child,
Growing still more rude and wild,
Till his chair falls over quite.
Philip screams with all his might,
Catches at the cloth, but then
That makes matters worse again.
Down upon the ground they fall,
Glasses, bread, knives, forks and all.
How Mamma did fret and frown,
When she saw them tumbling down!
And Papa made such a face!
Philip is in sad disgrace.

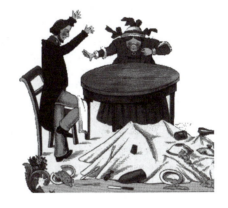

Where is Philip? Where is he?
Fairly cover'd up, you see!
Cloth and all are lying on him;
He has pull'd down all upon him!
What a terrible to-do!
Dishes, glasses, snapped in two!
Here a knife, and the fork!
Philip, this is naughty work.
Table all so bare, and ah!
Poor Papa and poor Mamma
Look quite cross, and wonder how
They shall make their dinner now.

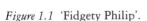

Figure 1.1 'Fidgety Philip'.

During the 1930s in Western Europe and the United States, the terms '*minimal brain dysfunction*', '*imbecility*' and '*idiocy*' came into clinical use due to the similarities shown by patients with central nervous system (CNS) injuries arising from head injuries, infection and toxic damage (Rafalovich 2001; Schacher and Tannock 2002). Later in the 1950s the diagnostic label was changed to '*hyperactive child syndrome*', or '*poor impulse control*', reflecting that no underlying organic damage had been identified. In 1968 the term was once again modified to '*hyperkinetic reaction of childhood*' and was included in the Diagnostic and Statistical Manual of Mental Disorders (DSM) (Spencer *et al.* 2007). The current definition of attention deficit hyperactivity disorder (ADHD) originates in the US and is in common use today. The ADHD debate continues all over the world, and is now much more informed by data from high-quality empirical studies of epidemiology, cause, pathophysiology and treatment than observational studies (Swanson 1998a; Barkley 2002).

How common is ADHD?

Determining prevalence rates for ADHD is far from straightforward and depends on a multitude of factors. These include the social and political attitudes of the day, the availability of service provision and cultural beliefs about the nature and management of childhood behaviour problems (Sayal 2008). As many problems of childhood and adolescence go unrecognised and untreated, prevalence estimates can only reliably be derived from epidemiological surveys. Several confounding factors make comparisons between existing prevalence reports difficult to make. First, rates vary depending on whether clinic, school or representative community samples are studied (Brown *et al.* 2001). Second, prevalence rates vary according to methodological differences, the assessment measures used and whether the ICD or DSM criteria are used. In North America and Australia, the DSM-IV is used and this primarily relates to the diagnosis of attention deficit/hyperactivity disorder, whereas the ICD-10 is used in Europe and refers to a more stringent definition of hyperkinetic disorder, which is a narrower and smaller subgroup of ADHD (Fonagy *et al.* 2002). When DSM-IV criteria are used, point prevalence rates of 5–10% are reported (Fergusson *et al.* 1993), and where ICD-10 criteria are used a prevalence of 1–2% is reported (Swanson *et al.* 1998a). The assessment tools and classification systems used to identify and diagnose ADHD are discussed in detail in the following chapters.

ADHD: a worldwide phenomenon?

Regardless of which classification system is used, there seems to be little doubt that more and more children are being diagnosed and treated for ADHD. In the UK in the 1980s, one in 2000 children were diagnosed with ADHD. Today, the estimates are closer to six in 2000. Some have reported that referrals of children with ADHD are now overwhelming specialist child and adolescent mental health services (CAMHS) in the UK (Salmon 2005). Rates of increase have been much steeper in the US, with 24 per 1000 children diagnosed in the 1980s, and estimates of 70 children per 1000 in the late 1990s (Olfson 2002). Various reports suggest that ADHD is the most common child mental health disorder in the US, and as many as half of all referrals to child and adolescent mental health services are related to this disorder (Barkley 1996; Greenhill 1998; Currie and Stabile 2006).

Despite the popular myth, there appears to be no evidence that ADHD is a by-product of American culture. It is not only in North America that rates of ADHD are reported to be high and rising. A review of studies from 50 countries across the world suggested that ADHD is at least as high in many non-US children as in US children (Faraone *et al*. 2003). In Australia, an increasing number of children with ADHD are being referred to child psychology and psychiatry clinics, with figures as high as 50% for some centres (Mellor *et al*. 1996) and rates of prescribing for stimulant medications mirror those in the US (Reid *et al*. 2002). Prevalence rates across European countries are significantly lower than those in North America (Anderson 1996; Timimi and Taylor 2004). However, an increase in the numbers of children being diagnosed with ADHD does not necessarily mean that the disorder is becoming more common. Rather, it may reflect differences in the definitions of ADHD, the diagnostic frameworks used, improved systems of identification and service delivery and changing attitudes towards disruptive behaviours of childhood and adolescence. Indeed, a large survey of the mental health of over 10,000 children in Great Britain found that there were no differences in the prevalence rates of hyperkinetic disorder in children aged 5–15 between 1999 and 2004 (Green *et al*. 2005). Similarly, a Scottish study compared children referred to a child guidance service and a group of control children matched for age, sex, socio-economic status and ability. All children were scored for hyperactivity using the Conners Teacher Rating Scale (CTRS) (Conners 1989). There were no significant differences in prevalence rates found as compared to US studies using the same measures (Gleeson and Parker 1989). This may suggest that apparent differences in prevalence of ADHD may be due to differences in diagnostic practice rather than true rates of the disorder itself.

Ethnicity and culture

There has been much research into the epidemiology of ADHD and treatments for ADHD, but little research into understanding the role of ethnicity (Gingerich *et al*. 1998). Despite this, ADHD has been variously referred to as a Western middle-class disorder of White boys (Olsfon *et al*. 2002). However, there are few high-quality research studies to qualify this rhetoric, and relatively little is known about how ADHD is experienced and manifested across ethnic groups. Across the world, there exists a range of perspectives held by parents, professionals and society about what constitutes socially acceptable and problematical behaviour (Weisz *et al*. 1991; Mann *et al*. 1992; Dwivedi and Banhatti 2005). Models of parenting, child rearing and behaviour management are each culturally bound and vary enormously across and within cultural groups. In addition, major differences exist in attitudes to help-seeking across ethnic groups (Eiraldi *et al*. 2006). Therefore, it is not surprising that there also exists significant variation in the way in which ADHD is recognised, understood and treated.

Much of the research about ADHD has come from North America and Europe, and it is only recently that the diagnosis has been investigated and recognised in different countries and cultures (Faraone *et al.* 2003). Several studies have illustrated widely differing rates of ADHD between countries and this may be partly due to the range of assessment processes and rating tools used, variations in the age range of children and young people in studies and differences in definitions of impairment which are also culturally determined. However, significant variations have been found even when the same rating tools have been used and these confounding factors have been controlled for. Mann *et al.* (1992) examined levels of hyperactivity in China, Indonesia, Japan and the US. They found that Chinese and Indonesian clinicians gave higher scores for hyperactive and disruptive behaviour than colleagues in the other countries (Mann *et al.* 1992). Dwivedi and Banhatti (2005) studied rates of ADHD in community samples and multi-site cohort studies as reported around the world. What seems evident from these reports is that it is very difficult to standardise views, attitudes and perspectives about ADHD and agree what constitutes acceptable or problematic behaviour (see Tables 1.1 and 1.2).

Does culture influence diagnosis?

The answer to this question is invariably yes, but how so is yet to be determined. Pastor and Rueben (2005) looked at parental reports of ADHD behaviours shown by children in the US to explore whether ethnicity played a

Table 1.1 Worldwide prevalence rates of ADHD

Country	Rate (%)	Assessment tools used	Year
Japan	7.7	DSM-II	1994
China	1.9–13	DSM-III	1992
Israel	5.0	Connors Teacher Scale	1981
Italy	3.9	DSM-III	1993
Spain	16.0	Connors Teacher Scale	1998
Iceland	5.7	DSM-IV	1999
Scotland	4.5	Connors Teacher Scale	1989
UK	16.6	DSM-III	1985
Netherlands	9.5	DSM-III	1985
Canada	5.8	Multiple checklists	1989
USA	7.1–12.8	DSM-IV	2003
Colombia	16.0	DSM-IV	1999
Brazil	5.8	DSM-IV	1999
Australia	12.0	Connors Teacher Scale	1984
New Zealand	15.0	Connors Teacher Scale	1976

Source: Dwivedi and Banhatti 2005

Table 1.2 Worldwide prevalence rates of ADHD

Country	Rate (%)	Assessment tools used	Year
Canada	5.8	DSM-III / parent/teacher rating scale	1989
China	5.8	DSM-III / teacher rating scale / interview	1985
Germany	6.4	DSM-III / rating scale	1995
Hong Kong	6.1	DSM-III / rating scale / interview	1996
India	11.2	DSM-III / parent rating scale / interview	1991
Netherlands	9.5	DSM-III / parent/teacher rating scale / interview	1985
UK	16.6	DSM-III / rating scale	1991
Finland	6.6	DSM-III-R / rating scale / interview	1998
Israel	3.9	DSM-III-R / interview	1992
Italy	3.9	DSM-III-R / rating scale	1993
Japan	7.7	DSM-III-R / rating scale	1994
New Zealand	3.0	DSM-III-R / interview	1993
Spain	14.4	DSM-III-R / interview	1994
Sweden	4.0	DSM-III-R / parent/teacher rating scale / interview	1996
Taiwan	9.9	DSM-III-R / rating scale	1993
Australia	9.9	DSM-IV / parent rating scale	1999
Brazil	18	DSM-IV / interview	2000
Colombia	16	DSM-IV / parent rating scale	1999
Iceland	5.7	DSM-IV / parent/teacher rating scale	1999
Ukraine	19.8	DSM-IV / interview	2000

Source: Faraone *et al.* 2003

role in diagnosis. Rates of the diagnosis of the disorder and use of prescription medication varied between White, Hispanic and African American children, and these differences could not be explained by racial and ethnic variables. Hispanic and African American children were less likely to be reported by parents to have ADHD symptoms and used less prescription medication compared to their White peers (Pastor and Reuben 2005). Similarly, Cuffe *et al.* (2005) used the Strengths and Difficulties Questionnaire (SDQ) (Goodman 1997) as an additional measure to estimate rates of ADHD in a sample of over 10,000 children aged 4–17 years. They found that 4.19% of males and 1.77% of females reached criteria on SDQ rating for ADHD. Rate of ADHD reported in Hispanic boys was 3.06% and girls 0.95%; White boys was 4.33% and girls 1.98% and Black boys was 5.65% and girls 1.87%. The researchers presented their findings with caution since it is known that the SDQ can give false positive and negative results and does not reflect full DSM-IV criteria. Furthermore, their study did not include other ethnic groups such as American Indian and Asian groups. Therefore, Cuffe *et al.* (2005) concluded that further cross-cultural studies are needed to prove that there are true differences in the rates of diagnosis in ADHD across different racial and ethnic groups.

In a large meta-regression analysis of over 100 research studies carried out in 21 countries, Polanczyk *et al.* (2007) found that the highest reported rates of ADHD emerged from Africa and South America. Corroboration came from the use of a dimensional ADHD scale. Children from Japan scored lowest, Jamaican and Thai children scored highest and children from the US scored about average (Polanczyk *et al.* 2007). This seems to cast doubt over claims made by Timimi (2004) and other critics that the phenomenon of ADHD is almost exclusive to Western societies. It is important to consider that most of the information about the impact of ethnicity in the diagnosis of ADHD is from the US and is not readily transferable to the UK. This is because the ethnic population mix is different, and sociological factors such as insurance-led healthcare in the US must be taken into consideration. However, it is clear that the reporting of symptoms by parents in different ethnic, racial and cultural groups is widely variable. It is therefore possible that diagnostic rates could be very different to actual prevalence rates of ADHD, and further high-quality cross-cultural research is needed.

Gender differences

Like all developmental disorders of childhood, ADHD is more common among boys than girls. ADHD has been conceptualised as a disorder of early and middle childhood, mainly affecting males. However, as interest and research into ADHD has grown researchers have felt it necessary to recon-ceptualise ADHD as a chronic disorder in both sexes (Willoughby 2003). Gender differences in the presentation of boys and girls in clinical popula-tions are evident. Brown *et al.* (1991) point out that the ratio of boys to girls who attend specialist treatment services is between 6:1 and 9:1, despite the ratio of boys with ADHD to girls with ADHD in the general population being somewhere in the region of 3:1. This can be partly explained by parental and professional attitudes towards disruptive behaviour. For example, mothers and fathers regard disruptive behaviour in different ways (Singh 2003; Singh 2004), and school-based professionals in particular are more likely to refer boys for assessment of ADHD (Maniadaki *et al.* 2006). Notwithstanding differences related to methodological issues, most North American and Euro-pean population studies concur that boys outnumber girls by at least 3:1 (Szatmari *et al.* 1989; Tannock 1998; Ramchandani *et al.* 2001; Fonagy *et al.* 2002; Voeller 2004; Green *et al.* 2005).

Various studies have suggested that ADHD is more likely to be regarded as problematic for boys (Gaub and Carlson 1997; Swanson *et al.* 1998a; Maras and Cooper 1999), and there are strong associations between hyperactivity and disruptive conduct disorders (Arnold 1996). By comparison, girls show greater skills in self-inhibition than boys, and are less likely to be regarded as 'troublesome' for parents and teachers (Stevenson and Williams 2000; Biederman *et al.* 2002a; Gershon 2002). This not only results in fewer girls referred for ADHD assessment and treatment services (Maniadaki *et al.* 2006) but it also means that there is a risk that girls with ADHD can be ignored or overlooked (Gaub and Carlson 1997; Hinshaw 2002). Largely due to this gender bias in clinical populations, the research base for ADHD has focused more on boys than girls. These factors mean that, just as cultural beliefs influence prevalence rates for ADHD, so too attitudes to behaviour may mask the prevalence of this disorder between the sexes (McGee and Feehan 1991; Reid *et al.* 2000). Further studies are required to focus on gender differences related to ADHD, behavioural and psychological manifestations, associated comorbidities and the developmental trajectory of this disorder in boys and girls. Nurses should be aware of this when providing school-based mental health services or assessing girls for ADHD and other disorders of childhood and adolescence.

What causes ADHD?

Defining disorders of childhood is generally far from straightforward. There is no single consistent causal theory of ADHD and it can be understood within biological, psychological and social domains. Researchers, academics and clinicians use various paradigms to recognise, describe and investigate the condition. For example, biologists investigate the neurological or genetic basis for the condition, psychologists investigate cognitive attributes and sociologists investigate family functioning which implicates both environmental and biological influences. Holistic theories, perhaps ambitiously, attempt to combine all of these together. Each of the domains of knowledge and understanding, both individually and collectively, enables a philosophy and causal model and generates a theory of understanding.

Despite the complexity involved, views have often been polarised in relation to the belief that ADHD is either a medical and developmental disorder, or that it is associated with poor parenting and child-rearing practices (Kendall 1999; Singh 2002; Singh 2004; Dean 2005). However, there is evidence to support genetic, neurochemical, neuropathological and cognitive mechanisms involved in ADHD (Schacher and Tannock 2002). More recently, hypotheses about the origins and predictors of ADHD have evolved from simple, one-cause theories to the view that it is a complex, multifactorial disorder caused by the confluence of many different types of risk factors. These often overlap, so that any one difficulty may act as a proxy for many other risks (Biederman and Faraone 2005; O'Connor *et al.* 2001). Most researchers, academics and clinicians now agree that genetic, biological, environmental and psychosocial factors all play an important part as they combine and interact to produce ADHD and that no single domain or causal factor is necessary or sufficient to initiate this disorder (Beiderman and Faraone 2005).

How can we distinguish ADHD from normal child development?

Where normal childhood behaviour stops and ADHD starts is an area of considerable international controversy and debate. It is generally agreed that hyperactivity, impulsivity and inattention each exist on a continuum of normal development, and there is no clear threshold between extremes of normality and truly abnormal degrees of these behaviours (Baughman 2001; Fonagy *et al.* 2002; International Consensus Statement on ADHD 2002; NICE 2008). Indeed, it has been argued that all children are hyperactive, impulsive and inattentive and that this is just part of being a child (Oas 2001). It is true that ADHD has no claims on the use of the word hyperactive. This term is commonly used to describe a child who is noisy, boisterous or full of energy. The activity level of a child may increase for many reasons including anxiety, fearfulness and as part of general behavioural difficulties (Jones 2003). However, when used to describe a child with ADHD, the term refers to something more serious, pervasive and impairing. The hyperactive child with ADHD will always be on the go. They are often noisy, restless and unable to sit still or quietly for more than a few minutes at a time. Difficulty controlling activity levels can mean that the amount of physical energy and activity they use in the classroom, for example, may be the same as that used in the playground. This is not only exhausting for the child concerned but it is also difficult to cope with for family and friends.

Similarly, inattention and poor concentration per se are not indicators of ADHD. It is not unusual for children to ignore what is going on around them. At one time or another, most children and young people will fail to concentrate or act without properly thinking, and this is a perfectly normal part of development and day-to-day functioning. However, for the child with ADHD concentration can be particularly difficult to sustain, particularly if there is lots going on around them to cause distraction. As a result they may become chaotic, disorganised and struggle to complete the developmental tasks of childhood and adolescence. As they enter adulthood, personal relationships and work commitments can be difficult to maintain and may often break down.

When does hyperactivity, impulsivity and inattention become ADHD?

The continuum theory described above is not unique to ADHD and can be applied to many physical disorders (Faraone 2005), most mental health problems (NICE 2008) and a range of developmental disorders such as diabetes, hypertension, anxiety and depression and autism (Furman 2005). For example, although blood pressure or serum cholesterol levels are continuously varying traits, few would argue that hypertension or dangerously high cholesterol are not medically urgent problems that require treatment (Faraone

2005). It is the impact of impairment in social, academic or occupational functioning that differentiates ADHD from ubiquitous symptoms or normal variations of behaviour (Taylor *et al.* 2004), and this is discussed further in the following chapter. The typical pattern is thus one of a highly energetic, impulsive, delay-averse, unfocused and behaviourally poorly controlled child who demands constant attention and redirection (Harrison *et al.* 2004). Arguably, ADHD can be distinguished from the normal continuum of child development by the number and severity of symptoms and their association with significant levels of impairment (NICE 2008). The younger the child is, the more difficult this distinction can be to make. The more severe forms of ADHD usually present when the child is two or three, but because infants of this age are normally active and have a short attention span, certainty about a diagnosis of ADHD can often be problematic (Fonagy *et al.* 2002).

Myth or reality?

For many researchers and clinicians, ADHD is an international disorder with a strong genetic and neurological basis. However, for the many critics of ADHD it is a powerful label of social control and a symbol of the medicalisation of childhood and misbehaviour (Searight and McLaren 1998; Conrad and Potter 2000; Timimi 2002; Cohen 2006). Since there is no 'gold standard' test to objectively prove that ADHD exists beyond the scope of normal childhood development, there has been debate about its existence and validity. Some have gone as far as to call ADHD a myth and a total, 100% fraud (Shrag and Divoky 1975; Armstrong 1995; Baughman 2006). The biological basis for ADHD has been rejected on the grounds that there is no positive test that proves its existence. This leads some to suggest that ADHD is little more than a social or cultural construction (Baldwin and Anderson 2000; Baldwin and Cooper 2000). In disputing the validity of ADHD as a diagnosis, Jackson-Brown (2005) argues that clusters of behaviour are only brought together in diagnostic terms if they are negative. Positive behaviours, he claims, such as stamp collecting or train spotting, do not warrant the same formulation and are not explained in terms of a diagnostic, biomedical model (Jackson-Brown 2005).

In an attempt to challenge the medical model of ADHD, many writers have suggested that the behaviour problems of children are rooted in social causes. Like children with disabilities, Davis argues, those with ADHD are represented as deficient, tragic, vulnerable and lacking agency (Davis 2007). Locating the origins of ADHD firmly in the social domain, other writers argue that the prescription of medication fails to treat the root social causes of this disorder which originate outside the child and in the world in which the child lives (Lloyd and Norris 1999). Davis goes further to argue that the medical discourse has enabled medical professions and drug companies to monopolise resources and create a culture of dependency (Davis 2007). Some even purport that ADHD has been invented in order to boost drug sales for the pharmaceutical industry (Charatan 2000). This has led to a popular belief that ADHD is overdiagnosed and too many children take medication for no good reason (McCubbin and Cohen 1997; Carey and Diller 2001; Timimi and Radcliffe 2005). However, a number of large population studies have sought to establish how many children are diagnosed with ADHD, what proportion is treated, how they are treated and whether they were prescribed stimulants. According to the Mental Health of Children and Young People in Great Britain report only about half of children with hyperkinetic disorder were taking medication (Green *et al.* 2005). This is supported by epidemiological data from the US which shows that only 12% of children with ADHD receive stimulants (Jensen *et al.* 1999). Perhaps controversially, this may suggest that ADHD is actually underrecognised and that medications are underprescribed.

ADHD: a social construction?

Despite there being widespread recognition of ADHD among health professionals, the validity of the diagnosis continues to be passionately challenged by critics (Faraone 2005; Timimi and Radcliffe 2005; Armstrong 2006). There is no doubt that clinical thresholds are socially and culturally influenced and determine how a child or young person's functioning is viewed as impairing or otherwise (Sonuga-Barke 1998). However, opponents have been concerned about an emphasis on a biomedical model of understanding and explaining children's behaviour (Brady 2005). This, Timimi (2005) argues, is a product of Western society where children and young people are all too often labelled as having psychiatric disorders, behaviour problems and special educational needs (Timimi 2004; Timimi 2005). This notion that ADHD is 'invented' is dismissed by many researchers who report the clustering of hyperactivity, impulsivity and inattention associated with significant impairment throughout the world (Ho *et al.* 1996; Lloyd *et al.* 2006).

Some argue that the concept of ADHD has evolved as a result of over-stressed parents and teachers and the increasing demands placed upon children and families to perform in competitive settings (McCubbin and Cohen 1997; Breggin 2001). Pressure on parents, particularly mothers, to ensure that their children meet societal norms fosters a culture of blame (Davis 2007). Some people claim that ADHD has become an explanation for bad behaviour or a decline in moral standards, implying that some children are simply naughty and do not know how to behave. Locating a problem within the child may be helpful to parents or teachers in understanding the difficulties, but the impact of being labelled for the child or young person themselves varies, and is not always a positive experience. Timimi and Radcliffe refer to this as 'problematising' children, and are concerned that societal influences and the impact of the environment on this process may become overlooked (Timimi and Radcliffe 2005). An international Consensus Statement on ADHD was published in 2002 by over 90 expert clinicians, academics and researchers from 12 countries including the UK (International Consensus Statement on ADHD 2002). This challenged the view that ADHD was a myth, fraud or benign condition, and set out compelling evidence for ADHD as a valid disorder with a strong genetic basis.

ADHD and genetics

The advent of genetically informative studies has had a major impact on knowledge about risk factors for childhood disorders. In order to understand the cause of ADHD as a neurological disorder rather than a socially created phenomenon the role of genetic studies has become increasingly important. Twin and adoption studies are generally the most precise means for estimating relative heritability of a trait (Kidd 2000), and such studies related to ADHD suggest a relatively high degree of heritability. There is strong and consistent evidence from family, twin and adoption studies from all over the world that ADHD symptoms are transmitted in families and influenced by genetic factors (Tannock 1998; Thapar *et al*. 1999; Sprich *et al*. 2000; Biederman *et al*. 1992; Biederman and Faraone 2005; Thapar *et al*. 2005; Faraone *et al*. 2005; Spencer *et al*. 2007).

Research shows that, if a parent has ADHD, there is a greater than 50% chance that at least one of their children will also have the disorder. Although the mechanism for inheritance remains unknown, the high population prevalence (5% to 10%) and modest risk to first degree relatives (about 15% to 20%) suggest that the process for transmission is complex and is likely to be mediated by environmental factors and gender (Plomin and Bergeman 1991; Faraone *et al*. 2001; Voeller 2004; Salmon 2005). Adoption studies have shown that the adoptive relatives of children with ADHD are less likely than their biological relatives to have ADHD or associated disorders (Thapar *et al*. 1999; Sprich *et al*. 2000). Further studies have highlighted a strong heritable component with hyperactivity and impulsivity and chronic antisocial behaviour persisting into adulthood (Hawkins *et al*. 1998; Farrington 2007; Thapar *et al*. 2007). Despite a number of contradictory findings, genetic links, particularly with the neurotransmitter chemical dopamine receptors D4 and D5 have been studied and replicated widely (Swanson *et al*. 1998b; Gill *et al*. 1997; Curran and Taylor 2000; Kirley *et al*. 2002; Holmes *et al*. 2002; Li *et al*. 2006). Notably, dopamine transporter (DAT) levels have been found to be increased in the striatum of children (Cheon *et al*. 2003) and adults (Krause *et al*. 2000) with ADHD.

Applying genetic knowledge to nursing practice

It is important to remember that high heritability for ADHD is not the same as genetic determinism (Taylor *et al*. 2004). Caution should therefore be exercised when discussing the cause of ADHD with parents and carers. In short, there is no specific ADHD gene. Rather, several genes are likely to be implicated, and those within the dopamine transmitter system are most likely to be involved (Kidd 2000). As with all other types of risk factor associated with ADHD, the individual genetic variants associated with the disorder are neither sufficient nor necessary to cause it, but contribute a small increase to the overall risk for ADHD. This helps to explain why some children who are genetically disposed to ADHD do not develop this disorder whilst others do (Johnson 1997; BPS 2000; NICE 2008).

As our knowledge about genetics increases, it is essential that nurses keep on top of developments to inform their practice. It is not only in the field of ADHD that knowledge is expanding. So too has our understanding about the genetic basis of a range of mental disorders including schizophrenia, bipolar disorder and panic disorder. The genetics white paper (Department of Health 2003) outlines how advances in knowledge about genetics are generating more accurate diagnosis, better personalised prediction of risk, new drugs and therapies, and improved targeted services (Department of Health 2003). Understanding the genetic influence on the development of ADHD may enable nurses to offer targeted interventions and inform specific pharmacologic and behavioural therapies (Kirk *et al.* 2006).

Pregnancy and birth

ADHD research concerned with biological adversities has explored difficulties during pregnancy and the immediate neonatal period. Toxaemia, foetal distress and exposure to drugs, alcohol and nicotine in utero have each been cited as associated risks for the development of ADHD. Long labour, prematurity and low birth weight have also been identified as risk factors (Linnet *et al.* 2003; Kent 2005; Linnet *et al.* 2006). The effects of maternal stress during pregnancy, foetal brain development, exposure to drugs and alcohol, obstetric complications and disrupted care during the early years are all thought to increase risks for neurobiological hazards (Schacher and Tannock 2002; Thapar *et al.* 2005; Mill and Petronis 2008). Research from the US and Finland suggests that small size at birth is a strong environmental predictor of ADHD (Bhutta *et al.* 2002; Lahti *et al.* 2006; Nigg and Breslau 2007). These are interesting findings given that foetal growth is known to be an indicator of the environmental exposures that programme foetal development (Mill and Petronis 2008).

ADHD and the brain

ADHD is often conceptualised as a neuropsychiatric or neurobiological disorder because of the close association with central nervous system manifestations. These include hyperkinesis, clumsiness and the higher prevalence of tics and epilepsy in children and young people with ADHD (Fonagy *et al.* 2002; Ford *et al.* 2005). It is thought that the genetic and environmental factors that lead to ADHD do so by altering the brain structures and functions associated with cognitive executive functioning (Salmon 2005). This has been supported by evidence from single photon emission computed tomography (SPECT) studies and magnetic resonance imaging (MRI) studies which show structural and functional differences in the brains of children and young people with ADHD (Zametkin *et al.* 1993; LaHoste *et al.* 1996; Amen *et al.* 1997; Adler and Chua 2002).

Recent research into brain imaging in the US suggests that whilst the brains of children with ADHD generally mature at a normal rate, some aspects of frontal brain development are delayed by up to three years (Shaw *et al.* 2007). This is most evident in the frontal cortex and temporal lobe areas, which play an important role in controlling and focusing thinking, attention and planning, suppressing inappropriate actions and thoughts and working for reward. These are all functions implicated in ADHD. In contrast, the motor cortex area of the brain is thought to mature faster than normal in children with ADHD, which explains their overactivity, restlessness and fidgetiness (Niedermeyer and Naidu 1998) (see Figure 1.2).

There have been significant advances in neuroimaging research in the last decade. Electrophysiological studies have identified abnormalities in the frontal cortex and basal ganglia. These have been associated with deficits of inhibitory and attentional control (Castellanos *et al.* 2002; Rubia *et al.* 1999). However, it is important to note that the conclusions of many brain imaging studies have been criticised because comparison groups have included children who are taking medication as well as those who are not (Castellanos *et al.*

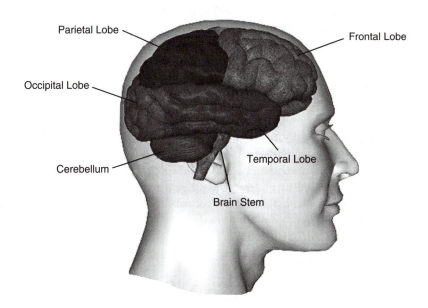

Figure 1.2 The human brain.

2002; Leo and Cohen 2003). This is a confounding factor since it is well known that the use of stimulant medication alters neural functioning and induces brain volume changes in children and young people taking medication (Volkow *et al.* 2002). For this reason, recent studies have differentiated children treated with psychostimulants and those who are medication naïve (Rubia *et al.* 2005).

Environmental factors

It is notoriously difficult to separate the influence of genetics and environment within the family context. The role of genetic influences in ADHD does not exclude the important role of environmental influences for several reasons. Individual differences in genetic risk factors are likely to alter the sensitivity of a child or young person to environmental risks. This may explain why some children seem vulnerable to psychosocial stressors whilst others are not (Caspi *et al.* 2002). Several comprehensive reviews exploring the environmental risks associated with ADHD have recently been published (Williams and Ross 2007; Banerjee *et al.* 2007; Mill and Petronis 2008). There is no evidence that environmental risk factors such as poverty, family chaos, diet or poor parental management directly cause ADHD (Sonuga and Balding 1993; Barkley 1990). However, the role of psychosocial adversity and dysfunctional family relationships in the mediation and maintenance of behaviour problems in children and young people cannot be underestimated. A range of psychosocial factors have strong links with the causes and maintenance of disruptive behaviour in general including poverty (Utting *et al.* 1993; McLoyd *et al.* 1997); poor parental supervision and discipline (Rutter *et al.* 1998); and family-based conflict (Dwivedi and Sankar 2004). Their influence on the development of ADHD as a discrete disorder is less clear and warrants further studies.

Research suggests that it is the aggregate of adversity factors rather than any single factor that leads to impaired child development (Rutter 1988; Institute of Medicine 1989; Rutter *et al.* 1998). Therefore, the greater the number of symptoms of ADHD, the greater the impairment is likely to be (Merrell and Tymms 2005). Several studies have used Rutter's Indicators of Adversity (Rutter *et al.* 1977) to explore the correlation between ADHD, psychosocial risk factors and impairment. After controlling for confounding factors such as parental mental health and gender, Biederman *et al.* (2002b) found that adverse psychosocial factors contributed to the risk of ADHD and its associated morbidity and dysfunction.

How important is diet?

There exists a popular misconception that hyperactivity is caused or exacerbated by food, particularly E numbers (Sonuga and Barking 1993; Wolraich *et al.* 1995). This is largely due to the media who have an interest in promoting controversial treatments, and the marketing of both exclusion and supplementation diets for children with ADHD has been widespread.

Restriction

Elimination diets have been suggested as a treatment for hyperactivity as early as the 1920s. Shannon (1922) noted that a group of children became less fretful, irritable and restless when one or more foods were removed from their diets. It was not until the introduction of the 'Fiengold diet' by a Californian allergist of the same name in the mid-1970s that elimination diets became part of popular culture. Fiengold advocated the restriction of some 3000 additives such as artificial colourings and flavourings as well as natural salicylates in the diets of hyperactive children (Fiengold 1975). However, this was not found to reduce symptoms of ADHD and his research and subsequent advice was later discredited (Conners *et al.* 1976; Mattes and Gittelman 1981; Pliszka *et al.* 1999).

More recently, a randomised, double-blinded, placebo-controlled crossover trial was conducted to explore the effects of artificial food colours and additives on children's behaviour (McCann *et al.* 2007). The study showed that additives commonly found in children's food increased the average levels of hyperactivity in a general population sample of children. The authors concluded that the adverse effects upon behaviour in terms of hyperactivity are not only seen in children with ADHD but in children in general. In other words, some additives make normal children hyperactive and hyperactive children worse.

It is generally accepted that some children may respond negatively to caffeine found in tea, coffee and carbonated drinks and become more active. The food dye tartrazine (E102) and food preservative benzoate can trigger behaviour problems in children (Rowe 1988; Rowe and Rowe 1994). Unfortunately, there is no way of knowing which children will be negatively affected. It is therefore good practice for nurses and other professionals to advise parents to conduct their own trial of restricting certain substances to see if behaviour improves or worsens. It is common sense for parents to restrict a certain food group if they consider that it makes the behaviour of their child worse (Spender *et al.* 2001). Furthermore, if there is thought to be a direct link between a particular food and a child's symptoms of hyperactivity this should be discussed and referral to a dietician should be considered (NICE 2008).

Supplementation

Various studies have explored the effects on hyperactivity caused by supplementing the diets of children with ADHD. Adding magnesium (Kozielec, and Starobrat-Hermelin 1997; Starobrat-Hermelin and Kozielec 1997), iron (Sever *et al.* 1997; Konofal *et al.* 2008) and zinc (Arnold *et al.*

1990; Akhondzadeh *et al.* 2004; Arnold and DiSilvestro 2005) have each been investigated. Perhaps more than any other supplement, there has been much interest in the effects of adding omega 3 fatty acids to the diets of children with ADHD (Richardson and Puri 2002; Voigt *et al.* 2001). Long-chain polyunsaturated fatty acids are essential for the development of nerve cells and their membranes. In addition to contributing to healthy eyes, omega 3 fats are needed for normal brain development and functioning and these are often lacking in modern-day Western diets (Ruxton 2004). Evidence indicates that fatty acid deficiencies may contribute to a range of adult psychiatric and neurological disorders, and to common neurodevelopmental disorders including ADHD, dyslexia, dyspraxia and autistic spectrum disorders (Richardson 2004).

Although this suggests that a diet rich in omega 3 or supplements may be of benefit to children with ADHD and other neurodevelopmental conditions, the few randomised controlled trials that have been published to date have yielded mixed results. The Oxford-Durham study investigated the effects of omega 3 fatty acids on a group of children with developmental coordination disorder. It was evident that there were no changes in motor skills but significant improvements in reading and spelling ages (Richardson and Montgomery 2005). However, whilst these results are promising, they were based on a group of children with dyspraxia, so caution must be exercised when making generalisations in relation to children with ADHD. There is currently not enough evidence-based research to support the restriction of diet as a cause or treatment for ADHD and no evidence for the benefits of adding vitamins, herbal remedies or metals. Parents should not be encouraged to make radical changes and implement major restrictions. Instead, healthy eating should be recommended. With support from nurses, healthy eating can be easily implemented by parents and carers and is likely to benefit the child's emotional wellbeing generally.

Understanding complex issues

It is now widely agreed that there are various developmental factors that impact on the way in which a child behaves. These are physical, cognitive, social, emotional, genetic, environmental and spiritual in origin, and the way in which these factors impact will vary from child to child. It is also generally agreed that developmental progress can vary between children of the same age. This evolving knowledge informs our understanding of what is considered to be appropriate or normal behaviour within expected and predictable developmental norms. Understanding the complex interplay of factors that combine to produce ADHD can be a daunting task, and it is important for nurses and other professionals to consider how ADHD is constructed and conceptualised. They must examine the evidence to validate diagnostic criteria and consider how the presenting behaviours and difficulties interact with genetic, environmental and social influences and evolve over time (Cannon *et al.* 2004). By looking at the interactive nature of adversity we can see how difficulties in one area can have a direct influence on another (see Figure 1.3, Figure 1.4 and Figure 1.5 overleaf).

The process of understanding ADHD is complex and relies on skilled

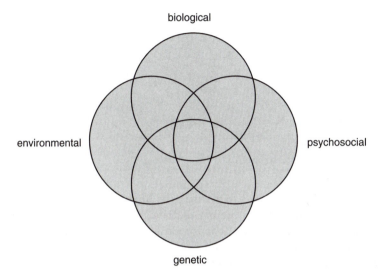

Figure 1.3 ADHD: multifactorial explanations.

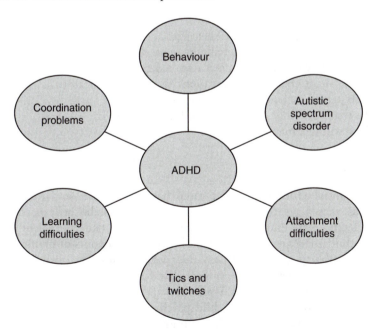

Figure 1.4 ADHD: associated problems.

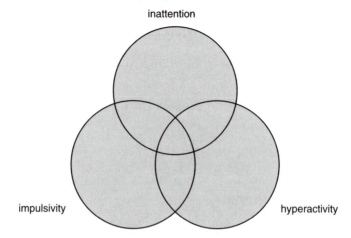

Figure 1.5 ADHD: core symptoms.

and experienced practitioners to evaluate the broad range of information and make sense of it within the context of the child's individual development and wider family functioning. It is important to try and conceptualise and understand what the core symptoms of ADHD (inattention, hyperactivity and impulsiveness) represent to the child and those who are around the child such as parents, siblings and teachers. Key questions to consider are whether the child's behaviours are:

- within the normal range for their age;
- associated with the child's temperament;
- explained by differences in maturational rates;
- the result of changing expectations in relation to reasonable behaviour from parents, school and wider society;
- the result of unmet emotional or educational needs;
- the result of a mental disorder.

Summary

The way in which childhood behaviour has been studied and treated over time has varied greatly. Child guidance clinics, established in the USA in the 1920s, were established to study the deviant and delinquent behaviour of children. Prior to this, the problematic behaviours of children were the responsibility of psychiatrists and paediatricians who were interested in the psychological as well as physical characteristics of children's disorders. Following the Second World War, the expertise of adult psychiatry and paediatrics combined to create child psychiatry, and child guidance clinics from the USA became established throughout Europe and the UK. Since then, ADHD has received much attention in research and in the media, and there exists significant debate about causation, over- and underdiagnosis, the medications used to treat this condition and the long-term outcomes for children, young people and families. With their knowledge of child development, routine contact with schools and an understanding of family relationships and dynamics, nurses are in key positions to make sense of childhood hyperactivity, impulsivity and inattention and begin to formulate the level of impairment that may associate these phenomena.

ADHD is characterised by high levels of inattentive, hyperactive and impulsive behaviours associated with significant impairment in psychological, social or academic functioning. However, there are many potential explanations for hyperactivity, impulsivity and inattention other than ADHD and these will be discussed throughout this book. Although our understanding of ADHD is becoming increasingly sophisticated, the exact causal pathways of ADHD remain unknown. International research suggests that a combination of biological, psychological and social factors together produce ADHD. Cultural variations exist in relation to the degree to which the symptoms generate impairment, and the extent to which ADHD is considered problematic. Ethnic variations in the diagnosis of children with ADHD and service use by their families appear to be the result of a combination of individual, cultural and societal influences, and barriers to access.

2 Diagnostic frameworks and ADHD

Key points

- ADHD is characterised by high levels of inattentive, hyperactive and impulsive behaviours associated with psychological, social or academic impairments.
- Impairments associated with ADHD are the consequences that occur from living with disabling symptoms related to limited self-control and self-regulation. To be diagnostically relevant, these impairments should be pervasive, occur across multiple settings and domains of functioning, and be at least of moderate severity.
- It is important to assess how much impairment experienced by a child or young person with ADHD can be explained by the disorder itself, and how much may be attributable to other personal, social or family-based difficulties.
- The ICD-10 is a multi-axial classification framework for diagnosing a range of mental disorders and is the preferred system used in the UK and Europe. The DSM-IV is a handbook for mental health professionals which includes standardised diagnostic criteria for a range of mental disorders and is used across North America.
- No single professional is likely to be able to provide the breadth and depth of assessment required to accurately diagnose ADHD, and input from the multidisciplinary team is essential.
- The diagnosis of ADHD should only be made by mental health or paediatric specialists following a full clinical and psychosocial assessment of the child or young person and their family.
- Nurses practise holistically and view children and young people who have ADHD as a whole. This does not minimise the potential for using diagnoses but illustrates the importance of providing care focused on individual needs rather than the description of the disorder the child or young person and their families or carers may be experiencing.

Introduction

There are no physical, neurological or laboratory tests that unequivocally correlate the symptoms of ADHD (Kidd 2000), and no matter how experienced or qualified the clinician, the diagnosis of ADHD is anything but straightforward. ADHD is a multifaceted disorder and no single discipline is likely to be competent to identify, assess and intervene alone (Williams and Salmon 2002). Diagnosis therefore becomes a mechanical feature in a holistic process involving a range of professionals (BPS 2000).

The issue of who is competent to make a diagnosis is an area of ongoing debate and controversy and will not be covered in any detail in this chapter. Suffice to say that many clinicians and researchers believe that it is necessary to have a way of grouping and classifying key symptoms, behaviours and abnormal functioning within a valid framework. This is in order to demarcate them from psychiatric 'wellness' and to help clinicians choose appropriate therapies (Robins and Guze 1970; Gowers and Glaze 2005). However, systems of diagnostic classification have not been without criticism. This has been within both the social care and education professions and amongst health professionals too. Debate continues about the usefulness of diagnosis, the rigidity of the psychiatric classification systems used to diagnose psychosocial difficulties and what are perceived to be the negative effects of labelling and stigmatisation of children and young people. This relates both to the criticism of diagnostic frameworks for ADHD specifically, and to psychosocial disorders of childhood in general. Timimi (2004), a passionate critic of ADHD, purports that the starting point for offering a holistic, integrated, multi-perspective model for helping children has to be the rejection of ADHD as a label that offers anything meaningful or useful to clinical practice.

Diagnostic frameworks

Various terms are used to describe and label the symptoms of ADHD. There are two classification systems in regular use to diagnose psychiatric and behavioural disorders in children and young people. These are the International Classification of Diseases (ICD) and the Diagnostic and Statistical Manual of Mental Disorders (DSM), and each identifies inattentive, hyperactive and impulsive symptoms. The DSM and ICD are both categorical models, meaning that minimum thresholds for symptoms must be met before a diagnosis of ADHD can be made. However, it is important to recognise that some children and young people may not meet the defined criteria but may nevertheless be experiencing significant difficulties in their day to day life. Some clinicians refer to such young people as experiencing 'sub-threshold' symptoms of ADHD (Faraone *et al.* 2006). Here, 'watchful waiting' or careful monitoring may be more appropriate than formal diagnosis.

Although diagnostic labels are primarily used as convenient shorthand among mental health professionals (American Psychiatric Association 1994), nurses should be aware that behaviours shown by children and young people rarely fit neatly into diagnostic boxes. Indeed, the majority of children with hyperactive, inattentive and impulsive behaviour are not impaired and should not receive a diagnosis of ADHD. There may be many explanations for each of these symptoms or experiences, and a full and comprehensive assessment is vital in gaining a full understanding about what may be going on for a child and their family.

Impairment

Studies of mental health problems in children and young people have consistently shown that assessing symptom counts alone produces highly inflated prevalence estimates (Roberts *et al.* 1998). Researchers exploring impairment associated with ADHD have also found that symptom count may be an unreliable proxy with poor predictive value (Spitzer and Wakefield 1999; Gordon *et al.* 2006). Despite this, the current world of research remains preoccupied with the objective measurement of symptoms rather than outcomes of treatment. We are aware that impairment also means different things to different people. Whilst researchers and clinicians tend to focus on psychological, social and educational functioning, impairment for children with ADHD is less academic. It is about impact, such as being the only child not invited to a birthday party. Symptom checklists, whilst useful as part of the assessment process, are extremely limited in what they tell us about the lived experience of ADHD (Landgraf *et al.* 2002).

We have heard that symptoms of hyperactivity, impulsivity and inattention exist on a continuum and range from being mild to extremely severe. ADHD affects each child and their family in its unique way. The symptoms vary in the severity with which they impact on the child and their family and social system. Many children experience symptoms without being adversely affected, whilst others become seriously debilitated. Recognised diagnostic criteria require that, in addition to a clinically recognisable set of symptoms or behaviours, a child must show distress or substantial interference with functioning for a diagnosis of ADHD to be made. While some omit this requirement for functional impairment (Pineda *et al.* 1999; Gadow *et al.* 2000), good practice in the UK dictates that a diagnosis of ADHD should only be made if there is clear evidence of clinically significant impairment in social, academic or occupational functioning. Use of the term impairment suggests that these symptoms occur more frequently and at a greater severity than is to be expected of the child's developmentally similar peer group (Taylor *et al.* 2004; Maughan *et al.* 2004; NICE 2008).

ADHD symptoms are not specific to any particular situation and impairments are experienced across multiple domains (Asherson 2005). Impairments associated with ADHD are the consequences that occur from living with disabling symptoms related to limited self-control and self-regulation.

To be diagnostically relevant, these impairments should be pervasive, occur across multiple settings and domains of functioning, and be at least of moderate severity. In addition, to be associated with a diagnosis of ADHD they should present a threat to general development or psychosocial adjustment that would be more likely than not to occur if specialist intervention was not to take place (NICE 2008).

It is not easy to measure impairment objectively. The impact of ADHD symptoms on family life, friendships and performance at school will wax and wane according to a number of risk and resilience factors. Assessment scales such as the Children's Global Assessment Scale (CGAS) (Shaffer *et al.* 1983) may be helpful in establishing baselines for impairment caused by ADHD. It is therefore important for the nurse to assess how much impairment experienced by a child or young person with ADHD can be explained by the disorder itself, and how much may be attributable to other personal, social or family-based difficulties. This understanding can only be achieved through careful assessment, observation and liaison with the family and other professionals.

International Classification of Diseases (ICD)

The ICD is a multi-axial classification framework for diagnosing a range of mental disorders (World Health Organisation 1993) and is the preferred system used in the UK and most European countries. The first edition, known as the International List of Causes of Death, was adopted by the International Statistical Institute in 1893. The ICD-9, published in 1975, referred to 'hyperkinetic syndrome of childhood', and the most recent version, ICD-10, was endorsed by the 43rd World Health Assembly in May 1990 and came into clinical use in 1994. Due to a lack of research primarily related to inattention, the term ADHD was not included in ICD-10, and the nearest equivalent diagnosis to ADHD is that of hyperkinetic disorder (HKD). In order to make an ICD diagnosis of hyperkinetic disorder (F90) there must be evidence of at least six of the following nine symptoms of inattention evident over the past six months. These symptoms must be maladaptive and inconsistent with the developmental level of the child (see Table 2.1).

There must also be evidence of at least three of the following five symptoms of disturbances of motor activity present for at least six months, which are maladaptive and inconsistent with the developmental level of the child (see Table 2.2).

Evidence must also be available of at least one of the following four symptoms of impulsivity present for at least six months, which are maladaptive and inconsistent with the developmental level of the child (see Table 2.3).

Table 2.1 ICD-10 criteria for inattention

- Poor attention to detail/careless errors
- Often fails to concentrate on tasks or play
- Often appears not to listen
- Often fails to finish things
- Poor task organisation
- Often avoids tasks which require sustained mental effort
- Often loses things
- Often distracted by external stimuli
- Often forgetful

Table 2.2 ICD-10 criteria for hyperactivity

- Often fidgets with hands or squirms in seat
- Often leaves seat when expected to sit still
- Excessive inappropriate climbing or running
- Is often unduly noisy in playing or has difficulty in engaging in leisure activities quietly
- Persistent overactivity not modulated by request or context

Table 2.3 ICD-10 criteria for impulsivity

- Often blurts out answers before the question is complete
- Often fails to wait turn in groups, games or queues
- Often intrudes into games or conversations
- Often talks excessively without response to social appropriateness

Diagnostic and Statistical Manual of Mental Disorders (DSM)

The DSM is a handbook for mental health professionals and includes standardised diagnostic criteria for a range of mental disorders (American Psychiatric Association 1994). Like the ICD, the DSM is a multi-axial system relating to different aspects of disorder or disability. The first edition of the DSM was published in 1952 and has since been updated four times by the American Psychiatric Association. The original DSM made no direct reference to disorders of hyperactivity or inattention. However, when the DSM-II was updated in 1968, the focus on mental disorders in general shifted from causes towards behavioural manifestations. There was a move away from unsubstantiated theories of brain damage to the behavioural aspects of psychiatric disorders. The DSM-II referred to 'hyperkinetic reaction of childhood', characterised by short attention span, hyperactivity and restlessness. As the understanding of ADHD evolved into the 1980s and the DSM-III was published, impulsive, hyperactive and attentional components were highlighted and the disorder became known as 'attention deficit disorder with hyperactivity'. The DSM-IV, published in 1994 and currently in use across North America, defines ADHD as an axis I disorder and describes symptoms of inattention (see Table 2.4), hyperactivity (see Table 2.5) and impulsivity (see Table 2.6).

In order for a diagnosis to be made using DSM-IV criteria, these symptoms must appear before the age of seven, persist for at least six months and appear in both the home and school environment. DSM-IV uses a more broadly defined set of symptoms and requires evidence of inattention and/or hyper-activity/impulsivity, thus leading to the possible diagnosis of:

a. ADHD combined type (symptoms of inattention and hyperactivity/ impulsivity criteria met);

Table 2.4 DSM-IV criteria for inattention

- Often fails to give close attention to details or makes careless mistakes in schoolwork, work or other activities
- Often has difficulty in sustaining attention in tasks or play activities
- Often does not seem to listen when spoken to directly
- Often does not follow through on instructions and fails to finish schoolwork, chores or duties in the work place (not due to oppositional behaviour or failure to understand instructions)
- Often has difficulty organising tasks and activities
- Often avoids, dislikes or is reluctant to engage in tasks that require sustained mental effort (such as schoolwork or homework)
- Often loses things necessary for tasks or activities (e.g. toys, school assignments, pencils, books or tools)
- Is often easily distracted by extraneous stimuli
- Is often forgetful in daily activities

Table 2.5 DSM-IV criteria for hyperactivity

- Often fidgets with hands or feet
- Often leaves seat in classroom or other situations in which remaining seated is expected
- Often runs about excessively in situations in which it is inappropriate (in adolescents or adults may be limited to subjective feelings of restlessness)
- Often has difficulty playing or engaging in leisure activities quietly
- Is often 'on the go' or acts as if 'driven by a motor'
- Often talks excessively

Table 2.6 DSM-IV criteria for impulsivity

- Often blurts out answers before questions have been completed
- Often has difficulty awaiting turn
- Often interrupts or intrudes on others (e.g. interrupts others' conversations or games)

b. ADHD predominantly inattentive type (six symptoms of inattention present, but criteria for hyperactivity/impulsivity not met);
c. ADHD predominantly hyperactivity-impulsive type (six of the symptoms of hyperactivity/impulsivity are present, but no evidence of inattention).

How do the ICD and DSM differ?

Over the last 20 years, the diagnositic criteria for ADHD have undergone several changes that impact on how this disorder is assessed. Significant differences exist between the European and North American diagnostic criteria for ADHD, particularly in relation to the role of inattention, the definition of pervasiveness of symptoms and the management of comorbidity (Schacher and Tannock 2002). This has had a major impact on prevalence studies which makes comparisons between ADHD in North America and Europe difficult to achieve (Lee *et al*. 2008). However, estimates put DSM-IV-defined ADHD as 20 times more prevalent than the narrower definition of hyperkinetic disorder in ICD-10 (Taylor *et al*. 1991). The main differences between the two frameworks are that:

*   ICD-10 defines a single disorder characterised by inattention, impulsivity *and* hyperactivity. By contrast, DSM-IV allows for the existence of sub-types of ADHD depending on the balance of symptoms and requires evidence of inattention *and/or* hyperactivity for the diagnosis.
*   ICD-10 includes a more rigorous criterion for pervasiveness than does DSM-IV. Whereas DSM-IV defines this as impairment in social, academic or occupational functioning from ADHD symptoms in two or more situations, ICD-10 requires the full syndrome to be evident in two independent settings (e.g. home and school).
*   DSM-IV provides a greater focus on inattention and offers less emphasis on hyperactivity.
*   Whilst ICD-10 allows the diagnosis of hyperkinetic conduct disorder, it discourages the use of multiple diagnoses. When other disorders are present, the clinician is encouraged to diagnose these separately. In comparison, DSM-IV permits multiple comorbid diagnoses to coexist with ADHD with few exceptions.

Despite differences relating mostly to symptom severity, weighting and pervasiveness, both the ICD-10 and the DSM-IV diagnostic frameworks recognise the symptoms of ADHD to be broadly similar. Each refers to increased levels of activity, impulsiveness and reduced concentration which lead to impairment in emotional, social and academic functioning (Biederman and Faraone 2005). In order for a diagnosis of ADHD to be made, the impairment must be pervasive, occur across multiple settings and be either moderate or severe (Hill and Taylor 2001; Taylor *et al*. 2004; NICE 2008).

The diagnosis of ADHD should only be made by mental health or paediatric specialists following a full clinical and psychosocial assessment of the child or young person. Although practitioners in the UK and Europe tend to use the ICD-10 to diagnose mental and behavioural disorders in children, it may be helpful to also consider the DSM-IV when making an assessment of ADHD (Taylor *et al.* 2004). In summary, both sets of criteria require that the symptoms of ADHD be:

- pervasive with symptoms occurring in two or more settings (e.g. home and school);
- present before the age of seven years, nearly always before the age of five years and frequently before the age of two years;
- persistent for more than six months;
- out of keeping with the child's developmental level;
- maladaptive and producing impairment in the child's social, academic or occupational functioning.

Although there is no gold standard test for ADHD, the diagnosis can be reliably applied when standardised assessment tools are used by clinicians with expertise in ADHD and researchers who are trained to use them and operational diagnostic criteria are applied. The current operational criteria for ADHD (DSM) and hyperkinetic disorder (ICD) are highly reliable when they are applied by trained professionals following the careful evaluation of reported behaviours and symptoms (NICE 2008). However, both diagnostic frameworks present with some shortcomings. Neither the DSM nor the ICD contains guidance to consider the developmental context of hyperactivity, impulsivity and inattention. This is an important factor to consider as the child matures and enters adolescence and adulthood. Barkley *et al.* (2007) advocates reducing clinical thresholds in the DSM-IV system from six to four, and to be less concerned about the domain of hyperactivity. It is important to remember that the ADHD diagnosis was developed for use in children and not adults, and the criteria do not take into account the maturational process of adolescence and adulthood.

It is therefore important to judge what may be developmentally appropriate or even expected, particularly in very young children, and how the criteria developed for children may be applied to adults. Today, our understanding of ADHD continues to evolve as diagnostic systems are further refined and the evidence base becomes more sophisticated. The DSM-V and ICD-11 classifications are due to be published in 2012 and 2014, and it is expected that there will be further revision to the criteria for ADHD to address outstanding issues such as subtypes of the disorder, age of onset and ADHD in adulthood.

DAMP

Some researchers and clinicians, primarily those from Scandinavia, refer to a syndrome called deficits in attention, motor control and perception (DAMP) (Rydelius 2000; Gillberg 2003). This concept was introduced in the early 1980s to relate minimal brain dysfunction (MBD) as defined in DSM-III, ADHD as defined by DSM-IV and hyperkinetic disorder as defined by ICD-10 (Gillberg 1981; Rasmussen 1982; Landgren *et al.* 2000).

Nursing diagnosis: friend or foe?

Over the years, passionate debate has existed about the use of diagnoses by nurses and other professionals (Nolan 1998; Crowe 2000; Ellis 2003). Those who support the use of nursing diagnoses claim that they provide consistency, visibility and efficiency. Proponents claim that if you can't name it, you can't control it, finance it, research it, teach it or put it into public policy (Hoyt and Cajon 1997). On the other hand, critics have been concerned about the labelling and stigmatisation of children with mental health problems, and some have argued that diagnostic classification systems all too easily box people into pigeon holes and convey meaning through professional shorthand (Frisch and Kelley 2002).

Since the 1970s, nursing diagnosis has been popularised by the North American Nursing Diagnosis Association (NANDA). This organisation has developed a number of products but is perhaps best known for its evidence-based classification of nursing diagnoses for use in practice and to determine interventions and outcomes. Unfortunately, NANDA was unsuccessful at including nursing diagnosis in the ICD-10, and international support for nursing diagnosis has been slow to develop as a result (Parsons 2003). Nursing diagnoses provide the basis for the selection of nursing interventions to achieve the outcomes for which the nurse is professionally accountable (Shoemaker 1984). A nursing diagnosis is like a medical diagnosis in that it is the classification of a group of phenomena or symptoms to convey meaning without the need for long descriptions.

Positively, a nursing diagnosis should be a statement about a child's health which can be validated by the young person and their family or carers. This should be achieved through information gathered from a comprehensive assessment, related to a problem or area of difficulty that requires a nursing intervention. It may therefore be helpful to think about nursing diagnosis as a narrative framework. This is to help make sense of what is happening, incorporate flexible approaches to meet the needs of individuals and to help children and young people and their families or carers to bring order to a chaotic situation in order to promote recovery (Parsons 2003).

Making a nursing diagnosis of ADHD

The diagnostic methods used by nurses to identify and classify ADHD are relatively understudied and research papers are few and far between (Vlam 2006). Nurses practise holistically and view children and young people who have ADHD as a whole. This does not minimise the potential for using nursing diagnoses which may provide a way for nurses to communicate complex issues. Instead, this illustrates the importance of providing care focused on individual needs rather than the description of the disorder the child or young person and their families or carers may be experiencing. Many registered nurses in both the US and UK diagnose ADHD. This is done by using diagnostic frameworks, completing standardised rating scales and undertaking comprehensive assessment interviews. In the US, nurses who diagnose ADHD are practising as family nurse practitioners, clinical nurse specialists and paediatric nurse practitioners (Vlam 2006). In the UK, specialist nurses such as nurse consultants diagnose ADHD after the assessment process and prior to initiating treatment (Ryan 2006; Ryan 2007).

Summary

No single professional is likely to be able to provide the breadth and depth of assessment required to accurately diagnose ADHD, and input from the multidisciplinary team is essential. An evaluation of ADHD typically includes diagnostic assessments with the child or young person, interviews with their family, behaviour-rating scales completed by parents or carers and teachers and direct observation of behaviour. This chapter has described the process for the identification and diagnosis of hyperactivity, impulsivity and inattention which cluster together to form ADHD and discusses the associated impairments required for a diagnosis of ADHD to be made by nurses.

3 Assessment and diagnosis

Key points

- Depending on the availability of local resources and the level of partnership working, the assessment of ADHD is undertaken by professionals in paediatric, mental health or a combination of both services.
- It is the combined breadth of skills and competencies provided by the multidisciplinary team which makes the whole greater than the sum of its parts. This means that the combined efforts of the multidisciplinary team when working with a child and family with ADHD are invariably much more effective than any single professional intervention.
- The process of assessment and diagnosis of children with ADHD should be extensive, dynamic, and should rely on several sources of information from parents or carers, teachers and other professionals and young people themselves.
- A range of clinical practice guidelines exist to help nurses improve standards of care, reduce variations in service quality and ensure that children and young people with ADHD receive care, treatment and monitoring that meet their needs.
- Several key tools to help assess and diagnose ADHD are available to nurses and other professionals. However, all assessment tools have their limitations and it is important that they are not used in isolation and should form part of a wider multimodal assessment or outcome evaluation process.
- Following a diagnosis of a child or young person with ADHD, nurses and other professionals should always ensure that general advice is given to parents or carers and teachers about positive parent–child contact, clear and appropriate rules about behaviour and the importance of structure in the child or young person's day.

Introduction

The process of assessment and diagnosis is as important as the outcome itself. A range of important factors need to be considered, such as the way in which the child functions, how they are parented and the impact of psychological, social and educational adversity. Just as it is important to assess risks and impairment, so too should nurses assess strengths and resilience factors in the child, family and wider community network. This is to inform decisions about whether the risks and benefits of professional intervention outweigh the risks of non intervention.

Most nurses in specialist CAMHS work within a humanistic framework and apply an eclectic and holistic approach to the assessment and treatment of children and young people and their families and carers (Woolley 2006). This means they see the young person as a whole and recognise that child and family needs are broad and varied. This insight is enabled by the nurse's well-developed communication skills and ability to engage with the young person and their family in a variety of ways and using a range of methods (Armstrong 2006). Before embarking on treatment or management, a thorough holistic nursing assessment is crucial, taking into consideration the individual characteristics of the child, the family and social situation in which they live, and the effects of the wider environment (Stevenson 2003; Leighton 2006). This should consider all aspects of the child's life and accommodate strengths, weaknesses and family dynamic factors in order to facilitate optimal outcomes (Ludwikowski and DeValk 1998). With their ongoing observations and evaluations, nurses are in key positions to help establish accurate diagnosis and monitor the effectiveness of care, treatment and management interventions (Porter 1988).

At the end of this chapter, three case studies are outlined to illustrate the process of assessment and diagnosis and the role of the ADHD nurse. These concern Stuart, a seven-year-old with ADHD and a simple motor tic; Paula, a 14-year-old with uncomplicated ADHD; and Phillip, a 15-year-old boy with hyperkinetic conduct disorder. The case studies are all real and are based on everyday clinical practice with children and families with ADHD. However, the names of the young people concerned and some of their details have been changed. This is to protect their identity and respect their confidentiality.

Multi-professional and multi-agency working

Most people are familiar with the question, 'how do you eat an elephant?' and the answer is of course 'in small bites'. This applies to working with children and families with ADHD where there are often many needs and several interventions to perform at the same time. It is the breadth of skills and competencies provided by the multidisciplinary team which makes the whole greater than the sum of its parts. This means that the combined efforts of the multidisciplinary team when working with a child and family with ADHD are invariably much more effective than any single professional intervention.

Many different agencies, services and professionals are involved in the care, treatment, education and management of children and young people with

ADHD. Both the English and Welsh National Service Frameworks for Children, Young People and Maternity Services (Department of Health 2004; Welsh Assembly Government 2005) state that multi-agency partnerships are essential in order to develop coordinated services for children and families including those with ADHD. The need to provide integrated services is also at the heart of the overarching change for children programme, Every Child Matters (Department for Education and Skills 2003). Children and young people who receive care and treatment from specialist child and adolescent mental health services (CAMHS) have multiple and complex needs. These needs are best addressed by the multidisciplinary team, most of which include nurses, child and adolescent psychiatrists, clinical psychologists, social workers and occupational therapists (Partridge *et al.* 2003; McDougall 2006; Ryan 2007a).

Although it is generally agreed that the assessment, treatment and management of children and young people is a multi-agency enterprise, the specific contribution of nurses (Brunette 1995; Brown 2003; Laver-Bradbury 2003; Osman and Parker 2003; Brown and Bruce 2004; Caldwell *et al.* 2005; Ryan 2006; Ryan 2007b); psychiatrists (Schacher and Tannock 2002; Taylor *et al.* 2004); paediatricians (Furman 2005; Keen 2005; Garcia-Jimenez 2006); occupational therapists (Chu 2003a; Chu 2003b), and psychologists (Power 1994; Hinshaw 1994) have each been published. Although many outline single professional responsibilities and attempt to define unique professional contributions, the majority recognise that multidisciplinary and multi-agency partnerships are essential for children with complex psychosocial disorders including ADHD.

Various guidelines and principles for successful multi-agency working with children and young people who have ADHD have also been published. These include those from the British Psychological Society (2000) which states the following principles in relation to assessment practices:

- The needs and best interests of the child are paramount.
- The child and carers should be involved and fully consulted at all stages.
- Systemic influences (e.g. in the family, peer group, school, interactions between family and school) should be considered in relation to the presentation of symptoms.
- Diagnosis should not be applied to a child primarily in order to meet the needs of others (e.g. carers, teachers).
- When a child is presented for formal assessment, the assessment process should enquire into the psychosocial background to the problem.
- It should be recognised that a positive response to medication is not an effective or appropriate assessment tool and does not justify abandonment of ongoing assessment, intervention, support and monitoring.
- It is unlikely that a single clinician and/or a single consultation will constitute an effective assessment procedure.
- It should be emphasised that the symptoms and other presenting

problems that make up a diagnosis of ADHD can be mimicked as a result of a wide range of physical, social and psychological conditions and circumstances.

- Diagnosis of ADHD should only be made after other possible explanations for the existence of the problem are fully considered.
- Cultural factors should be considered at all stages of identification, assessment and intervention.

What is the nursing contribution to children and young people with ADHD?

Whilst many nurses have attempted to define their specific contribution to the mental health and wellbeing of children and young people, this may be a pointless endeavour. There is no single definition of a CAMHS nurse, and there is huge variation in the background, qualifications and roles of nurses working in specialist services (Jones and Baldwin 2004; Jones 2004). New ways of working for health professionals have enabled advanced and extended roles for nurses to emerge (Department of Health 2006; Department of Health 2007), and the role continues to evolve to meet the constantly changing demands of service users and the profession as a whole (McDougall 2006).

Nurses who have specialised in the care and treatment of children with ADHD include nurse consultants, practice nurses, ADHD liaison nurses and nurse specialists in ADHD. In many areas of the UK, nurses are leading services for children and young people with ADHD. As well as spearheading nurse-led clinics (Harding 2006; Ryan 2007a), they are prescribing medicines for children and young people with ADHD (Ryan 2007b) and establishing ADHD care pathways (Laver-Bradbury 2003). Specialist ADHD nurses provide follow up for complex cases and work with hard-to-reach families. In addition, they play a vital role in supporting primary care professionals such as health visitors and school nurses who work on a daily basis with children and young people who have ADHD. It is not only specialist ADHD nurses that are improving services for children and young people with ADHD. School nurses have also developed services that benefit children and young people, including drop-in clinics (Richardson-Todd 2003) and school-based monitoring systems for pupils taking medication (Kelly and Rounsley 2004).

In many areas of the UK, it typically takes several weeks from referral to the child receiving a diagnosis of ADHD (NICE 2008). This is a concerning issue for most parents who understandably want their child's difficulties to be addressed in the shortest possible time. The growth of extended and advanced roles for nurses provides opportunities to improve access, offer increased choice and reduce waiting times for children and families requiring ADHD assessment services.

What is the nurse's role in assessment?

Like the role of the nurse in general, the role of the nurse in assessing children and young people with ADHD is wide and varied and they play a pivotal part in multidisciplinary team-working (Ryan 2006; 2007a). As Leighton (2006) suggests, the nature of the assessment depends on the context in which the nurse practises. For example, a specialist CAMHS nurse would be expected to complete a more thorough, holistic assessment than a school nurse with limited mental health experience working in a primary setting (Leighton 2006). With their knowledge of child development, nurses in paediatric settings, schools and CAMHS are in key positions to identify and recognise symptoms of ADHD, support children and young people in primary settings and refer those who are struggling with more pronounced levels of hyperactivity, impulsivity or inattention for specialist services. Teachers and other school-based professionals often seek the advice of school nurses and specialist CAMHS nurses in relation to disruptive or inattentive behaviour in the classroom, and this is discussed further in Chapter 9.

As previously discussed, levels of impairment in day-to-day functioning of young people and their families can be great, creating distress and disharmony in social interactions and relationships. Nurses are in good positions to help young people live with or overcome these distressing times in their lives. By providing support during periods of distress children and their families can be enabled to develop strategies to modify or contain incidents that have caused and maintained such distress (Wilkin 2003). This notion of care is at the heart of nursing and is a delicate interaction requiring sensitivity and compassion. Being with the young person and family, assisting them to create their own answers to their distress and difficulties and not taking over is likely to be more helpful than acting as the 'expert' in the search for solutions (Barker 2003a).

What makes a thorough nursing assessment?

The process of assessment in nursing is generally straightforward and involves the collection of information from several multi-agency sources. This is primarily in order to paint a picture of what may be happening for the child or young person concerned. The nursing assessment should therefore focus on the child's interaction with their psychosocial world and on the key relationships they have formed with parents and siblings, friends, teachers and the wider community. The assessment should generally be structured to allow individual time for the child or young person, time for parents or carers to discuss their concerns alone and a combined family interview.

Where the process of assessment becomes more complicated is the point at which the nurse makes a formulation or draws a conclusion about what the information they have gathered means. This is due to the variability of accounts and judgements, and the validity of the information that has been gathered. For this reason, it is important that the nursing assessment is seen as a continuous, iterative process where the gathering of information remains ongoing (Keen and Keen 2003). A comprehensive assessment goes beyond examination of hyperactivity, impulsivity and inattention and includes exploration of the problems that led to referral and impairments in functioning which follow or are associated with ADHD (Hill and Taylor 2001).

The cornerstone of any nursing assessment is to carefully gather a detailed history that embraces the presenting difficulties and the concerns of the child or young person and their family or carers. The assessment of a child or young person should therefore include both historical and current information about the family and its functioning. A thorough history of physical health, motor coordination, cognitive development, family functioning and school performance should be included. It is important for nurses to remember that the assessment should be considered within the context of normal expected developmental milestones. As Leighton (2006) states, the nursing assessment should always be holistic and focus on:

- establishment of a therapeutic relationship with the child and their family or carers;
- identification of the problems including duration, intensity and frequency;
- the effects on everyday life and functioning;
- identification of any intrinsic family and environmental factors which trigger and maintain the problem;
- analysis of the relationship between different variables;
- identification of specific risk factors;
- assessment of the child and family's capacity to participate in treatment.

Many children and young people will have been subjected to numerous assessments by professionals in the various agencies they have come into contact with, and will have had many encounters with paediatric, mental health and education services (Young and Bramham 2007). Commentators such as Salmon *et al.* (2006) suggest that this is because services in the UK are often compartmentalised, and children are referred for assessment via a 'labelling route' rather than considering the child as a whole. This results in the child seeing numerous professionals, at various times and in different places (Salmon *et al.* 2006). When considering the needs of a child with ADHD, it is likely that assessment of the child's educational, social needs or mental health needs may well have been undertaken. However, these may have been completed in isolation and an integrated understanding about how such needs impact on the child's overall functioning is often lacking. Holistic assessment of need is important in order to understand how an unmet need in one domain such as mental health may affect need in another domain such as education (Mitchell 2006).

Methods of assessment

A comprehensive nursing assessment is detailed, structured, comprehensive and based on multiple sources of information. Enabling children and families to feel comfortable enough to participate in the assessment process requires the nurse to call upon all their skills of engagement, observation and communication. These are essential in order to assess motivation, identify barriers to change and evaluate family dynamic factors. There are various methods of assessment that can be used to evaluate development, behaviour and family functioning (Scahill and Ort 1995; Barker 2003b). These include:

- interviewing;
- personal accounts;
- questionnaires and rating scales;
- direct observation.

Interviewing

Face-to-face interviews with children and young people, parents or carers and other significant adults and teachers are intended to clarify the key issues including the thoughts, feelings, beliefs and views of the young person and their family. They can be structured or unstructured and paced according to the developmental needs of the child. Motivational interviewing (Prochaska and DiClemente 1982) is a directive, client-centred, goal-directed approach which focuses on current concerns and perspectives. It is often useful with adolescents and young adults and aims to make the connection between problems and solutions. Miller and Rollnick (2002) identify various stages of change that underpin motivational interviewing, and nurses should bear these in mind when assessing children and young people and their families and carers (see Table 3.1).

Change comes from within and must be generated by children and young people themselves. This means that nurses should always fully involve children and families in the identification of problems and the planning for change. Whilst used most often in the field of addictions, the principles of motivational interviewing can be extremely helpful in understanding the key issues for people with ADHD, and assessing the potential for positive change at an individual and family level (Safren *et al.* 2005; Christner *et al.* 2007; Wagner 2008).

Personal accounts

It is important for nurses to remember that family remembers are each likely to have different perspectives about the problem at hand and different ideas about what needs to change for things to improve. Encouraging all those involved to keep diaries or personal records about behaviours or symptoms

Table 3.1 Stages of motivational interviewing

- *Pre-contemplation*: people at this stage do not believe that they have a problem and are unaware and unready. The task of the nurse during the pre-contemplation stage is to raise doubt and awareness and highlight discrepancy.
- *Contemplation*: people at this stage recognise that they may have a problem, but may be ambivalent about doing something about it. The task of the nurse during the contemplation stage is to tip the balance towards preparation. This can be assisted by inviting the young person or family member to make a list of positives and negatives, as well as benefits and losses.
- *Preparation*: people at this stage recognise that they have a problem and want to sort it out. The task of the nurse during the preparation stage is to assist the family to choose the most appropriate course of action. Here, goal-setting and recording plans can be helpful.
- *Action*: people at this stage have started to implement their plans and work towards their goals. The key role of the nurse during the action stage is to support children and families in their steps towards achieving positive change and recognise that this can be a difficult process.
- *Maintenance*: people at this stage have managed to achieve positive change and the key task is to help them identify and use relapse prevention strategies to remain on track.

that concern them can assist the assessment process and help monitor change throughout the treatment period.

Questionnaires and rating scales

Research-based questionnaires and standardised rating scales can be helpful in assessing age- and sex-matched relative symptom severity (Conners 1998a). They can provide specific detail about particular problem areas which can be used by nurses to assist with the process of formulation and treatment monitoring. Standardised assessment tools and rating scales offer a convenient way of obtaining information from several different domains (Barkley 1991; Scahill and Ort 1995). A range of so-called broad- and narrow-based assessment tools, rating scales and questionnaires have been established to assist nurses and other professionals to assess ADHD and track treatment effectiveness. Narrow scales specifically measure ADHD symptoms, whereas broad scales measure additional dimensions including comorbidity (Achenbach 1995).

As well as to assess the core symptoms of ADHD, assessment scales enable clinicians to monitor the impact of impairment and evaluate other associated issues such as self-esteem, side effects and general quality of life. Those that have been applied specifically for use in school and those that have been designed for use with adults are discussed later in the book.

Strengths and Difficulties Questionnaire

Two of the most widely used behavioural screening questionnaires are the Strengths and Difficulties Questionnaire (SDQ) (Goodman 1997) and the

Child Behaviour Checklist (CBCL) (Achenbach 1991). Although the SDQ does not rate ADHD specifically, the focus on conduct problems, emotional symptoms, hyperactivity, peer relationships and pro-social behaviour can assist practitioners to assess behaviour and negative pathology in general. The SDQ can also be used by children aged over eleven as a self report measure (Goodman *et al*. 1998). This is often valuable in helping to assess the perceived differences between parents and children, which can often be marked (Lahey *et al*. 1987; Safer 2000; Furman 2005). A teacher measure also provides the opportunity to measure the child's functioning in school, which can be particularly beneficial in terms of understanding peer relationships. The impact measures can also be helpful in determining the perceived implications of ADHD on school and academic performance.

Child Behaviour Checklist

The CBCL can be used with children aged 4–18 and is usually completed by parents. However, a teacher version and youth self report are also available to compare ratings. Whilst the CBCL does not specifically measure ADHD, there is a focus on activities at home and in school, externalising problems and a total behaviour problem scale. Although both the SDQ and the CBCL are used widely, they are not always sensitive to change so have limitations when evaluating response to treatment.

Conners Rating Scale

Perhaps the most widely used assessment tool is the Conners Rating Scale (CRS), with versions for children and young people aged 3–17 and adults, and adapted for parents and teachers separately (Conners 1997a). The Conners rating scales each have established reliability and validity and are available in both long and short form. The long form includes assessment of DSM-IV symptom subscales and comorbid disorders and takes 15 to 20 minutes to complete. The short form can be scored based on number of symptoms or in comparison to established norms. In addition, the Conners Global Index provides information about restless-impulsive factors and emotional lability in childhood (Young and Bramham 2007).

Brown Attention Deficit Disorder Scale

The Brown Attention Deficit Disorder Scale (BADDS) (Brown 1996) and the Home Situations Questionnaire (HSQ) (Barkley and Murphey 1998) are both narrow-band scales that specifically measure ADHD symptoms. The BADDS focuses on executive cognitive functioning deficits and impairments. The domains covered in the scale include those related to organising and prioritising; focusing; sustaining and shifting attention; regulating alertness and processing speed; managing frustration and modulating emotions; and utilising working memory (Brown 1996).

ADHD Rating Scale IV

The ADHD Rating Scale IV is a behaviour questionnaire to be completed independently by parents and teachers (DuPaul *et al*. 1998). It is based on the DSM-IV criteria for ADHD and includes empirically derived subscales for inattention and hyperactivity-impulsivity. The ADHD Rating Scale IV is used much more in the US than in the UK.

What are the limitations of assessment tools and rating scales?

For any assessment tool to be used effectively, it is important that the nurse administering the tool has been trained to use it. The inter-rater reliability of assessment tools for ADHD has been shown to be only moderately good (Verhulst and Van der Ende 2002), and nurses should be aware that all measures have weaknesses and limitations. Therefore, the relative strengths and weaknesses of particular assessment tools should be understood by nurses and other professionals before drawing conclusions about their results or application.

Importantly, many tools only focus on symptoms and do not measure impairment, and the developmental status of the child or young person will affect the rating. Just as it is not good practice to make a diagnosis on the basis of observation alone, the use of rating scales in isolation is not sufficient to make a diagnosis of ADHD. This is because the use of rating scales alone may generate both false positive and negative diagnoses, and undermines the importance of a full clinical assessment and psychosocial evaluation (NICE 2008). Good assessment tools should not disempower nurses or stifle individual clinical judgement. Indeed, where an assessment tool produces an outcome that the nurse considers to be unrealistic or inaccurate, it is important that clinical judgement prevails and discussion with the multidisciplinary team is considered as part of the evaluation of the assessment. It is the combination of an experienced nurse using a structured, validated tool which is likely to produce the most reliable outcomes (Mitchell 2006).

Observation

Direct assessment of the child or young person in both structured and unstructured situations can be helpful. This may include the clinical interview and classroom setting as well as the home and playground environment.

The family interview

The assessment processes for ADHD are often complex, drawing on the nurse's skills of observation, communication and therapeutic engagement.

This process of family engagement is of fundamental importance and is the bedrock on which positive therapeutic change rests (Reder and Fredman 1996; Flaskas 1997; Lewer 2006; Higgins and McDougall 2006). There is little point discussing treatment options before the family is positively engaged by the nurse. It is usually parents who provide the authority for the assessment to take place, and who also give permission for any subsequent treatment of their child. For many parents, the family interview may provide a supported opportunity to 'tell their story' for the first time.

The importance of involving parents in care and treatment began in the 1900s when child guidance clinics emphasised that the problems of children were embedded in a family context (Broderick and Schrader 1991). The aim of the family assessment is to establish an understanding of overall family functioning. This is achieved by asking specific questions, collecting information from various sources and through direct observation. The family assessment can take place with the whole family, individual family members or groups of members. It not only acts as a medium for gathering relevant clinical information but also sets the context for the development of a collaborative, therapeutic relationship. This trusting alliance is a crucial part of the overall assessment process and enables the nurse to consider which problems may be amenable to change, and provides an opportunity to foster a working relationship with the child and family to empower them to change (Barker 1997). For this reason it is essential for the nurse to identify and focus on family strengths as well as difficulties.

The assessment of a child should include an observation of their interaction with the family. During the family assessment the interview room should be well equipped with toys that are suited to the developmental needs of the child. This facilitates play as a medium for engaging the younger child, whilst allowing parents or carers to describe their concerns (Joseph 1998). Observing how the child uses and interacts with toys will provide important information about how able they are to occupy themselves and for how long. The family assessment room should be private, quiet and free from external distractions such as telephones. This is to keep impingements to a minimum and to reduce the level of stimulus during the assessment. The room should be uncluttered with furniture, and chairs should be positioned to avoid creating barriers and to maximise observation. During the family interview the nurse should take note of the following:

- the child's activity levels, interactions in the family group and on a one to one;
- the child's ability to concentrate and focus on the task in hand;
- levels of hyperactivity and impulsivity that are out of keeping with the developmental stage of the child;
- verbal and non-verbal interactions between family members;
- strategies used by family members to manage behaviour during the assessment interview.

The verbal component of the family assessment also provides an opportunity to exclude concerns about other difficulties the child may be experiencing related to mood or anxiety, specific learning disabilities and problems related to speech and language. These may exist instead of ADHD or may be those commonly experienced by children and young people with ADHD, such as conduct disorder

Family history

The purpose of taking a detailed family history is to formulate an understanding about communication, functioning and parenting as well as gain information about health and illness in the immediate and extended family unit. A genogram is a pictorial display of a person's family relationships and medical history. It goes beyond a traditional family tree by enabling the user to visualise hereditary patterns and psychological factors that impact on relationships. Use of a 'genogram' or family tree can be a helpful way of enquiring about the family and can assist with building a picture of family relationships and support (McGoldrick and Gerson 1985). Trans-generational patterns may emerge that assist the nurse in locating the child's difficulties within a historical context. The genogram is created using simple symbols to represent gender and with various lines to illustrate family relationships.

During the course of taking the family history other psychosocial problems rather than ADHD may emerge that may help to explain the child's difficulties. This can include parental conflict, financial worries and major life events that have adversely affected the family. Although these factors do not cause ADHD, they may sustain or exacerbate difficulties and impact negatively on the capacity for positive change. It is vital for the nurse to gain an understanding of how parents, carers and siblings respond and cope with pressures. It is also important for nurses to determine how language, emotion and behaviours are transacted within the family and whether support from the extended family or wider community is available. This is because any subsequent parenting strategies will need to be tailored to the needs of individual parents or carers. As a minimum, the family history should generate information about:

- who is in the family and who lives at home;
- contact with divorced, separated or absent parents;
- family relationships and communication styles;
- coping styles;
- internal and external family support systems;
- domestic violence;
- positive and negative key life events.

Cultural factors

Nurses who are undertaking a family assessment of ADHD should always be sensitive to cultural differences. The cultural background of the family directly affects its views of normative family structure, communication style, world views and philosophies and models of child development (Canino and Inclan 2001; Parke 2000; Moncher and Josephson 2004). Culture also influences the meaning that people impart to their 'illness' (Bussing *et al.* 2003). The involvement of extended family members, the ways in which emotion is expressed and beliefs about health and illness are all culturally influenced and will vary from family to family. At the millennium, there were at least three million people living in the UK who were born in countries where English is not the national language, and over 300 languages were spoken by London schoolchildren (Baker and Eversley 2000). These figures are likely to have increased further during the last decade, making the need for culturally sensitive services for children and families even more of a priority. This means that there is no simple solution to providing culturally competent assessment and treatment interventions for children and families with ADHD. Cultural presentations are too complex to be addressed by standardised assessment protocols or care plans. Instead, a systemic understanding of each family culture is required and nurses will need to explore the unique needs of each child and their family in detail (McMorrow 2006). This is essential before drawing conclusions about the assessment process or formulating a diagnosis and treatment plan.

Developmental history

The need for a comprehensive account of the child's development from parents or carers is of fundamental importance when nurses are making an assessment of ADHD or any other disorder of childhood. If parents have difficulty recalling information about early years development, it may be necessary to seek permission to request records from other professionals such as GPs, health visitors, school nurses or paediatricians. Taking a comprehensive developmental history involves asking about:

- maternal health during pregnancy, including information about conception, antenatal development, foetal growth, toxaemia and threatened miscarriage;
- maternal use of medication including illicit drugs, alcohol and nicotine;
- labour, delivery and birth including any perinatal complications and need for special care;
- postnatal development including attachment relationships;
- developmental milestones including motor development, language acquisition, growth and sleep;
- temperament;

- medical history including other developmental disorders, physical illnesses, injuries, epilepsy and tics;
- progress at school including learning difficulties, ability to separate from parents or carers and comparison to peer group of same age and developmental status.

Neurodevelopmental assessments

Nurses in the US are much more routinely involved in performing and evaluating neurodevelopmental assessments than nurses in the UK. This is largely a result of historical and cultural factors rather than policy or good practice, and such assessments in the UK have traditionally been undertaken by medical or psychologist colleagues. This is in contrast to the US where nurse practitioners administer and score neurodevelopmental examinations and tests with children and young people who are being assessed for ADHD (Ludwikowski and DeValk 1998). New ways of working in mental health (Department of Health 2007) and the development of new and advanced roles for nurses (Department of Health 2006) provide an opportunity to review whether nurses with appropriate training and supervision should undertake neurodevelopmental assessments as part of their extended, advanced and expert roles.

Child interview

Regardless of their age and understanding, it is always important to directly involve children at every stage of the assessment and treatment process (Tan and Jones 2001; Wright *et al.* 2006). Of course, the younger the child is the more their parents are likely to be directly involved in the interview process. In contrast, older children and adolescents who are becoming more independent often want more of a direct role in the assessment and value the opportunity to meet with the nurse alone. However, it is important for the nurse to establish consent for treatment whatever the age of the child or young person and this is discussed further at the end of this book.

Just as the interview should contain toys for younger children to play with, so too should careful attention be given to setting a developmentally appropriate context for older children and young people who may feel patronised if the room is furnished in a childish fashion (Wilson 1991). When engaging with adolescents and young people the nurse should provide a statement about confidentiality and explain their duties in relation to confidentiality and safeguarding vulnerable children. This is to set the scene for a positive therapeutic relationship to form where the young person feels able to trust the nurse and feel safe. During the child interview, particular note should be taken of levels of inattention, hyperactivity and impulsivity. However, in a novel and arousing setting hyperkinetic symptoms may not be evident. It is therefore essential that the assessment of core ADHD symptoms is performed across a range of structured and unstructured settings. As a minimum, the nurse should seek to obtain information about the following factors during the child interview:

- ability to separate from parents or other care givers;
- physical appearance;
- motor functioning and coordination;
- speech and language comprehension;
- age appropriate social interactions;
- mood and cognitive processes.

For older children, it can often be helpful to use standardised rating scales to gain information about the lived experiences of ADHD and to detect emotional difficulties. These include the Child Strengths and Difficulties Questionnaire (SDQ-S) (Goodman 1997; Ronning *et al.* 2003) and the Conners Adolescent Self Report (CASR) (Conners 1997b).

Parent or carer interview

The parent or carer interview provides an opportunity to discuss concerns at an adult level with the nurse. Parents and carers often find this helpful because they may wish to discuss negative or problematic behaviour privately without their child listening. This is to be supported since the self-esteem and self-image of children and young people with ADHD is often fragile, and because parents also need a space to talk freely about the challenging behaviour of their children. Nurses should expect that parents and carers will sometimes describe their child negatively and with hostility. This may be because they have struggled for many years with difficult behaviour and feel frustration and resentment that family relationships have been strained or damaged (Hinton and Wolpert 1998; Harborne *et al.* 2004).

A separate parent or carer interview also provides an opportunity for the nurse to assess whether there are additional family-based problems such as parental conflict, financial difficulties or domestic violence that may be relevant and require further assessment or signposting. However, focusing on wider family-based difficulties may sometimes cause resistance in parents who have come for help ostensibly because of their child's difficulties. Here, it is important for the nurse to tread carefully when obtaining information about the family as a whole, and the parents as individuals or as a couple (AACAP 2007).

Prior to or during the parent or carer interview, a range of questionnaires can be completed which assists the overall assessment process. These include the Revised Conners Parent Rating Scale (CPRS-R) (Conners *et al.* 1998b); the Strengths and Difficulties Questionnaire (SDQ) (Goodman 1997); and the Child Behaviour Checklist (CBCL) (Achenbach 1991). Parenting rating scales are useful as a supplement to the interview, but should not be regarded as a replacement. They have the advantage of systematic cover but the disadvantage of uncertainty in relation to how parents or carers make the ratings. This is referred to as adaptation or 'halo effects' (Taylor *et al*. 2004).

Information from other sources

When assessing ADHD it is important to gather as much information as possible. This is to obtain a comprehensive account of historical factors and to understand the appraisals that different people may have about the child's presenting difficulties. Multiple sources of information also produce comparisons that may reveal contradictions or inaccuracies not previously recognised by other professionals. Sometimes such inaccuracies are propagated from one report to another until the original source material is verified. It is easy to see how myths about diagnosis and needs can be generated and perpetuated. Once in circulation, these can easily distort formulations about the assessment of needs and the type of service a young person receives as a result (Mitchell 2006). It is therefore vital that nurses seek to corroborate or verify the information they gather when making an assessment of ADHD.

Nurses require appropriate consent to seek information about the children and young people they are working with. Schools often provide a rich source of information to assist the assessment process. With permission from parents or carers, educational reports and completed questionnaires can be requested. Nurses should attempt to meet with the child's teacher and observe the child in both the structured and unstructured educational environment. This is to compare functioning in school with information obtained during the individual and family-based components of assessments undertaken in the clinical setting. Meeting teachers and professionals such as school nurses also provides an opportunity to discuss school-based strategies to manage disruptive behaviour.

Use of standardised rating scales such as the revised Conners Teacher Rating Scale (CTRS-R) (Conners *et al*. 1998c) and Strengths and Difficulties Questionnaire Teacher Report (SDQT) (Goodman 1997; Koskelainen *et al*. 2000) may provide useful information about the child's functioning in school. If necessary, more detailed accounts about academic progress should be sought from speech and language therapists, educational psychologists and voluntary services who can often be helpful in supporting the child in the classroom setting (Law and Garnett 2004). School-based interventions for children and young people with ADHD are discussed in detail in chapter 9.

Reaching a conclusion: formulation and diagnosis

In making a formulation, assessment of resilience factors and the child or young person's strengths are as important as describing their difficulties (Bird and Emond 2007). The care and attention the nurse gives to detail during the assessment of a child with suspected ADHD is crucial. Where there are concerns that a child or young person may have ADHD, it is necessary to evaluate the range of information obtained during the assessment and consider this in the context of what is expected for their age and development. The child or young person's symptoms and behaviours should also be evaluated against the criteria described in the ICD-10 and DSM-IV diagnostic categories described in chapter 2. The presence of comorbid mental health problems or psychosocial difficulties should be considered and discussed with the child and their family or carers as well as the multidisciplinary team. After the initial assessment and before starting treatment, it is important to measure baselines. This is to understand the child or young person's current level of psychosocial functioning, and also to measure this against response to any treatment that may be implemented following the assessment. Hill and Taylor (2001) suggest that during baseline monitoring, information in the following areas should be documented:

- presenting complaints and problems;
- core ADHD symptoms as described in DSM-IV or ICD-10 frameworks;
- level of academic achievement;
- social and interpersonal relationships with peers, parents and teachers;
- parental attitudes to their child.

Nurses and other professionals should recognise that not all children and young people with symptoms of hyperactivity, impulsivity and inattention will receive a diagnosis of ADHD, and it is the degree of impairment or adversity associated with their symptoms which leads to a diagnosis. Applying a diagnosis of ADHD to a child or young person is a serious matter, and there needs to be clear evidence of clinically significant impairment in social, academic or occupational functioning. Furthermore, this impairment should be caused by symptoms of hyperactivity, impulsivity and inattention and be interfering with the child or young person's day-to-day activities with family, friends and at school. Once a diagnosis of ADHD is made and this has been discussed with the child or young person, parents or carers and teachers, the nurse should begin the process of care planning and delivery of interventions to help manage the presenting difficulties arising from hyperactivity, impulsivity and inattention. This is discussed elsewhere in this book.

Summary

Nurses do not practise in isolation from the wider multidisciplinary team. On the contrary, nurses who work with children and young people who have ADHD do so in a multi-professional and multi-agency context, and have much to learn from and share with their colleagues (McDougall 2006). No single professional is likely to be able to provide the breadth and depth of assessment required to accurately diagnose ADHD, and input from the multidisciplinary team is essential. As well as nursing and psychological interventions, children and young people usually require medical assessments and may often need psychometric tests from psychologists. The impact of global learning disabilities, particularly with hyperkinetic disorder, and specific learning difficulties such as dyspraxia or speech and language problems needs to be fully understood. This is both in terms of assessing inattention and in terms of planning treatment and management which is developmentally appropriate. This will require the combined skills of a range of professionals.

Case studies

The following case studies are outlined to illustrate the process of assessment and diagnosis and the role of the ADHD nurse. These concern Stuart, a seven-year-old with ADHD and a simple motor tic; Paula, a 14-year-old; and Philip, a 15-year-old.

Stuart, aged 7

Referral information

Stuart was referred to the specialist ADHD nurse by his GP. This followed a letter from Stuart's teacher who had expressed concern that Stuart could not sit still and was preventing other pupils learning. The referral letter stated that Stuart's parents had always found his behaviour challenging, but felt that they had adapted their parenting style to manage their son's behaviour. Parents were concerned that he was not achieving in school, was falling behind with his work and had few friends. His parents described him as a warm and loving child and a pleasure to be with.

Family history

Stuart lives at home with his mother Susan, aged 27, and father Matthew, aged 27 (see Figure 3.1). The family lived with maternal grandparents for the first 18 months of Stuart's life and these remain an important source of support to the family. Paternal grandparents retired and went to live in Spain, and Stuart and his parents rarely see them. Susan suffered with postnatal depression following Stuart's birth, but did not receive treatment for this. During this time, Matthew and maternal grandparents were alternative positive care providers for Stuart and it was thought that he made a good attachment to all the adults in the family. There was no reported mental disorder on either side of the family, but Susan reports that her mother believes that Stuart is very like Susan was as a child. When asked about this further, Susan explained that she was 'always on the go', struggled to make friends and did not do well at school.

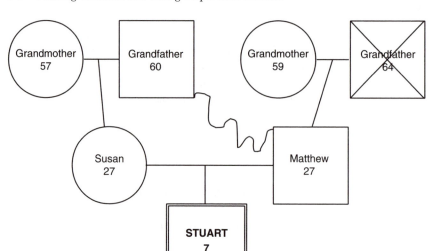

Figure 3.1 Genogram of Stuart's family.

Developmental history

Stuart was a planned pregnancy and was born full-term normal delivery, following a threatened miscarriage at 31 weeks gestation. There were no reported developmental concerns. Stuart walked at 14 months and talked fluently by two and a half years. When Stuart started nursery at aged three, he separated readily from parents and there was no anxiety or distress. However, nursery staff regularly commented that he appeared to be more hyperactive than his peer group and found it more difficult to settle on a chosen activity. Stuart's family struggled to manage his demanding behaviour, but Susan felt it was normal as she had no other children to compare him with. When Stuart joined the reception class his teachers described him as hyperactive and excitable. He would run around the classroom, be frequently off task, found friendships troublesome and stood out from the other boys in his class. By Year 1 the following observations had been included in his reports. 'Stuart cannot sit still and disrupts the class'; 'He is restless, always on the go and stands out from his peer group'; 'Stuart lacks concentration, is always racing ahead and can't remember what to do next'; 'Although he is kind and sensitive to his peers, Stuart has failed to form positive relationships with peers and adults'.

Assessment

During the interview, Stuart found it difficult to occupy himself with age-appropriate toys, and sought the assistance of the adults in the room to play with him. He was loud, noisy and interrupted the interview frequently by talking over the adults. During the individual assessment, Stuart separated easily from his family and did not appear shy or timid. He was active and restless during the interview. It was difficult to gain his eye contact and attention for any period of time. Stuart found it hard to follow a train of conversation or complete an activity, choosing to report information about a recent school project that he was interested in. He hurriedly drew a picture of himself, showing little interest and including only minimal detail. Although Stuart was warm and sociable, he was a little overfamiliar. Stuart was observed to have a slight facial motor tic during the assessment.

Diagnosis

Attention deficit hyperactivity disorder and simple motor tic.

Management plan

1. Psycho-education to parents and teachers about the symptoms and treatment of ADHD, through verbal discussion at school meeting and written information.
2. Consultation to educational psychologist and behaviour support service to assist school in helping Stuart access his education fully.
3. Conners questionnaires given to parents and teachers to record baseline behaviours.
4. Continued behaviour management advice to parents.
5. Trial of non-stimulant medication atomoxetine (Straterra) in view of facial motor tic following routine health screening and discussion with parents about contra-indications and potential side effects.

Evaluation

The trial of atomoxetine treatment was unsuccessful in terms of reducing hyperactivity, impulsivity and inattention. A trial of stimulants (methylphenidate) was discussed with parents as the next treatment option as follows:

1. Methylphenidate 2.5 mg three times a day for seven days
2. Methylphenidate 5 mg three times a day for seven days
3. Methylphenidate 7.5 mg three times a day for seven days
4. Methylphenidate 10 mg three times a day for seven days

After evaluation, it was agreed that the positive benefits from stimulants outweighed the possible side effects of exacerbating the facial motor tic. The trial was later reviewed at a school-based meeting convened by the nurse and including Stuart, his parents, the SENCO, Stuart's class teacher and the specialist behaviour support teacher. Conners questionnaires completed by parents and teachers and verbal reports demonstrated an improvement in hyperactivity, increase in concentration and reduction in impulsivity. Stuart produced more work of a better quality as the doses of treatment increased, and there was no evidence of increase in facial motor tics. However, the higher dose of methylphenidate 10 mg three times a day had produced significant loss of appetite and sleep disturbance, without any greater treatment effect. Therefore, it was agreed that Stuart should reduce back down to methylphenidate 7.5 mg three times a day with later review in the nurse-led clinic.

Outcome

Stuart continues to take methylphenidate without any side effects. He is growing and gaining weight appropriately. Stuart's performance in school has improved; he produces more work and of a better quality and he is more sociable and included by his peer group. His parents have been pleased with his progress and they have made changes to their parenting style and feel more consistent in their approach to his behaviour management.

Paula, aged 14

Referral information

Paula was referred to the local Tier 3 child and adolescent mental health services (CAMHS) following a letter from the school's special educational needs coordinator (SENCO). There had been concerns about Paula's learning and behaviour and she had previously been placed on the Special Needs Register. Paula was reportedly unable to concentrate for more than a few minutes at a time and this was causing many disruptions in the classroom. Paula continued to make poor academic progress and displayed very immature behaviour. By the time Paula had reached Year 4 her behaviour was much more unacceptable and she was unable to follow any direct instruction, constantly fidgeted and chattered throughout classes. The SENCO noted that Paula's parents were also experiencing great difficulties at home with her behaviour.

Assessment

Following on from a comprehensive assessment by CAMHS, Paula was assessed by the ADHD nurse specialist. At interview she was restless, unable to settle to any constructive activity and was extremely talkative in a very loud voice.

Family history

Paula lives at home with both her parents who regard themselves as older than the average parents (see Figure 3.2). She has a younger brother, aged

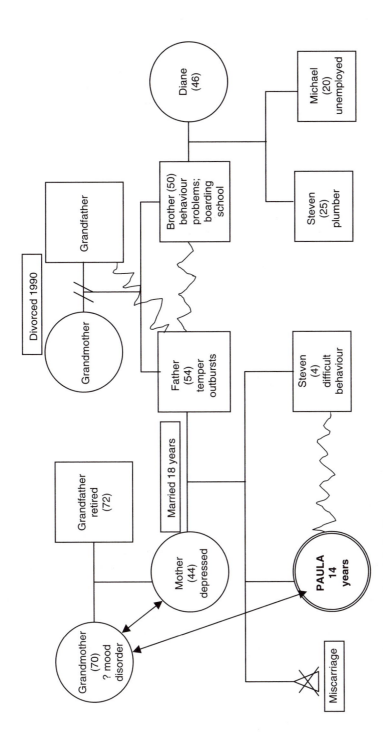

Figure 3.2 Genogram of Paula's family.

four, and, prior to Paula's birth, her mother suffered a miscarriage at about four months into her pregnancy. Both parents gave brief unremarkable accounts of their own history and family, although on the father's side there was a history of one of his siblings attending boarding school for 'behaviour problems'. Mother described herself as being very close to her parents as she is an only child. Maternal grandmother suffers from anxiety and mother has depression and poor physical health. Fathers' parents separated when he was grown-up, and he no longer has any contact with his father or brother, both of whom he had a volatile relationship with.

Developmental history

There were various concerns during mother's pregnancy with Paula. She was admitted to hospital on several occasions with threatened miscarriage and Paula was delivered at 38 weeks by emergency caesarean section due to foetal distress. Although the neonatal period was reportedly uneventful, mother suffered from postnatal depression and Paula was given a nursery place early. It was thought that Paula settled in school relatively quickly without any evident difficulties.

Diagnosis

Attention deficit hyperactivity disorder.

Treatment interventions

After discussion with Paula and her parents, a trial of methylphenidate was undertaken. Although Paula showed a positive response to medication, she experienced some unpleasant side effects. After the dose was reduced, it was reported that Paula was much better able to sit and concentrate. During the trial of medication, she also gained an academic certificate and was better able to get on with her peers in the classroom and her brother at home.

Parents were offered a Parents Skills Intervention Group to help them manage difficult behaviour at home. Paula was also referred to a voluntary-sector-run social skills group to help with her peer relationships. Although on the initial trial of medication Paula suffered significantly from unwanted effects of medication, as she has grown up and grown older she has been able to tolerate the modified-release preparation of methylphenidate very successfully. Paula made a successful end to her high school career completing her GCSE examinations and going on to further education at college doing childcare.

Planned withdrawal

Throughout Paula's care she has undergone periods of planned withdrawal of treatment. However, this has resulted in an increase in overactivity and inattention which has impaired Paula's ability to focus and concentrate in the school setting.

Philip, aged 15

Referral information

Philip was referred to the nurse consultant in ADHD by his GP. This followed increasing concerns about antisocial behaviour, recent exclusion from high school due to abusive and threatening behaviour, and problems with anger and aggression. Philip has also recently been cautioned by the police after damage to his family home. Parents were concerned that Philip had undiagnosed ADHD.

Family history

Philip lives at home with his parents and is their only child (see Figure 3.3). He has a half-sibling by his father's previous marriage who has a history of drug misuse and mental health problems. Philip also has a half-sister who works for a living. There is very little contact between Philip's siblings and relationships are reported to be poor. Philip's father divorced from his first wife acrimoniously and now has little contact with his children who are both grown-up. Mother has contact with both her parents and maternal grandmother is very close to Philip. Father's parents have both died and he did not have a good relationship with either of them.

Developmental history

Philip was an unplanned pregnancy to his mother when she was aged 17. He was born full-term normal delivery weighing 7 lbs and his immediate neonatal period was satisfactory. He was described as being a perfect baby and there were no developmental problems with his hearing, talking, toilet training or sight. He attended nursery from three years of age, settled in well, and there were no complaints about his behaviour. Around the age of five when Philip started school, there were reportedly difficulties with his sleep pattern, and he found it difficult to settle into the routine of school. Philip presented with behavioural problems and there were concerns about his learning. It was initially thought that he might need a statement of special educational needs, but the statementing process was never initiated. Parents report that over the years they have had concerns about hyperactivity, poor concentration and impulsivity. Philip's physical health is good and his appetite and mood are unremarkable.

It was difficult to elicit from the parental interview the extent of Philip's inattention. However, there was clear evidence of hyperactivity and impulsivity. When Philip was seen on a one-to-one he became increasingly restless

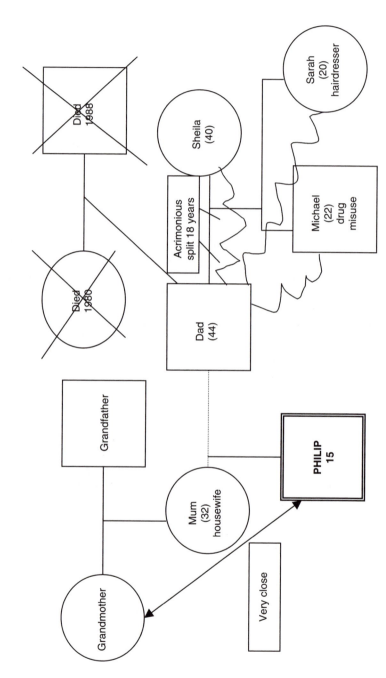

Figure 3.3 Genogram of Philip's family.

and bored as the interview progressed. He presented as being very fidgety and restless in the chair and was very softly spoken with good eye contact. There was no oppositional behaviour observed in the clinic setting. Philip highlighted his own difficulties with inattention, not being able to sit still and being unable to focus and concentrate. He reported that the smallest thing would distract him. He feels that he is always in trouble with his parents and claimed that friends had complained that he fidgets and does not see things through to the end. This clearly impacted upon Philip's mood and made him feel worthless. He felt that his school career had been very poor, and was concerned that the problems he is having are making his mother ill.

Diagnosis

Philip was given a diagnosis of hyperkinetic conduct disorder. As he was quite old when he was referred to CAMHS there was clear evidence of antisocial and criminal behaviour. There was developmental and historical evidence of hyperactivity, reduced concentration and increased impulsivity. Whilst this did not manifest as difficulties in his very early years in primary school, since mid-primary school there have been increasing difficulties with motor restlessness, fidgetiness, poor tolerance, learning problems and antisocial behaviour.

Interventions

A trial of atomoxetine was started to provide 24-hour management of his symptoms. Philip expressed no particular views about starting medication, and the decision to use medication was based on parental choice of the treatment options available. Parents were offered a place in the Triple P Teenagers Group to help them to review their strategies to manage Philip's antisocial and oppositional behaviour in the home setting.

Outcomes

After a trial of medication, Philip's performance in school changed dramatically. There have been major improvements in his academic performance and teachers praised his positive behaviour. Parents report that the temper outbursts at home have all but disappeared. Philip is less restless and able to sit down to complete jigsaws, and is undertaking tasks and activities under his own volition. Parents are pleased that they now only have to complain about typical adolescent behaviours such as not getting up in the morning and staying out late.

4 What are the costs of ADHD?

Key points

- The symptoms of ADHD are associated with a range of impairments in personal, family, social, psychological, academic and occupational functioning. Nursing interventions should be carefully tailored not only to improve core symptoms of hyperactivity, inattention and impulsivity but also to focus on improving functional outcomes for young people.
- Failure to interrupt the developmental trajectory of ADHD can lead to educational failure, family-based difficulties, social exclusion, low self-esteem and increased risk of mental disorder in adult life. Nurses and health visitors in particular are in key positions to intervene early and help reduce the costs and burden of ADHD and improve the quality of life for children and their families.
- Children, young people and adults with ADHD place a significant financial burden on health, social care, education and criminal justice agencies. Childhood hyperactivity and impulsivity are risk factors for accidents and injuries, substance misuse and antisocial or offending behaviour in adolescence and adulthood.
- Psychosocial factors can either foster resilience and personal strength or increase risk and failure. The strongest risk factors for children with ADHD are poor outcome are family history of ADHD, psychosocial adversity and comorbidity with conduct problems, mood disorders and anxiety.
- Not all children with ADHD have poor outcomes as adolescents or adults. Protective factors include early intervention, a supportive family and social network and fewer difficulties with hyperactivity and impulsivity than attentional problems.

Introduction

Little is known about the specific costs of ADHD in childhood, the costs to families in coping with a child with this disorder, long-term outcomes in adulthood and the costs of untreated ADHD in general. However, the adverse social, familial and personal consequences of ADHD cannot be overstated. Many children with ADHD and their parents or carers and siblings develop emotional, social and family-based difficulties as a direct consequence of their primary difficulties (Kidd 2000). Various studies demonstrate that children and young people with ADHD are more likely to experience educational failure, low self-esteem and are at increased risk of mental disorder in adult life (Fischer *et al.* 1993; Searight and McLaren 1998; Schachar and Tannock 2002; Swenson *et al.* 2003; Maughan *et al.* 2004). Compared with other groups of children and young people those with ADHD are more likely to:

- show poor educational attainments and drop out of school;
- have poorer early work histories with higher risks of unemployment;
- leave their homes and families at younger ages;
- enter romantic and sexual relationships earlier, and experience more difficulties and breakdown in those relationships;
- become pregnant or father children earlier than their peers;
- be involved in crime;
- have poorer general health in their adult lives.

This chapter aims to illustrate how the costs of both treated and untreated ADHD can be perpetuated and affect all domains of functioning for children and families. Problems with hyperactivity, impulsivity and inattention can lead to a range of negative outcomes which, if left untreated or unmanaged, can lead to a cycle of escalating difficulties and a negative downward spiral for young people and their families. This means that assessment should be holistic, planning should be multi-dimensional and intervention should be provided at a multi-agency level.

Financial costs

The headline figures suggest that the economic burden of ADHD is extremely high and falls to health, education, social care and youth justice economies. In England and Wales alone, approximately £66 million is spent on ADHD services for children and young people each year. Approximately £23 million is spent on specialist ADHD assessment services, £14 million on follow-up care and nearly £30 million is spent on drug treatments for ADHD (King *et al.* 2006; NHS Information Centre 2006). These are escalating costs. It has been estimated that by the end of the decade expenditure on pharmacotherapy in England will have trebled to nearly £80 million (Schlander 2007). These figures do not necessarily mean that children and young people are being overtreated. Rather, more children and young people with ADHD are being diagnosed, and drugs such as slow-release preparations are becoming more sophisticated and more expensive to buy. This trend in prescribing and escalating costs has also occurred across North America and in other European countries (International Narcotics Control Board 2003), but comparisons are difficult to make due to differences in healthcare systems and rates of diagnosis, particularly for very young children.

Health costs

The costs of both treated and untreated ADHD are substantial. It is not possible to address all the negative health outcomes associated with ADHD in one chapter but these are generally associated with the risk of accidents, the impact of substance misuse and the mental health services required to treat psychological problems and cormorbid mental disorders. Increased use of health services is also apparent in parents or carers of children and young people with ADHD (Harpin 2005). This is particularly associated with higher rates of stress, mental illness and alcohol use (Cunningham *et al.* 1988; Brown and Pacini 1989).

Accidents are the leading cause of death among children and young people in Great Britain (Department for Education and Skills 2006). In children and young people generally, these are caused by road traffic accidents or by injuries or accidents caused at home or in school. Due to difficulties with visuomotor problems, impairment of executive functioning, high distractibility and hyperactivity, children and young people with ADHD are at greater risk of injuries than those without ADHD (Bijur *et al.* 1986; Taylor *et al.* 1991; Swenson *et al.* 2004). They more frequently attend accident and emergency departments following injuries caused by impulsive, aggressive or risk-taking behaviours (Rosen and Peterson 1990; Gerring *et al.* 1998; DiScala *et al.* 1998; Swenson *et al.* 2003).

Substance misuse

Whilst children and young people with ADHD are more likely to smoke and take drugs, they are no more likely than those without ADHD to drink alcohol (Green *et al.* 2005). Research shows that young people with ADHD are at heightened risk of developing substance misuse disorder as adults (Biederman *et al.* 1991; Molina and Pelham 2003; Harpin 2005), and this places an additional burden on the health economy. Substance misuse rarely exists in isolation, but occurs in the context of other problems that affect young people in modern society (Melrose and Brodie 2000). At one end of a continuum it can be seen as part of growing up in modern society. It can be seen as a method of coping with negative emotions or bringing on a 'buzz'. At the other end of the continuum it is linked to a range of mental health problems and disorders including serious mental illness (Cantwell *et al.* 1999; King *et al.* 1996; Young *et al.* 1995).

The relationship between substance use and mental health problems in general is not straightforward. Whether substance use triggers mental ill health in people who would not have experienced problems otherwise, or whether a predisposition to mental disorder existed all along is an area of debate (Bukstein *et al.* 1989; Wilens *et al.* 1999; Crome 2004). The relationship between ADHD and substance misuse is even more complex and relatively understudied. Young people with ADHD are at heightened risk of substance abuse due to impulsivity, a tendency to mix with peers who may not be doing well at school and self-medication. However, there is some longitudinal follow-up data showing that treatment with stimulants for children with ADHD protects against substance misuse disorder in adulthood (Biederman 2003).

Emotional health and wellbeing

Good self-esteem is fundamental to self-actualisation and healthy psychological and emotional development. The way in which we perceive ourselves forms part of our identity, and helps shape our self-image. Low self-esteem and perception has been the focus of attention in various studies of children and young people with ADHD. Children are much more likely to describe themselves in negative rather than positive terms. These include being 'bad', 'mad', 'naughty' and 'weird' (Kendall *et al.* 2003). They are more likely to be demoralised, have low confidence and suffer peer rejection than their non-affected peers (Flicek 1992; Kreuger and Kendall 2001). This may arise from peer group difficulties, academic problems and social exclusion.

We often hear people with good self-esteem making positive self-motivating statements such as 'I can do this'. In contrast, those with low self-esteem doubt their abilities and are more likely to say 'I can't do this'. Perhaps not surprisingly, research shows that, if children view themselves negatively, they tend to behave in negative ways. Negative self-statements are closely associated with low self-esteem and it is easy to see how a negative spiral can escalate and lead to further difficulties for a child or young person with ADHD (Haynes 1990). It is widely agreed that there is a reciprocal relationship between self-esteem and a range of negative outcomes including academic underachievement and delinquency. Low self-esteem fosters delinquency, and delinquency improves self-esteem (Rosenberg *et al.* 1989). It is essential that nurses and other professionals take every opportunity to support the child with ADHD to develop confidence, emotional resilience and good mental health. This is because low self-esteem is a strong predictor of future mental health problems and disorders, and because good self-esteem is known to be a strong protective factor (Rutter 1990; Fergusson *et al.* 2000; Fryers 2007).

Mental health problems and disorders

Children and young people with ADHD often have additional mental health problems and disorders. Like ADHD, if these are left untreated, they can contribute to educational failure, family and social problems, crime and anti-social behaviour. As well as placing demands on specialist mental health services, these also place a burden of responsibility and cost on social services, schools and the youth justice system. Many unresolved mental health problems during childhood continue into adulthood, disrupting personal, social and occupational functioning. Again, it is easy to see how untreated mental health problems and disorders in children and young people with ADHD can lead to a cycle of difficulties across all domains of functioning. Major mental health problems and disorders are discussed further in the next chapter.

Sleep

Good physical and emotional health depends on regular, quality sleep. Although many children with ADHD appear not to need much sleep, daytime behaviour is often worse when sleep is affected (Harpin 2005). Whether they are coexistent sleep disorders, difficulties associated with inattention and arousal or the unwanted effects of stimulant medication, sleep problems are extremely common in both children and young people and adults with ADHD (Stein 1999; Lecendreux *et al.* 2000; Brown and McMullen 2001; Owens 2005). Sleep difficulties not only cause or exacerbate difficulties for children and young people themselves but also affect families who may have sleep disrupted by the hyperactivity and restlessness of their child with ADHD (Effron *et al.* 1998). As well as higher levels of nocturnal activity per se, sleep latency, nightmares, insomnia and restless legs are all very common. Young and Bramham (2007) illustrate how dysfunctional sleep cycles affect children and young people with ADHD (see Figure 4.1).

Nurses can support families to manage the sleep problems associated with ADHD in a number of practical ways. This can include helping families understand sleep patterns by keeping sleep diaries, and through advice on how best to manage sleep problems and disorders. It is important to encourage parents or carers to implement a night-time routine that is consistent. This should involve going to bed and getting up at about the same time each day, keeping the bedroom a dark, quiet place and ensuring the room is at a comfortable temperature. Parents should encourage their children to avoid engaging in stimulating or arousing activities before bed such as watching TV or playing computer games.

Education costs

The costs for education economies are also higher for children and young people with ADHD. This is due to the higher cost of special education, the increased prevalence of learning difficulties, and the added costs of classroom support and school health services (Guevara and Mandell 2003). ADHD in the school setting often impacts negatively upon learning. Pupils with ADHD produce less work than their peers and struggle to keep up, both academically and socially. This compounds their sense of being different and can lead to disillusionment with learning. All too often, pupils with ADHD are

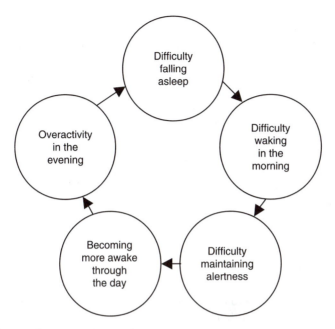

Figure 4.1 Dysfunctional sleep cycle.

Source: Young and Bramham 2007

excluded from the education process and exclusions from school damage the young person's education attainment. Parents may then need to take time off work to supervise their child. Where this is difficult to manage, young people who are excluded from school are sometimes left unsupervised and bored. This places them at higher risk of engaging in petty criminal behaviour leading to contact with the youth justice system. Once again, we can see how the costs associated with ADHD can transgress multiple domains and lead to snowballing of problems for both the young person and their family.

Social functioning

A large survey carried out by the Office for National Statistics on behalf of the Department of Health and Scottish Executive focused on a range of difficulties associated with hyperkinetic disorder including social aptitude and difficulty with friendships (Green *et al.* 2005). Parents were asked to assess the ability of their child to empathise with others and over four-fifths (83%) were reported to have significant difficulties in this area. Over half of those with ADHD found it more difficult than average to keep friends compared with only 5% of other children (Green *et al.* 2005).

Difficulties recognising and interpreting subtle social cues and feedback make it difficult for children and young people to learn from and modify their behaviour. Even when they learn to rein in their intrusive or aggressive responses, children and young people with ADHD continue to behave in socially inappropriate ways. In other words, they can learn the scripts but they don't learn the nuances (Henker and Whalen 1999). This inability to self-regulate in terms of successful planning, problem-solving and being able to accommodate social responses sustains the poor relationships so often experienced by people with ADHD.

Peer relationships

Children and young people with ADHD often stand out from their peers due to their limited ability to socialise. It has been suggested that they fail to read social situations effectively, and do not readily pick up verbal and non-verbal cues from others about the impact or appropriateness of their behaviour (Hall *et al.* 1999; Charman *et al.* 2001). Selikowitz (2006) suggests that they are 'socially tone deaf'. Due to difficulties with executive functioning such as poor working memory, many children and young people have difficulties with self-regulation and self-control. They are consequently less receptive to feedback from adults and peers which is a necessary part of modifying social behaviour. This can lead to their being unpopular and becoming isolated.

Not surprisingly, children and young people with ADHD experience significant difficulty forming and sustaining positive peer relationships. Same-age friendships are difficult to maintain due to difficulty reading social situations and intrusiveness. Consequently, children and young people with ADHD may become loners, or form friendships with those younger or older than themselves. With younger children, they may blend in because of immaturity, and with older children, more allowances may be made for their inappropriate behaviour (Selikowitz 2006). Some children and young people get bullied because they stand out as being different. As they get older, many gravitate towards peers with similar difficulties and engage in antisocial or criminal behaviour (Fryers 2007). Girls with ADHD are reported to experience greater difficulty in forming and maintaining positive friendships than boys with ADHD. This may be due to the more pervasive range of social dysfunction experienced by girls than boys, and higher rates of aggression and oppositional behaviour shown by boys (Blachman and Hinshaw 2002; Young *et al.* 2005).

A lack of positive peer relationships compounds difficulties for children and young people with ADHD who fail to benefit from the opportunity to be in social situations where appropriate social skills are used and developed. This creates a circular problem and generates a 'self-fulfilling prophecy' (Merton 1968). That is, the interpersonal behaviour of children with ADHD isolates them from their peers. At the same time, their isolation from peers prevents the acquisition of social skills necessary to form and sustain positive peer relationships. It is not that children and young people with ADHD disregard the rules of social interaction; rather they just have difficulty following them (Shattell *et al.* 2008).

People with ADHD often experience significant difficulties with social functioning and this may contribute to exclusion, peer group rejection and isolation (Hinshaw 1991; Greene *et al.* 1996; Greene 2001; Scott *et al.* 2001). Indeed, as many as half of children with ADHD also have difficulties with friendships and in relationships with their parents, siblings and teachers (Nixon 2001). This can lead to a diminution of social networks and a negative cycle of social exclusion. All nurses and other children's professionals share a responsibility for improving social inclusion and reducing the stigma associated with ADHD. This is to help prevent the escalation of impairment that all too often accompanies this disorder.

Parenting and family costs

Children with ADHD do not exist in a vacuum and are part of a complex multi-system, the most significant component of which is the family. Children and young people who have problems with attention, overactivity and impulsivity often struggle to conform to parental expectations. At the same time, growing up sometimes brings with it rebelliousness and risk-taking, particularly as children enter the unpredictable period of adolescence. Without thoughtful consideration, this combination of factors may be a recipe for family-based conflict and relationship difficulties. These have been well documented in relation to children and young people with ADHD and their families (Anastopoulous 1992; Anastopoulous *et al.* 1993; Johnston and Mash 2001; Edwards *et al.* 2001). It is perhaps not surprising that parents may sometimes need support to differentiate what can be explained by their child's ADHD and what is part of normal growing up. After all, their child is first and foremost their child, and the ADHD is secondary. This can be a difficult line to tread for parents and carers. At the same time they are expected to be firm but be flexible, and to set limits but make allowances. Not all parents manage to achieve this careful balance on their own, and many will require support and guidance from professionals. Some parents attribute all their child's difficulties to ADHD, whilst others try to separate out those behaviours that they attribute to ADHD and those which are part of growing up.

There is consistent evidence to show that parenting a child or young person with ADHD is more difficult than parenting children and young people without ADHD. It has been suggested that those with ADHD require a unique style of parenting with a particular need for consistency (DuPaul *et al.* 2001). Parents of children and young people with a diagnosis of ADHD report that they feel they have fewer parenting skills and strategies to draw upon, lower confidence in their parenting abilities and higher rates of depression, self-blame and social isolation than parents of children without ADHD (DuPaul *et al.* 2001). Parents and carers of young people with ADHD describe experiencing a range of emotions and difficulties. These are associated with feeling overwhelmed by the pressures of caring for their ADHD child, and insensitive remarks from partners, teachers and friends about their child's behaviour. This can leave many parents feeling embarrassed, unable to manage and worried about what the future holds for their child.

A large survey of parents and carers painted a distressing picture of how ADHD can affect family life. Almost two-thirds of the parents had divorced, separated or experienced marital distress due to their child's ADHD. Almost 80% of families had been offered no help from Social Services, despite the fact that 15% of the parents had lost their job as a direct result of caring for their ADHD child and almost half had been treated for depression due to dealing with ADHD in their family (ADDISS 2006). These costs to the family were replicated in a recent population survey of children and young people in Great Britain. This showed that parents of children with hyperkinetic disorder were more likely to be single or previously married and living alone and to be unemployed (Green *et al.* 2005). In addition, almost half of parents of children with ADHD also had a score on the General Health Questionnaire (GHQ) indicative of an emotional disorder (Green *et al.* 2005). Higher rates of stress, relationship difficulties and marital breakdown have been reported in parents of children with ADHD (Mash *et al.* 1983; Murphy *et al.* 1996; Harpin 2005).

Social exclusion

It is not only the child with ADHD who experiences difficulties, and we have heard that their behaviour can have a wide-ranging and negative impact on family life and relationships with friends. There is mounting international evidence of the discrimination experienced by people with mental health and psychosocial problems (Repper and Perkins 2001; Muthukrishna 2007; NICE 2008). In a population survey of mental health in children and young people, over half of all children aged between five and 15 scored in the bottom quartile on a scale measuring the extent of the network of family and friends to whom the child felt close (Green *et al.* 2005).

Due to concerns about their child's behaviour, parents, carers and siblings of those with ADHD often report feeling restricted in what they are able to do in terms of social activities. They report feeling anxious about what people think, embarrassed and worn out (Dean 2005). Events such as planning and organising a day out can be demanding because they require a break from the predictable routine that children and young people with ADHD come to depend on. This means that preparing for days out, special occasions or even shopping trips can often result in having to tolerate greater levels of activity and boisterousness prior to the event. This can create dilemmas for families as they strive to promote social and family inclusion for children with ADHD, and at the same time risk perpetuating social exclusion by experiencing negative comments and feedback from family members and the general public about their child's behaviour. Parents can be left choosing whether to give the child with ADHD one-to-one positive time, or forgo the positives of family-based activities because it is so difficult to do both at the same time. Siblings can become upset or disappointed when special occasions are disrupted. The social exclusion experienced by children and families with ADHD is promoted and maintained by unhelpful popular media coverage which portrays children with ADHD as naughty and their parents as uncaring. Philo *et al.* (1993) showed that negative media reports can and do override the evidence gained from personal experience.

Antisocial and offending behaviour

The costs to the youth and criminal justice systems of treated and untreated ADHD are substantial and arise from mental health comorbidity and antisocial behaviour. Young people with ADHD, particularly the subgroup who also have conduct problems or comorbid social aggression, are at higher risk of developing antisocial or criminal behaviour (Barkley *et al.* 2004). It has been suggested that the prevalence rates of this disorder in delinquent adolescents and young people range from 4% to 72% (Wexler 1996; Vermeiren 2003). Their impulsivity, oppositional and defiant behaviour and tendency to mix with a peer group who have similar problems put children and young people with ADHD on a developmental trajectory towards crime and delinquency (Mannuzza *et al.* 1998; Rasmussen *et al.* 2001; Black *et al.* 2004). Not surprisingly, this combination of factors makes young people with ADHD more likely to be arrested (Satterfield *et al.* 1994), and juvenile prison populations in the UK and in other European and North American countries contain young offenders with high rates of ADHD and other mental health and psychosocial disorders (Rosler *et al.* 2004)

How can nurses help reduce costs and improve outcomes?

One of the fundamental aims of nursing children and families with ADHD is to help improve quality of life and produce positive outcomes. Of course, measuring quality of life associated with ADHD is no easy task, and often the outcome measures will be anecdotal rather than scientific. However, some researchers have attempted to evaluate quality of life as it is affected by ADHD by developing outcome measures. One such evaluation tool is the ADHD Impact Module designed by Landgraf *et al.* (2002). This measures the impact of hyperactivity, impulsivity and inattention on emotional health and social wellbeing.

Putting the difficulties of measurement to one side, there is much that nurses can do in their public health roles to improve health outcomes for children and young people with ADHD. 'Choosing Health', the Government's white paper on public health (Department of Health 2004b), is a strategy to enable all people including children to make informed and healthy lifestyle choices through prevention and early intervention. Primary health prevention refers to those interventions that are aimed at the general population and are intended to preclude the possibility of psychosocial disorders occurring in the first place. Secondary prevention, otherwise called early intervention, is intended to prevent psychosocial problems evolving into disorders that are impairing. Nurses across all settings must weave prevention strategies into their everyday work with children and young people who have ADHD. School nurses are highlighted as key players in improving health outcomes for all children and young people including those with ADHD. We have heard that young people with ADHD are at greater risk of accidents, substance misuse and mental health problems, and impulsivity can lead to lifestyle choices which are often ill considered and reckless. Through their contact with children and young people, nurses in schools, hospitals and prison settings are well placed to encourage children and young people with ADHD to choose not to smoke, not to use alcohol and drugs and to engage in healthy sexual behaviour (Department of Health 2004b).

Improving mental health and psychological wellbeing

'Choosing Health' recognises that good emotional health is of fundamental importance and aims to ensure that children have access to opportunities to nurture their mental health and emotional wellbeing. All nurses and other children's professionals share a responsibility to ensure that every child is given every opportunity to reach their fullest potential and to enjoy good mental health. This is to give them the best start in life. Good mental health involves the ability to enter into and sustain mutually satisfying personal relationships. It is about having emotional resilience, good self-esteem and the skills to cope in the face of stress and adversity. Interventions that enhance self-esteem are therefore crucially important in the treatment of children and young people with ADHD. Nurses should take every opportunity to help children and young people with ADHD build positive self-esteem. Guidance is available for nurses to help enable children and young people to develop positive emotional health and psychological wellbeing (Department of Health 2004a).

Achieving positive outcomes

Psychosocial factors can either foster resilience and personal strength or increase risk and failure. It is important to note that for many people with ADHD, outcomes can be positive. Although the nature of association is not clear, links have been made between creativity, giftedness and brilliance in both children and adults with ADHD (Webb and Latimer 1993; Kutner 1999; Cramond 1994). A review of longitudinal studies noted that by their mid-twenties, two-thirds of those diagnosed with ADHD in their childhood showed no evidence of mental disorder in adulthood. Furthermore, nearly all those with ADHD were gainfully employed and some held higher or professional occupations (Mannuzza and Klein 2000). Further research is required to better understand why some children and young people appear to thrive in the face of stress and adversity.

Summary

The symptoms of ADHD are associated with a range of impairments in personal, family, social, psychological, academic and occupational functioning. Compared with their peers, children with ADHD experience more difficulties in structured settings, struggle in social and academic settings and are more likely to suffer serious psychological impairment throughout their development. Nursing interventions should be carefully tailored not only to improve core symptoms of hyperactivity, inattention and impulsivity but also to focus on improving functional outcomes for young people.

5 Major mental health problems and ADHD

Key points

- ADHD rarely exists as a single disorder. High coexistence with mental disorders, specific learning difficulties and a range of psychosocial problems generates the need for multidisciplinary assessment and treatment strategies.
- ADHD often exists alongside other mental health problems, psychosocial difficulties and developmental disorders. A diagnosis of ADHD may not explain all the difficulties a child or young person is experiencing and it is crucial to explore other reasons for hyperactivity, impulsivity and inattention. Professionals who work with children and young people with ADHD should be aware of these alternative explanations in the course of their assessment and formulation.
- Since children and young people with ADHD and comorbid disorders have greater cognitive, psychological and social impairments, early recognition and intervention is crucial.
- Behavioural problems including conduct disorders, mood disorders such as bipolar disorder and emotional problems such as depression and anxiety can sometimes appear similar to ADHD, and should be considered as a differential diagnosis.
- A better understanding of ADHD comorbidity is required to guide practitioners during the assessment and treatment process, and to inform research and the future classification systems for mental health and behavioural disorders.
- Following diagnosis and before embarking on treatment, healthcare professionals should undertake a comprehensive assessment of comorbidities, parental mental health and the child's or young person's social, familial and educational circumstances.

Introduction

ADHD rarely exists as a single disorder and coexistence or comorbidity is very common (Jensen *et al*. 1997; Dalsgaard *et al*. 2002; Gillberg *et al*. 2004;

Hurtig 2007). Indeed, as many as two-thirds of children and young people with ADHD will have one or more other mental health, neuropsychiatric or developmental disorders (Kaplan *et al.* 2001; Green *et al.* 2005). Some have gone as far to say that ADHD without additional comobidity is rare and may not exist at all (Salmon *et al.* 2006). This means that the process of assessment is rarely straightforward and can often be complex. In particular, the interpretation of hyperactivity can be difficult and treatment decisions may sometimes be controversial. This is both in terms of the high potential for differential diagnosis, and the risks of over- and underdiagnosis of ADHD.

It has been argued that the average primary care professional without a specific mental health background is not sufficiently trained or experienced to identify, differentiate or diagnose most conditions that are comorbid with ADHD (Furman 2005). It is therefore important that nurses and other professionals understand the most common psychosocial disorders that can be experienced by children and young people with ADHD. Whilst the most common of these are conduct disorder, depression and bipolar disorder, a range of developmental and psychosocial problems can also be experienced by children and young people with ADHD. It should never be assumed that a child or young person has ADHD until a full and comprehensive assessment has been undertaken by a multidisciplinary team of professionals. This team will usually include specialists from mental health and paediatric health services, teachers and other school-based professionals and parents or carers.

Conduct problems

Mental health and child care professionals use a range of terms to describe conduct problems. These include disobedient, aggressive, antisocial, challenging, oppositional, defiant and delinquent behaviour. Much more than mischief, rebelliousness or temporary behavioural changes, persistent conduct problems involve the violation of social norms, persistent rule-breaking and a pervasive disregard for authority (Higgins and McDougall 2006). The Diagnostic and Statistical Manual of Mental Disorders (DSM-IV) describes conduct disorder as a repetitive and persistent pattern of behaviour involving aggressive behaviour that causes or threatens physical harm to others; non-aggressive conduct that causes property damage; and deceitfulness or theft and serious violations of rules (American Psychiatric Association 1994). Similarly, the ICD classification of mental and behavioural disorders (ICD-10) focuses on conduct disorder as repetitive and persistent patterns of dissocial, aggressive, oppositional or defiant behaviour (World Health Organisation 1993). The prevalence of conduct disorders in the general population of 11- to 16-year-olds is about 8.1% for boys and 5.1% for girls (Green *et al.* 2005). The criteria for ADHD and conduct disorder are similar and caution must be exercised when assessing and diagnosing both.

Comorbidity for conduct problems with ADHD is high, with as many as half of all children with ADHD also having conduct disorder (Biederman *et al.* 1991; Jensen *et al.* 1997; Nolan and Carr 2000). The causal mechanisms for this are not well understood, and further research is required to improve the classification of these disorders, improve treatment decisions and examine whether ADHD and conduct disorder share similar or different developmental trajectories (Thapar *et al.* 2001; Hyun-Rhee *et al.* 2006; van Lier *et al.* 2007). Longitudinal evidence shows that ADHD contributes to and predicts the persistence of conduct problems and that ADHD usually precedes conduct disorder (Taylor *et al.* 1996). In contrast, there is no evidence that conduct problems in the absence of ADHD lead to the later development of ADHD (NICE 2008).

Oppositional defiant disorder (ODD) is associated with ADHD and is thought to arise from the difficulties associated with executive functioning and self-regulation. Children with this disorder cannot effectively regulate their emotions which can lead to anger, hostility, aggression and defiance. ODD is relatively benign in early childhood where ADHD is not present. When it is comorbid with ADHD there is a high correlation with this developing into conduct problems in later development. Whilst there is some evidence that oppositional defiant disorder is related to disruptive parenting (Farrington 2007), there is no evidence that adequate treatment of ADHD can prevent the onset of conduct problems. The potential for misdiagnosis both ways is high when assessing for conduct problems and ADHD, particularly when assessing younger children where an apparently inattentive pattern of failing to complete activities is instead due to defying adult expectations of the child to conform (Taylor *et al.* 2004).

Children and young people with ADHD experience more difficulty in school, suffer greater relationship difficulties with peers and encounter higher levels of conflict with family members (Hinshaw 1994; Khune 1997). This is discussed in greater detail in chapter 4. Children and young people with ADHD who also have conduct problems are at even greater risk of psychosocial adversity. The combination of conduct problems and ADHD has been shown to predict and co-occur with later persistent substance misuse (Crome and Gilvarry 2005). Children and young people with difficult or challenging behaviour can be problematic for parents and teachers to manage. It is important for nurses to be aware that behaviour problems and ADHD can occur separately or together. When children are younger it is easier to differentiate the two problems, but this becomes more difficult as the child becomes older and the behaviour problems more severe. It is therefore important not to exclude either ADHD or conduct problems without a comprehensive and thorough assessment. Where ADHD and conduct problems coexist, European clinical guidelines recommend that the ADHD should be treated first, since the conduct problems are often secondary (Taylor *et al.* 2004).

Depression and anxiety

When children and young people are anxious or depressed they are often preoccupied with their thoughts and are easily distracted by worries. This can lead to 'off task' behaviours and a deterioration in academic and social functioning. This is also evident in children and young people with obsessive compulsive disorder who may be preoccupied by their behaviour or thoughts and appear to have poor concentration. It is important to assess whether the distractibility and poor concentration of a child or young person can be explained by depression or anxiety, ADHD or a combination of these. This is because comorbidity with ADHD and both depression and anxiety is high. A large survey of the mental health of children in Great Britain showed that one in eight children with ADHD also had an emotional disorder (Green *et al*. 2005).

The common denominator in emotional disorders and ADHD is poor emotional regulation (Loeber *et al*. 1994; Spencer 2001). Depression and anxiety can also be explained in terms of low self-esteem and conflict arising from interpersonal relationship difficulties and poor educational attainment. Both disorders can result in children and young people appearing agitated and preoccupied (Taylor *et al*. 2004). A large multimodal treatment study in the US showed that as many as a third of children and young people with ADHD also have cormorbid emotional disorders such as anxiety or depression (MTA Cooperative Group 1999). The most common of these were simple phobias or separation anxiety. Simple anxiety, generated by difficulties in succeeding academically, vocationally or socially is also very common in children and young people with ADHD.

Depression in childhood can manifest as low self-esteem, irritability, social withdrawal and somatic complaints and is common in children with ADHD (Butler *et al*. 1995; Spencer 2001; NCMH 2006). During adolescence this may present as major clinical depression similar to that experienced by adults. Children and young people with comorbid emotional disorders appear to have a later onset of ADHD, fewer learning difficulties and are less responsive to stimulant medication than children without comorbid emotional disorders (Taylor 1994). It has been suggested that those who meet the criteria for hyperkinetic disorder are more likely to experience behaviour problems and conduct disorder. By comparison, those who have ADHD without hyper-activity are more likely to experience anxiety and depression (Barkley *et al*. 1990).

The decision to treat comorbid anxiety or depression discretely depends on the wishes of the child or young person, their capacity to use a cognitive behavioural therapy approach, the relative severity of the symptoms and the degree of functional impairment associated with both disorders. In many cases, if the ADHD is appropriately treated, the anxiety or depression becomes less problematic for the child or young person. However, this is not always the case, and nurses should be aware that the child or young person may continue to be anxious or depressed even if their ADHD is adequately treated. Good practice guidance on the identification and management of anxiety and depression in children and young people is available, and nurses should consider this when considering whether a child with actual or suspected ADHD is depressed or anxious (National Institute for Clinical Excellence 2004; National Institute for Health and Clinical Excellence 2005).

Bipolar disorder

The hallmarks of bipolar include elated mood, grandiosity, flight of ideas and racing thoughts (Geller at al. 2002; Post *et al*. 2004). These can appear very similar to behaviours associated with ADHD and accurate diagnosis is further complicated by very high comorbidity rates (Geller and Luby 1997). Indeed, the younger the child is, the more difficult the two disorders can be to distinguish. This is because symptoms such as distractibility, overactivity, restlessness over talkativeness and emotional instability characterise both disorders. This makes the potential for misdiagnosis high. However, studies of ADHD and bipolar disorder suggest that the two disorders exist as discrete entities in many young people (Biederman 1998).

The most common shared symptom between ADHD and bipolar disorder is irritability (National Collaborating Centre for Mental Health 2006). However, ADHD will normally have become evident during childhood, whereas bipolar disorder is more common during adolescence, which means the development of new symptoms can be relevant in distinguishing the disorders. However, a number of factors distinguish the two disorders. Unlike ADHD which is persistent and stable, bipolar disorder follows an episodic or cyclical course. In addition, mania and inappropriate or impairing grandiosity are present in bipolar disorder and are not part of ADHD (see Table 5.1).

Nurses and other professionals can be assisted to distinguish ADHD from bipolar disorder by using specific diagnostic tools such as the Washington University Kiddie Schedule for Affective Disorders and Schizophrenia (WASH-U-KSADS) (Geller *et al*. 1996) which contains specific items for ADHD and can be completed separately by children and parents or carers. Although diagnostic tools are not sufficient to distinguish one disorder from another with absolute certainty, they can be useful to inform the wider multidisciplinary and multimodal assessment process.

The medical management of bipolarity should usually be addressed before managing ADHD symptoms with ADHD medication (Gellet at al. 2002). Children and young people with bipolar disorder and ADHD are particularly at risk of developing a manic episode, and caution must be exercised when using stimulants to treat their ADHD. Good practice guidance on the assessment, treatment and management of bipolar disorder is available for nurses and other professionals and this includes a section on children and young people (National Collaborating Centre for Mental Health 2006). Nurses should always consult this guidance when differentiating between the

Table 5.1 Differentiating ADHD and bipolar disorder

Symptom	ADHD	Bipolar disorder
Overactivity	✓	✓
Impulsivity	✓	✓
Hyperactivity	✓	✓
Inattention	✓	✓
Decreased need for sleep	✓	✓
Fatigue	✓	✗
Poor concentration	✓	✓
Psychomotor agitation	✓	✓
Irritability	✓	✓
Distractibility	✓	✓
Restlessness	✓	✓
Overtalkativeness	✓	✓
Persistence	✓	✗
Low self-esteem	✓	✗
Pressured speech	✗	✓
Racing thoughts	✗	✓
Flight of ideas	✗	✓
Hypersexuality	✗	✓
Labile mood	✗	✓
Elation	✗	✓
Euphoria	✗	✓
Suicidality	✗	✓
Grandiosity	✗	✓
Psychosis	✗	✓
Cyclical	✗	✓
Episodic	✗	✓

presentation and needs of those with ADHD and bipolar disorder either separately or in combination.

Psychosis

Psychotic disorders are very rare in children and relatively rare in adolescents. However, when making an assessment of a young person who appears easily distracted and who has poor concentration, psychosis should be considered in the formulation and differential diagnosis. Children and young people who are psychotic or who are suspected to be psychotic will require urgent assessment or treatment from specialist mental health services.

Autistic spectrum disorders

Children with autism and autistic spectrum disorders sometimes exhibit hyperactive behaviour, and children with ADHD often have autistic traits (Gillberg and Billstedt 2000; Fitzgerald and Corvin 2001; Banaschewski *et al.*

2005). The relationship between these two disorders, if indeed they are two discrete disorders, is not well understood. Children and young people with autistic spectrum disorders are often aloof, preoccupied with their own interests and not always on task with group activities. They may appear to be inattentive and experience motor restlessness. Clark *et al.* (1999) studied the rate of autistic symptoms in a sample of children with ADHD and found that between 65% and 85% of parents reported significant difficulties in their child's social interaction and communication. The difficulties that parents reported related to non-verbal communication, imaginative play, empathy and peer friendships (Clark *et al.* 1999).

Separating autistic behaviours from hyperactivity is not based on excluding hyperactive features but on detecting the presence of autistic types of impairment (Taylor *et al.* 2004). Young people with both ADHD and autistic spectrum disorder experience difficulties with executive functioning. However, problems with self-regulation are more closely associated with ADHD, whilst difficulties associated with the theory of mind, that is, the cognitive capacity to attribute mental states to oneself and others, are more closely associated with autism (Baron-Cohen *et al.* 1993). In addition, the cognitive impairments shown by children with autistic spectrum disorders tend to be global, whereas in ADHD they are related more often to how demanding or rewarding the task is to the individual. DSM-IV and ICD-10 guidance categorically states that ADHD should not be recognised in the presence of pervasive developmental disorders or autistic spectrum disorders. However, best practice guidance and research recommends that a diagnosis of ADHD can be made in a child with these disorders (Reierson *et al.* 2007; NICE 2008)

Tic disorders

Due to the strong neurological basis of ADHD, some children with this disorder also develop tics or Tourette's syndrome (Rothenberger *et al.* 2004). Tics are common in childhood and most are mild, transient or episodic. Unless they bother the child, tics do not usually require medical attention. If tics significantly affect social functioning, behaviour therapies or pharmacological management may be indicated (NICE 2008). Tourette's syndrome is characterised by involuntary motor and vocal tics of varying frequency and severity. Treatment depends on the impairment caused by the tics and the quality of life experienced by the child or young person concerned. It is likely that there is a one-way comorbidity for Tourette's syndrome in children and young people with ADHD. This means that although less than 2% of children with ADHD meet the criteria for Tourette's syndrome, ADHD occurs in at least half of those with a diagnosis of Tourette's. The use of stimulants can exacerbate tics in some children with ADHD, and for this reason atomoxetine is often used as it does not adversely affect tics (NICE 2006).

Attachment and separation

The first five years of a child's life are vitally important in forming and sustaining key relationships. Attachment disorders can occur where children have experienced adverse life events or disrupted attachment relationships. This can lead to indiscriminate clinging to adults, overly outgoing and indiscriminate relationships and difficulty in forming long-standing, trusting relationships (O'Connor and Rutter 2000; Taylor *et al*. 2004). Children who have been physically or sexually abused may be hypervigilant, have behaviour problems and present as disorganised in their attachments to significant others. Early negative life experiences, separations from parents and early relationship difficulties can produce behaviours similar to ADHD. Children with attachment disorder can appear overactive, disinhibited, appear to have low tolerance and frustration levels suggestive of poor concentration and have poor self-control. It is difficult to distinguish attachment disorder and ADHD and they may exist together (NICE 2008).

Learning difficulties and disability

Mental health and developmental disorders are much more common in children with learning disabilities than in other children (Emerson 2003). Attentional difficulties may be the result of global or specific learning disabilities and are common in children and young people and adults with ADHD (Rasmussen and Gillberg 2000; Fox and Wade 1998). In reporting on the Ontario Child Health Study, Szatmari *et al*. (1989) stated that approximately one-third of those diagnosed with ADHD also had specific problems with reading, spelling and mathematics which were unaccounted for by low intelligence. Not surprisingly, specific learning difficulties can lead to lower grades and poorer overall academic performance when compared with non-affected peers at school (Mannuzza *et al*. 1998; Willoughby 2003).

Understanding the child's level of learning, ability and attainment is an integral part of understanding the symptoms they present. Nurses and other professionals should consider whether poor achievements at school are a result of learning difficulties, inattention or a combination of the two. Similarly, psychomotor abnormalities and overacivity are common in both learning disabilities and ADHD. In learning disability this may be caused by brain damage and the need for sensory stimulation. Furthermore, behaviour problems characterise both ADHD and learning disabilities (Chadwick *et al*. 1998). However, the reasons for these and the process for how they are maintained are different. Conduct disorders are less directly associated with learning disabilities than ADHD. The sleep patterns of children and young people with ADHD and those experienced by people with learning disabilities are often disrupted (Quine 1991; Quine 1992; Quine 1993), and nurses should consider this as part of their assessment and formulation.

Assessing children and young people with learning disabilities

Nursing assessments must always be developmentally appropriate and take into account the child's level of ability. For example, if a child has a chronological age of ten years, yet functions at the academic level of a five-year-old, the presenting symptoms should be assessed in the context of what is expected of a five-year-old. It is also important to adapt the assessment process to suit the child's developmental abilities. Some children and young people with learning disabilities struggle to label their emotions and articulate subjective experiences in abstract language. Obtaining accurate information about their thoughts, feelings and internal world can therefore be a challenging process for the nurse and the potential for miscommunication can be great (Levitas *et al.* 2001; Hardy and Bouras 2002; McDougall 2006). Prior to the assessment of a young person with a learning disability and suspected ADHD, the nurse should prepare their assessment strategy and may wish to plan some of their questions in advance. They should be aware of any communication needs associated with hearing or vision, and the interview should be paced according to level of understanding and attention span. Open-ended rather than closed questions should be used and the nurse should avoid using jargon or abstract language, particularly when the young person is suspecting of having or has been diagnosed with Asperger's syndrome (Atwood 1998).

In summary, learning disability can coexist with ADHD and does not exclude the diagnosis. When making a differential diagnosis, the nurse must consider whether the disturbance of activity and attention is too severe to be explained in terms of the child's developmental abilities in the context of their learning disability. This is often a complex process and nurses should always consult with their multidisciplinary colleagues when formulating conclusions and making diagnoses.

Substance misuse

Much has been made in the media about the similarities between methylphenidate and cocaine, and both drugs work by blocking the dopamine transporter (Taylor *et al.* 2004; Quist *et al.* 2003). The effects of illicit substances, particularly drugs such as amphetamine and cocaine, can produce inattention, impulsivity and irritability. These are all behaviours experienced by children and young people with ADHD. As it is not unusual for young people to take illicit drugs, professionals should be aware of the signs and symptoms of substance misuse and how these might be recognised in a young person with ADHD.

Other disorders of childhood

It is not only mental health disorders that produce behaviours which can be similar to those shown in a child or young person with ADHD. A range of developmental and psychosocial factors may help to explain a child's hyperactivity, impulsivity or inattention. Many children with ADHD experience neurodevelopmental delays including language acquisition problems and sensory motor coordination deficits (Taylor *et al.* 1991; Gillberg 2003). In addition, speech and language problems (Love and Thompson 1988; Hinshaw 2002), poor hand–eye coordination and clumsiness (Losse *et al.* 1991; Hallgren *et al.* 1993; Rasmussen and Gillberg 2000), hearing impairment (Hindley and Kroll 1998) and difficulties with reading and writing (August and Garfinkel 1990; McGee *et al.* 1992; Gillis *et al.* 1992; Fonagy 2002; Marzocchi *et al.* 2008) are all very common.

Epilepsy is a common neurological disorder of childhood and children with epilepsy are at risk for symptoms of ADHD (Dunn *et al.* 2003; Hesdorffer *et al.* 2004). As with other difficulties, children with epilepsy can appear restless, preoccupied, distracted and off-task. Behaviour problems are not unusual in children with epilepsy. Due to the impulsivity and hyperactivity of children with ADHD, they are more prone to serious injury including brain injury, thus contributing to existing ADHD symptoms if the injury was severe. Some children may appear to have ADHD symptoms following head injury where there were no primary concerns. The results of brain injuries per se can also mimic ADHD symptoms, and excluding one from the other and assessing comorbidity requires specialist assessment.

Summary

It is important that professionals who work with children and young people with ADHD understand that ADHD rarely exists as a single disorder, and that comorbidity with a range of psychological, developmental and psychosocial disorders is common. Nurses should therefore be aware of the most common disorders and symptoms that can overlap with or mimic ADHD. Since children and young people with ADHD and comorbid disorders have greater cognitive, psychological and social impairments, early recognition and intervention is crucial. Cormorbidity leads to significant impairment in everyday functioning at home, in school and with peers. The prognosis and outcomes for children and young people with ADHD and cormobid disorders can often be poor, and nurses should help ensure that treatment strategies are multimodal and address psychological, educational, family and social functioning.

6 What do children, young people and families tell us about living with ADHD?

Key points

- High-quality research about the views and opinions of children with ADHD and their parents or carers is lacking. A small number of phenomenological studies have sought to understand how children and young people feel about being labelled with ADHD, what they think about taking medication, and their experiences of stigma. Since most of the research comes from the US, nurses should be cautious when applying findings to the UK, where education, social care and health services are different.
- The experiences and views of children and young people with ADHD and those of their parents or carers will be vastly different and often inconsistent. It is vitally important that nurses routinely explore narratives and enquire about the lived experience of ADHD. This is in order to provide holistic, child- and family-centred care and to help ensure that interventions are tailored to produce optimal outcomes.
- Children and young people report that having ADHD makes them feel different. This can impact negatively on self-perceptions, self-esteem and self-confidence. Nurses should take every opportunity to help children and young people with ADHD build positive self-esteem.
- It is not only the individual child or young person who suffers from the negative impact of ADHD. Living with a child who has ADHD is no easy task, and parents and carers, brothers and sisters, friends and teachers are also affected. Nurses should always consider the wider impacts as part of their assessment and management strategies. This may sometimes require a formal assessment of family needs focusing on personal, social and mental health needs, and liaison with other professionals will help ensure that families receive the support they require.
- Nurses should educate young people about ADHD and listen to their views about diagnosis and treatments.
- Gaining a subjective understanding of the everyday experiences of living with ADHD may lead to improved assessments and better treatment outcomes for all family members affected by this disorder.

Introduction

There have been numerous studies regarding the epidemiology, cause and treatment of ADHD, but little research into the lived experiences of those who are living with this disorder on a day-to-day basis. The aim of this chapter is to summarise what children and young people with ADHD, their siblings and parents or carers tell professionals about their experience of living with ADHD. What is known about how children and young people feel about having ADHD, what they think about being diagnosed and labelled and what their experiences are of taking medication will be explored. In addition, the challenges of parenting children with ADHD and the different perceptions of mothers, fathers and siblings will also be described. Finally, what parents and carers think and feel about the professional services they receive from healthcare providers and schools will be discussed. It is important to note that the views of children, parents or carers about ADHD are not always the same and can often be disparate.

What does research tell us?

High-quality research about the views and opinions of children with ADHD and their parents or carers is woefully lacking, and rarely are children and young people's voices heard in relation to their experiences of ADHD (Pryjmachuk 1999; Kendall *et al.* 2003). Existing research has focused on the views of children and young people (Baxley *et al.* 1978; Efron *et al.* 1998; Krueger and Kendall 2001; Meaux *et al.* 2006) and on those of their parents or carers (Singh 2004; McElearney *et al.* 2005; Hansen and Hansen 2006). A relatively small number of studies and focus groups have sought to understand how children and young people feel about being labelled with ADHD (Kendall 1997; Hinton and Wolpert 1998; Cooper and Shea 2000; Shattell *et al.* 2008), how they feel about taking medication (Meaux *et al.* 2006), and their experiences of ADHD in school (Muthukrishna 2007). Most of these studies have been qualitative in design and have used semi-structured interviews to evaluate the lived experience of ADHD. This is not a criticism, since qualitative healthcare research enables us to study selected issues, cases or events in people's lives in a level of depth and detail that quantitative strategies cannot provide. Quantitative approaches also allow for large-scale measurement of ideas, beliefs and attitudes (Paton 2002) and are ideal for evaluating the lived experience of ADHD. A small number of evaluation tools have been developed in the US to assist practitioners to seek service user views about ADHD. These include the ADHD Knowledge and Opinion Scale Revised (AKOS-R) which is a 43 item scale used to evaluate opinions about psychological and pharmacological treatments for ADHD (Rostain *et al.* 1993).

Whilst developing the practice guideline for ADHD, the National Institute for Health and Clinical Excellence (NICE 2008) explored personal accounts from young people, adults and their families about their day-to-day experience of living with a diagnosis and symptoms of ADHD. It is important to remember that the experiences and views of children and young people with ADHD and those of their parents or carers will often be inconsistent and sometimes vastly different. Views evolve from individual experiences and are shaped by unique life stories and personal accounts. Contact with health service providers, teachers, social workers and other professionals will all influence views, both positively and negatively. These views and beliefs can remain fixed or may change during the course of the assessment and treatment process. It is therefore important for the nurse to remain aware that views and opinions may change throughout the course of treatment, and this is an important factor when we consider consent for treatment. The views of children, young people and parents or carers can be sought in a number of different ways including:

- service user testimonies and personal accounts;
- qualitative studies of children, young people and family views;
- service user involvement in service planning and evaluation.

It is vitally important that nurses routinely explore narratives, enquire about the lived experience of ADHD and ask about the quality of the services that children, young people and families or carers receive. This is in order to provide holistic, child- and family-centred care and to help ensure that interventions are tailored to produce optimal outcomes.

Being labelled

Studies about the experience of living with ADHD have attempted to identify the core beliefs that children and young people hold. Just as there are various academic explanations for how ADHD is caused, so too do young people hold differing beliefs. It is clear from many studies that children have little understanding about what ADHD is and how it may be caused. As Judy Kendall, a professor of nursing from Oregon who has written prolifically about the lived experience of ADHD points out, many children and young people report having 'no idea' why they have ADHD, or conclude that it is just part of who they are (Kendall 2003). Children and young people report a range of views about being labelled, and being diagnosed with ADHD appears to carry benefits as well as risks. In a study of adolescents with a diagnosis of ADHD, Krueger and Kendall (2001) focused on how young people with ADHD perceived themselves and their diagnosis. Interestingly, this study suggested that young people often internalise their diagnosis of ADHD and do not resist being described as having ADHD. Themes suggested that girls were much more likely to describe themselves as inadequate, whilst boys framed themselves as being angry and defiant. This was surprising to the researchers who had expected the group to describe feeling misunderstood, frustrated or fed up and to associate these feelings with difficulties at school or at home. Instead, the young people identified themselves with ADHD, as this in fact was who they were (Krueger and Kendall 2001).

The experience of being diagnosed with ADHD can also be negative. In a small study of 39 children and young people with ADHD, Kendall *et al.* (2003) heard that participants generally associated their diagnosis with adversity. These included problems with day-to-day living, and problems at school such as difficulty thinking caused by distractibility, and feelings of confusion arising from poor listening skills. Problems with behaviour, difficulties following rules and boundaries and not getting along with other people were also recurring themes. Adolescents in particular were aware that they had problems with disinhibition, impulsivity and aggression which made forming and sustaining peer relationships problematic. Various terms were used to describe having a diagnosis of ADHD. Young people consistently talked about feeling 'sad', 'mad', 'bad', 'weird' and 'ashamed'. They felt responsible for the impact of their behaviour on family and friends and told researchers that this made them feel sad and angry (Kendall *et al.* 2003).

Taking medication

Research has focused on the experience of taking medication much more than any other aspect of living with ADHD. This may be no coincidence since the pharmacological treatment of ADHD has received more research attention and media coverage than any other aspect of the management of this disorder (Coghill 2003; Banaschewski *et al.* 2006). Children and young people appear to hold a range of views about the use of medication, and these often vary from those of their parents and teachers. Effron *et al.* (1998) sought the views of over 100 young people about taking methylphenidate and dexamphetamine. Just over 30% reported that they felt much better; 28% described feeling better; 25% did not feel any different on medication; 11% reported feeling worse and 5.5% said that they felt much worse while taking medication. Young people were also asked to rate how helpful they thought the medication was for their ADHD symptoms. 42% reported that it was very helpful, 26.5% a bit helpful, 20% were unsure, 4.5% not very helpful and 6% did not think that medication was helpful at all (see Table 6.1 and Table 6.2).

In the study by Effron *et al.* (1998), young people who were interviewed made various positive statements about taking medication. These included 'It felt much easier to sit down and do my work' and 'Everyone plays with me now, because they know I won't get them into trouble'. Young people also reported negative responses in relation to taking methylphenidate or dexamphetamine tablets including 'They stop me getting to sleep', 'They give me a headache' and 'They make me feel funny' (Efron *et al.* 1998). These

Table 6.1 How young people felt whilst taking ADHD medication

Young people's views	Percentage
Felt much worse	5.5
Felt worse	11
Felt same as usual	25
Felt better	28
Felt much better	30

Source: Effron *et al.* (1998)

Table 6.2 Young people's views about the effectiveness of ADHD medication

Young people's views	Percentage
Very helpful	42
A bit helpful	26.5
Unsure	20
Not very helpful	4.5
Not helpful at all	6

Source: Effron *et al.* (1998)

are interesting findings which have implications for nurses caring for children and young people with ADHD. On the one hand, children and young people complained of side effects and negative feelings about taking medication, yet two-thirds felt that taking medication was either helpful or very helpful. This illustrates the need to get the balance right between achieving the positive benefits of medication and tolerating unwanted side effects. Amongst other things, this is because the unwanted effects of medication are associated with high rates of non-compliance.

In a similar study, McElearney *et al.* (2005) looked at a cohort of 40 children with ADHD and 40 children with epilepsy to understand their views about taking medication. Information was gathered using questionnaires which explored the attitudes of both children and parents towards medication. The results for the ADHD children showed 60% of children and 95% of parents knew the name of their medication; 92.5% of children and 92.5% of parents knew what the medication was for; 60% of children and 87.5% of parents were compliant with treatment regime; 32.5% had told a friend they were taking medication and 82.5% of parents would give medication in front of another family member. Overall 60% of children and 90% of parents reported good things about taking medication; whereas 15% of children reported negative aspects about medication whilst only 42.5% of parents reported this (see Table 6.3).

Table 6.3 Comparison of parents' and young people's attributes and knowledge of medication

	Young people (%)	Parents (%)
Name of medication	60	95
Purpose of medication	92.5	92.5
Concordance with treatment regimes	60	87.5
Tell a friend or family member	32.5	82.5
Good things about taking medication	60	90
Bad things about taking medication	15	42.5

Source: McElearney *et al.* (2005)

Once again, it is interesting that it is parents more than young people them-selves who consider the effects of medication to be positive. Young people reported that they adhered to treatment regime less than parents' reports. Parents who reported less concordance to treatment regimes also reported more unwanted effects. Young people with ADHD were reluctant to talk to friends about ADHD and medication use compared to young people with epilepsy, suggesting the awareness of the stigma associated with having ADHD (McElearney *et al.* 2005). Again, whilst this was only a small study, the results highlighted the differences in the reported positive effects of treatments with stimulants in young people and their parents, illustrating the importance of discussing treatment and unwanted effects with all family members.

Medication was a common theme in a study by Kendall *et al.* (2003). Children and young people who were interviewed said that medication helped control hyperactivity, increased concentration and improved perform-ance in school. Whilst they considered medication to be the most helpful aspect of treatment, young people in the study said they didn't want to take pills. They reported that ADHD medications tasted bad and highlighted unwanted effects such as headaches and stomach aches. Worryingly, young people expressed shame and fear about having to take medication to control their behaviour and felt reluctant to share this information with others. While reports varied, some young people said that medication made them feel different, while others felt depressed or lacking in motivation (Kendall *et al.* 2003).

Research suggests that many young people have realistic expectations about the value of medication for their ADHD. Consistent with high-quality controlled trials, they report that medication controls disruptive behaviour and helps bring about improvements in friendships, but does not improve schoolwork and academic functioning (Meaux 2006). Indeed, the positive outcomes from taking medication to help manage ADHD have been reported to be largely social and associated with better peer relationships. Some children and young people say that taking medication helps them think clearly, understand better and feel in control. This, they say, helps them get on better with family and friends. The negative outcomes are reported to include reduced appetite and difficulties with sleep, and the effects of stigma (McElearney *et al.* 2005). Although children and young people frequently report that they do not like taking medication, they are able to recognise the 'trade-off' involved in tolerating negative effects and benefiting from the positive effects (Meaux *et al.* 2006).

When views about medication differ

Children and young people as well as their parents and carers report positive and negative feelings about taking stimulant medication for their ADHD. However, in various studies related to perceptions about stimulant medication views about benefits and costs have differed. Parents often consider medication to be more helpful than children and young people do themselves (McNeal *et al.* 2004). The study by Effron *et al.* (1998) also highlighted perceptual differences that often occur between young people and parents. Whilst parents and teachers reported that medication had produced positive effects, the young people themselves often felt that there was no difference on or off treatment. This is not a usual finding in clinic situations where it is difficult for young people to report objective changes in their own presentations. Young people's views are important even when they find it hard to express what they think and feel, and these should always be sought by nurses when making decisions about continued treatment with medication for ADHD. Therefore, it is important to acknowledge that children's views may well be different from those of their parents or carers.

Difficulties at home

We have heard that the experience of ADHD affects not only the individual child but also their whole family and sometimes the wider community. Children and young people with ADHD are often aware that their impulsivity, hyperactivity and intrusiveness can be annoying or feel overwhelming to others (McElearney *et al.* 2005). Both scientific studies and the growing service user literature about ADHD consistently demonstrate that children and young people with ADHD experience difficulties and suffer impairment at school, at home and with peer relationships (Kendall *et al.* 2005). However, we know little about how this makes them feel. A consistently recurring theme in qualitative studies involves struggling to get on with parents, siblings and partners. Young people report that arguments with parents and difficulties with friendships are common. Children with ADHD perceive that their parents are less patient with them than with their siblings. However, when parents are able to be supportive of young people by acknowledging their positives, highlighting their strengths and affirming their love for the young person, this is reported to be a powerful mediator in terms of their self-esteem and place in the family.

Difficulties at school

Young people often talk negatively about their experiences of having ADHD in school. Numerous studies demonstrate that the symptoms of hyperactivity, impulsivity and inattention present children and young people with a range of academic and social challenges in the school setting (Muthukrishna 2007). Service user testimonies consistently support research findings by confirming that school presents children with ADHD with a range of difficulties. Many describe feeling frustrated because the school is unable to accommodate their needs. Children and young people consistently highlight difficulties with paying attention, listening and concentrating. Feelings of frustration caused by the class moving on to other topics just as they were understanding concepts often result in young people feeling inadequate.

As well as reporting that it is difficult to cope with ADHD in school, pupils are able to identify measures that teachers take to make things easier. Children and young people with ADHD report that when teachers take time to help them with classwork or go over homework this helps with feelings of isolation in the classroom and improves learning (Shattell *et al*. 2008). Asking for extra time, sitting in quiet areas of the classroom to reduce distractions, using a computer and recording lectures to be listened to again are all reported as being helpful (Shattell *et al*. 2008).

Feeling different

We have heard that children and young people use a range of terms to describe themselves and these are often negative. For many, the experience of being told they are stupid, lazy or disruptive is internalised and has a detrimental effect on self-concept and self-esteem. Barber *et al*. (2005) looked at perceptions of children with ADHD versus non-ADHD children. They discovered that young people with a diagnosis of ADHD scored less positively than non-ADHD children overall and in particular in areas related to school performance, social skills, physical appearance and self-worth.

Research consistently shows that children and young people with ADHD perceive themselves to be different from their non-ADHD peer group (Kendall *et al*. 2003; Shattell *et al*. 2008). This common theme has also been highlighted in studies of adults with ADHD (Young and Bramham 2007). This highlights the need for nurses in clinical practice to be aware of issues of low self-esteem, lack of self-confidence and the potential need for peer support. Frame *et al*. (2003) demonstrated that school-based peer support groups for children with ADHD have positively increased self-worth. School nurses in particular should consider the impact of a diagnosis of ADHD on the young person's life and review whether further assistance would be helpful in improving self-esteem and self-confidence. Whilst feeling different can impact negatively on self-perceptions, self-esteem and self-confidence, it may not be an adverse experience for all children and young people with ADHD. However, school nurses and other professionals should take every opportunity to help children and young people to build positive self-esteem through whole-class or whole-school interventions. This is in keeping with the spirit of Every Child Matters (Department for Education and Skills 2003) and the current social inclusion agenda.

Stigma

Service user feedback demonstrates that stigma is a widely experienced negative consequence of being given a diagnosis of ADHD (Hinshaw 2005; Muthukrishna 2006). For some children, this is associated with taking medication or being laughed at (Kendall *et al*. 2003), whilst for others the stigma is due to feeling different (Barber *et al*. 2005; Shattell *et al*. 2008). In a study by Meaux (2006), children with ADHD wished for a better understanding of their disorder by society as a whole, and felt stigmatised for having to take medication. Although they felt less stigmatised by the diagnosis of ADHD, this often led to low self-esteem and poor self-confidence (Meaux 2006).

Despite the rather widespread knowledge about ADHD, those who are hyperactive, impulsive or inattentive are frequently the targets of blame. This is not only by parents and carers but also by professionals who attribute intentionality to children and young people with ADHD (Tollefson and Chen 1988; Hoza *et al*. 2000; Blunt-Bugental 2003). In holding them accountable for their inability to pay attention, sit still or remain quiet, it has been suggested that those who regard the symptoms of ADHD as being under the child's control are less motivated to try and help (Tollefson and Chen 1998). Helping to remove the stigma associated with ADHD is no easy task. Some nurses have suggested that deconstructing ADHD as an illness or disability, and instead building on strengths may better serve the child involved (Ludwikowski and DeValk 1998).

What do parents tell us?

Little is known about the views of parents and carers about their children with ADHD (Hoza *et al*. 2000). From the available literature, parents describe the impact that ADHD has on the family system as a whole, how it affects them themselves as parents and the impact they believe ADHD has on their affected and non-affected children. Kendall and Shelton (2003) and Jackson (2003) each describe this simply as 'chaotic'. A small number of studies have explored the role of parental schemata in the management of children with ADHD. This refers to the unconscious cognitive structures that organise experiences by providing scripts and goals (Bull and Whelan 2006). Understanding the core beliefs that parents hold about ADHD is crucially important if nurses are to engage parents and provide meaningful and sensitive interventions. This is because the way in which children are parented has a direct effect on treatment outcomes for children and young people with this disorder (Winsler 1998).

Accessing help

Parental accounts of living with ADHD are eloquently described in the NICE guidelines (NICE 2008). These are 'snapshots' of personal accounts and summarise the difficulties that some parents face when trying to not only understand the behaviour of their own child but also get someone else to understand it too. Like young people themselves, parents commonly believe that their child is innately different. Mothers in particular often recall feeling this to be true from a very early age (Colley 2005; Bull and Whelan 2006). They describe how they question their own parenting abilities and wonder if they have failed their child. The NICE guidelines describe how all too often parents struggle to access a service that is appropriate, caring and thoughtful. Typically, their journey from assessment to diagnosis is long and arduous, and this depended to some extent on where they live, whether their GP understands ADHD and whether treatments and ongoing supportive care are available.

Fighting battles

Harborne *et al.* (2004) undertook a small study of nine families in the UK with a child with ADHD and other comorbid problems such as mild learning difficulties, Asperger's syndrome and statement of special educational needs to look at parental views of their child being diagnosed with ADHD. A range of themes emerged focused around blame, battles and emotional distress. Blame was associated with poor parenting and was particularly levelled at mothers. Overwhelming experiences of frustration were themed as 'battles', where parents disagreed with teachers and other professionals about the nature, cause and appropriate treatment and management strategies for ADHD. Emotional distress was a common theme in the study, where mothers had suffered profoundly as a result of their child's difficulties. Low self-esteem, a lack of confidence and a poor sense of self-worth were all common experiences for parents (Harborne *et al.* 2004).

Parents living with a young person with ADHD report that it is stressful on an ongoing basis. Douglas (1999) describes life prior to diagnosis as chaos and torment with each everyday task seeming like an uphill struggle. The added responsibility and burden placed on parents and families caring for a child or young person with ADHD are often well understood and acknowledged, yet there is very little real understanding and support from society as a whole. In describing the impact upon the family system, Douglas (1999) reports that relationships and friendships involving the child become fraught, and parents become isolated and lonely, wondering where they are going wrong (Douglas

1999). Feelings of loneliness and isolation have also been described by Shattell *et al.* (2008). Parents report mixed views about the usefulness of a diagnosis for their child. Some regard this as a positive experience (Klasen and Goodman 2000), others feel guilty and somehow responsible (Singh 2004). For many parents, particularly mothers, these feelings of guilt can quickly transform into feelings of inadequacy, blame and shame (Singh 2003; Hansen and Hansen 2006). In a small study of 29 families living with ADHD, beliefs about impairment varied between GPs and parents (Klasen and Goodman 2000). GPs were less likely to view hyperactivity as a medical problem than parents. Whereas parents reported that labelling the problems was a generally helpful process, GPs felt that diagnosing hyperactivity was potentially harmful. However, parents and GPs agreed that living with ADHD caused dysfunction and family stress. They also agreed that backup services and specialist help were difficult to find and that information provided by professionals was often conflicting and ambiguous (Klasen and Goodman 2000).

Medication

Perhaps not surprisingly, parents frequently have ambivalent feelings about their child taking medication (Cohen and Thompson 1982; Liu *et al.* 1991; Bennett *et al.* 1996). This is not unique to ADHD medication and similar concerns have been expressed by parents whose children have asthma (Peterson-Sweeney *et al.* 2003), epilepsy (Gordon *et al.* 2001) and chronic pain (Foreward *et al.* 1996). Some parents expect that medication will fix all the problems associated with their child's ADHD (Ludwikowski and DeValk 1998). Others are sceptical about its effects on behaviour (Bussing *et al.* 2003; Bull and Whelan 2006). The majority appear to experience dilemmas associated with the positive and negative effects that medication may potentially or actually bring to their children. In a phenomenological study about attitudes to stimulant medication, Hansen and Hansen (2006) described parents as being caught in a balancing act as they considered the desirable and undesirable effects of medication at home and in school. It is important that a realistic understanding reached about the purpose of treatment with medication, and those difficulties which treatment with medication will not directly address.

Mothers and fathers

It has been suggested that mothers and fathers of children with ADHD have different core beliefs and attitudes to parenting (Tallmadge and Barkley 1983). Whilst the popular misconception that ADHD is caused by poor parenting is reported to be upsetting for both mothers and fathers, the way in which this experience is internalised appears to vary. In many reports about parenting children with ADHD, mothers in particular describe their own mental health problems such as being depressed, stressed, not sleeping, gaining weight and feeling they are going mad (Faraone *et al*. 1995; Harborne *et al*. 2004; Bull and Whelan 2006). Interestingly, in a study by Kendall *et al*. (2003), young people expressed little insight into the impact of ADHD on the family as a whole but recognised the important role of their mother in supporting and caring for them.

In a study of fathers' perspectives on ADHD, Singh (2003) found that of 22 fathers, only four thought their son's behaviour required medical attention. They all agreed that their children were badly behaved, but attributed this to poor motivation, falling behind at school and being spoilt by overindulgent mothers. Fathers, it was concluded, were more likely to believe that the difficulties their sons were experiencing were inevitable and part of 'boys being boys' (Singh 2003). Interestingly, in a focus group study by Bussing and Gary (2001) parents offered an alternative explanation for not taking their daughters with ADHD symptoms to see a doctor. They expressed a view that their daughter's behaviour was just a sign of being a 'tomboy'. They felt the girls would eventually outgrow this behaviour and become more 'lady-like' (Bussing and Gary 2001). It is of note that many of the fathers in Singh's study had not been involved in the assessment of their son's behaviour. Only seven had any involvement and 13 thought that treatment with medication was a good idea. It has previously been observed that fathers are much less likely to participate in research studies and participate less than mothers in the healthcare assessment process and parent support groups (Schmidt-Neven 2000; Petersson *et al*. 2003; Singh 2003; Bull and Whelan 2006; Hurt *et al*. 2007). This illustrates the importance of involving fathers as well as mothers in the assessment and treatment processes for young people. Assessment strategies may need to be different, and the process of engagement with mothers and fathers may evolve at different rates.

Blame

Many parents have a long history of feeling blamed, and blame themselves, for the behaviour problems of their children (Taylor *et al*. 2004). It is not unusual for judgements to be passed in relation to parenting children and young people with ADHD. Accusations about poor parenting, an inability to manage bad behaviour and a lack of control are common. Yet at the same time, such parents may be raising other children with no difficulties with behaviour or compliance. Guilt is almost synonymous with parenting a child who has ADHD, and it is rare that a parent will resist such blame and challenge it, particularly if it is levelled by a professional (Myttas 2008).

It is mothers who are more likely to feel directly blamed and personally responsible for their child's difficulties (Singh 2002; Singh 2004). This finding has been replicated elsewhere, where mothers describe feeling blamed by partners and professionals in contact with their child (Sobol *et al*. 1989; Gerdes *et al*. 2003; Harborne *et al*. 2004; Cronin 2004). Not surprisingly, this may lead mothers to doubt or question their own parenting skills and many conclude that they have failed their children or done wrong (Colley 2005). For many mothers, receiving a diagnosis of ADHD brings a sense of relief. It is a liberating experience which enables them to feel differently about the causes of their child's difficulties and their own role as a parent (Singh 2003; Harborne *et al.* 2004). Core beliefs associated with blame can have a profound emotional impact upon the self-concept and emotional wellbeing of parents, and it is easy to see how the negative cycle of blame can be perpetuated. It is essential that nurses seek to understand parental attributions about ADHD. This is to help break unhelpful cycles of blame by enabling parents to discuss their beliefs about ADHD and dispelling the unhelpful myths that add to the already challenging task of parenting a child with ADHD. Parents who feel blamed are likely to be sensitive to criticism. It is therefore important that nurses build a trusting relationship to address issues of blame and guilt as part of the wider treatment and management strategy. Where parents have developed mental health problems of their own, nurses should ensure that they discuss how help can be accessed to address these.

Experience of service use

Service user satisfaction can be difficult to measure and is often a subjective opinion. A small number of studies have explored satisfaction with diagnostic services and overall management of children and young people with ADHD. In a survey of attitudes about ADHD services, Hazell *et al.* (1996) found that 69% of parents were satisfied or very satisfied with their child's care and treatment. This compares to 55% of parents who were satisfied or very satisfied with their management in a study by Concannon and Tang (2005). What parents appear to value most is having sufficient time to discuss their child with a professional who is knowledgeable about the diagnosis and treatment for ADHD. All too often the research literature highlights an overwhelming sense of frustration with professional services. They report disagreements with teachers and health professionals about the nature of ADHD, the origins of their child's behaviour and how best to help. Some feel overwhelmed by conflicting or contradictory opinions about the relative benefits of medication, discipline and other management strategies (Klasen and Goodman 2000). Other parents report coming into contact with uncaring professionals who leave them feeling patronised and unsupported (Harborne *et al.* 2004). Nurses are in a good position to provide care and support to parents in understanding ADHD and discussing options for intervention and care.

It should be of major concern to nurses and other professionals that some parents struggle to access a service that they consider is appropriate, caring and thoughtful. Depending on where they live or on the attitudes of local professionals, the journey from assessment can be long and arduous for families (Pryjmachuk 1999; Litner 2003; NICE 2008). Parents consistently report that primary care professionals such as GPs, teachers and health visitors have little understanding about ADHD and that they feel misunderstood and unsupported. They are often left unaware of the treatment options, whether supportive care is available and what the monitoring process is likely to involve. Parents of children and young people with ADHD have reported that, more than any other aspect of living with ADHD, professionals focus on medication management and that this is to the exclusion of other important issues impacting on their child and family (Meaux 2006). It has also been suggested that professionals spend too much time training family members to be better parents or carers. Issues that are important to families themselves, such as respite, emotional support and family-centred mental health services rarely get the attention they deserve, it is said (Kendall 1998).

A common denominator in much of the qualitative research into the experience of living with ADHD is of children and young people, parents and carers and siblings feeling misunderstood and unsupported by professionals. This illustrates the need for nurses to bring about service improvements through more effective engagement, an increased focus on child and family care and better service evaluation strategies. As the largest single professional group in healthcare services, nurses are in key positions to help deliver improvements consistent with published best practice guidelines.

What do siblings tell us?

The experience of having a brother or sister with ADHD has received only scant attention in the research literature (Jones *et al.* 2006). Research exploring the effects of childhood illness or disability on brothers and sisters appears to show that outcomes can be both positive and negative, and that impairment arises due to a combination of factors and mediating variables (Stocker *et al.* 1989; McHale *et al.* 1995; Seligman and Darling 1997; Harpin 2005). These factors include the following:

- number, ages and gender of children in the family;
- the nature of the child's illness or disability;
- temperament of the children involved;
- the amount of information and knowledge the sibling has about the illness or disability;
- the degree to which a sibling adopts a caretaking role;
- restriction on the sibling's social life;
- degree to which parental time and resources are monopolised;
- the extent to which siblings are involved in communication and decision-making within the family.

The available research focusing on the experiences of living with a brother or sister with an illness or disability highlights a number of common themes which can be applied to living in a family with ADHD. Some siblings report feeling 'forgotton' when another child is ill or disabled (Rolland 1994). Others describe perceived favouritism of one child over another by parents or carers (Brody *et al*. 1996). As Barclay (1995) pertinently states, 'How do we get our other kids to understand why their sibling acts the way she does and is different from them? They think she is lucky for the all help she gets'. Siblings become tired and exasperated living with their brother or sister with ADHD, swinging between love, resentment and envy (Barclay 1995). Furthermore, many siblings of children who are chronically ill or disabled become ill themselves. Negative effects have been reported including depression, somatic complaints and aggression. In addition, the impact has also been reported to cause resentment, embarrassment and guilt (Faux 1993; Stoneman and Berman 1993). Kendall (1999) reports how the overwhelming experience of siblings of children with ADHD is one of general and pervasive disruption. In talking about how it felt to live with a brother or sister with ADHD, siblings described family life as chaotic, conflictual and exhausting. Considerable energy was spent on coping with daily disruption which they expected to be never-ending (Kendall 1998). Some reported being hit or victimised by their brother or sister with ADHD, whilst others felt intimidated by aggressive or threatening behaviour arising from hyperactivity and impulsivity (Kendall 1999).

How can nurses help siblings?

These narratives highlight the importance of directly including siblings in the nursing assessment process of a child with ADHD. All too often so-called 'non-affected' children are overlooked when a child with ADHD is in contact with healthcare services (Kendall 1999). Just as it is crucial to empower parents to support their child who has ADHD by providing information and understanding management strategies, so too should the nurse engage and support siblings. This is in order to both optimise outcomes for children with ADHD and to acknowledge and address the individual support needs of siblings who are living with them on a day-to-day basis. This is not always easy or appropriate to do with a sibling who may already feel overwhelmed. Of course, most siblings care about their brothers or sisters with ADHD and this can have a beneficial effect on all those concerned. Increased self-esteem, pride, empathy, maturity and resilience have all been reported as positive impacts linked to living with a child who has ADHD (Stoneman and Berman 1993; Faux 1993). However, for most siblings, caring does and should occur at an emotional rather than practical level. Where siblings are acting as 'young carers' and fulfilling a caretaking role more appropriately suited to a parent than a child, this will need to be formally addressed by the nurse. Here, the involvement of voluntary sector services may be helpful.

Safeguarding vulnerable children

Reports of violence should always be taken seriously. Where brothers or sisters feel intimidated or threatened this should be regarded as a safeguarding children matter. This is not to say that all concerns expressed by siblings should be processed as a child protection matter. Rather, nurses should consider the individual needs of siblings as part of the management plan and wherever possible ensure that these needs can be met in conjunction with parents or carers, other professionals and the voluntary sector. It is important to address the needs of siblings with parents, and individual support for the children in the family may sometimes be required. Where parents are unable to keep siblings safe from their brother or sister with ADHD, social services may need to be involved to support the family and ensure that all family members can feel safe and secure in their family home. Guidance for nurses and other professionals related to safeguarding and protecting vulnerable children is available to help them address this issue sensitively and competently (Department for Education and Skills 2006). Families with one or more children with ADHD often require social support including family-based support. However, a lack of resources in children's services can sometimes mean that such support is difficult to access.

Summary

Research about the cause and treatment of ADHD has largely been quantitative and led by medical professionals or academics. In contrast, most investigations into the lived experience of ADHD have been qualitative and appear to have been carried out by nurses. This is perhaps not surprising when we consider that the role of the nurse is fundamentally about engaging, understanding and caring. However, much of this research has taken place in North America and some studies are now somewhat dated. Caution must therefore be exercised when extrapolating good practice recommendations. This is because attitudes to ADHD have changed drastically over recent years, the medications used to treat this disorder have become more sophisticated and parental expectations of healthcare providers and other services have increased. In addition, significant differences exist regarding the role of the nurse on both sides of the Atlantic in relation to scope of professional practice.

It is not only the individual child or young person who suffers from the negative impact of ADHD. Parents and carers, brothers and sisters, friends and teachers are also affected. Gaining a subjective understanding of the everyday experiences of living with ADHD may lead to improved assessments and better treatment outcomes for all family members affected by this disorder. Nurses should always consider the wider family impacts as part of their assessment and management strategies. This may sometimes require a formal assessment of family needs focusing on personal, social and mental health needs, and liaison with other professionals will help ensure that families receive the support they require. Nurses should pay special attention when working with young people with ADHD to help build self-esteem, educate young people about ADHD and listen to their views about diagnosis and treatments. Helping young people and their families manage a chronic condition such as ADHD will impact upon outcomes for young people, acknowledging that ADHD is a complex disorder presenting with other difficulties. Parents of children with ADHD often feel blamed for their children's behaviour and difficulties, and nurses should remain aware of this throughout the assessment and treatment process. Sensitive and empathic communication is essential, and providing consistent care is necessary.

7 Treatment and management strategies

Key points

- Before embarking on any treatment or management strategy it is essential to complete a thorough and comprehensive assessment of the child or young person. This should be complemented by an assessment of family functioning which will provide helpful information about how best to intervene.
- The therapeutic relationship is the bedrock on which successful treatment and management strategies are based. Through their holistic approach to care and treatment, nurses have a long tradition and history of creating strong therapeutic partnerships with service users.
- Although multimodal treatment strategies are heralded as the winning combination, all too often children with ADHD and their families or carers receive little more than stimulant medication. Nurses are in key positions to help ensure that the treatment and management of ADHD becomes more holistic and focused on outcomes.
- Medication should only be used as part of a wider multimodal treatment strategy and alongside psychosocial interventions that include individual and group parenting programmes, social skills training and self-instruction.
- It is not only the child or young person with ADHD that needs support. Parenting or caring for a child with this disorder can be a challenging task, and nurses should always consider family support needs as part of any assessment, treatment and management strategy.
- A range of alternative therapies including dietary restriction and supplementation have been used in the management of ADHD. At present there is insufficient evidence to recommend these interventions as mainstream treatments.
- Difficulties with hyperactivity, impulsivity and inattention evolve across the life course. This means that the needs of infants, children, adolescents and adults are different, and the help and support nurses provide must be developmentally appropriate.

Introduction

Most parents bring their children to public services because they want help, advice, guidance or answers. There are many treatment interventions that can help relieve the core symptoms of ADHD and support parents or carers to manage their child's behaviour effectively. As well as medication for the core symptoms of ADHD, these include psychosocial interventions such as cognitive behavioural therapy, social skills training, anger management, family and systemic therapy, coaching and counselling approaches. The purpose of these interventions is to address impairment, social exclusion and the comorbidities that are associated with ADHD.

It is crucially important that treatment interventions are collaborative, involving children and young people, their parents and carers and other professionals such as teachers as fully as possible. Single treatment interventions are rarely effective with children and young people who have ADHD. Instead, it is a combination of interventions that can help make a difference and produce positive outcomes. Those for the treatment of ADHD are varied and nurses usually provide these in the context of a multimodal treatment strategy. This typically comprises psychoeducation, parent training and behaviour management, school-based interventions and psychopharmacology (Ryan 2006). Treatments for ADHD which are discussed in this chapter are broadly:

- Pharmacological
- Psychosocial
- Psychoeducational.

The therapeutic relationship is the bedrock on which successful treatment and management strategies are based. Through their holistic approach to care and treatment, nurses have a long tradition and history of creating strong therapeutic partnerships with service users.

What are the objectives for treatment?

One of the primary objectives for treatment is to promote and facilitate normal development, autonomy and self-reliance (Wood and Hughes 2005). Another important purpose of treatment for ADHD is to reduce unwanted behaviour, increase desirable behaviour and improve personal, social and academic or occupational outcomes for children and young people. Whilst some have suggested that treatment plans should be problem-orientated (Wood and Hughes 2005), others believe that the objectives for treatment should be focused on needs (Mitchell 2006). When working with children and young people with ADHD positive outcomes are likely to be maximised when the goals of treatment reflect a combination of both problems and needs. This is particularly important when we consider that ADHD is associated with a high level of unmet need (Steer 2005).

The range of treatments and interventions that are offered to children and young people, their families and other professionals who work with them depends upon a combination of factors. This includes service user choice, the severity of the ADHD symptoms, the degree of developmental or psychosocial impairment and the presence of any comorbid difficulties. It is crucial to understand the evidence base for those interventions that work and which are known to be effective (Fonagy *et al*. 2002). This is so interventions can be targeted and tailored to individual children and young people. It is usually necessary to provide a combination of interventions in order to produce positive outcomes for children and their families (Hinshaw 1994). However, consensus has not been reached on what constitutes evidence in child and adolescent mental health services (CAMHS). New service models are constantly evolving and the effectiveness of many CAMHS interventions have yet to be evaluated (Roberts and McDougall 2006). The evidence for short-term interventions is routinely reviewed (Skuse 2003), and it is unfortunate that longer-term evaluations of medication and psychosocial interventions have not been undertaken to provide a clearer understanding of the relative benefits and risks of treatments over time. Availability of service also depends on whether local services are commissioned to provide ADHD interventions. Unfortunately, in some areas of the UK ADHD is not even recognised among professionals as being a valid disorder that requires resources.

Treatment with medication

It is now widely recognised that pharmacological treatments have a central role to play in the management of complex psychosocial disorders. There has been more research into the use of medication for ADHD than into any other area of child and adolescent psychopharmacology, and about half of all papers published about psychoactive medication and children are on the subject of ADHD (Coghill 2003; Banaschewski *et al*. 2006). As part of a wider review to explore what works for children and young people with ADHD the National Institute for Health and Clinical Excellence (NICE) has reviewed the use of pharmacological as well as psychosocial interventions. This was to evaluate the effectiveness of the treatments methylphenidate, dexamphetamine and atomoxetine (NICE 2006a; NICE 2008). NICE (2006a) concluded that methylphenidate, dexamphetamine and atomoxetine were each effective treatments for ADHD. However, based on a review of the available research, no firm conclusions could be drawn in relation to the superiority of one treatment over another. NICE recommended that the clinician should base their decision about which medication to use on their professional judgement, knowledge about the child or young person concerned and service user choice.

Stimulants

Although the first reported use of stimulants to treat ADHD was in 1937 (Goldman *et al*. 1998), they did not come into general use until the 1960s. Stimulants act on the central nervous system by producing a dopamine-agonistic effect similar to that generated by amphetamine or cocaine (Volkow *et al*. 1998). This is why there is concern about stimulant misuse or abuse and so-called 'diversion', where medication prescribed for ADHD is sold on the streets (Indiana Prevention Resource Center 1998; Hall *et al*. 2005). Stimulants affect parts of the brain that are responsible for consciousness, control of attention and activity. There are two principal stimulant medications used to treat ADHD. These are methylphenidate and amphetamine. A third stimulant, pemoline, is generally no longer used due to the risk of toxic hepatitis (Smyth and Gowers 2005). Stimulants are used as first-line treatments to increase attention and decrease restlessness and hyperactivity (Santosh and Taylor 2000). The exact mechanism that leads to an improvement in symptoms of ADHD is not fully understood and is the subject of ongoing research.

Multiple studies have demonstrated the short-term efficacy and safety of stimulants in treating the core symptoms of ADHD by improving attention span, increasing impulse control and reducing hyperactivity and restlessness (Greenhill *et al*. 1999; Kratochvil *et al*. 2002; NICE 2008). However, despite widespread prescription and an extensive literature surrounding their use, there remains a lack of consensus about the risks and benefits of stimulants for children and young people with ADHD (Spencer *et al*. 1996). Various commentators have suggested that ADHD is overrecognised and too many children and young people are taking stimulant medications (Safer *et al*. 1996; Timimi and Radcliffe 2005). However, in a large-scale survey of children in the UK, less than half of those identified as having hyperkinetic disorder, the most severe form of ADHD, were taking medication. This suggests that, despite a large increase in the numbers of children prescribed stimulant medication in recent years, concerns about overprescription are unfounded. Moreover, the reports of this survey suggest that a large proportion of children and young people are failing to access an evidence-based treatment for ADHD.

Short- and long-acting preparations

Before prescribing stimulants it is important for nurses or other clinicians who prescribe to consider the preparation and pharmacological effects of the available medications and broker these with the individual needs of the child or young person. Immediate-release stimulants are available, which are short-acting drugs and their action lasts approximately four hours. This means that the relief from hyperactivity, impulsivity and inattention from immediate-release stimulants can also be short-lived. Many children and young people who take immediate-release stimulants experience what is referred to as a 'rebound effect' as serum blood levels of the stimulant decrease over time. This can cause children and young people to become more irritable and symptoms of ADHD to become more pronounced. Rebound effects can be particularly problematic in schools as the medication levels and effects are usually at their lowest during the most unstructured times of the day such as lunchtime, break and after school. Therefore, sustained-release preparations that are taken once a day can have positive effects in terms of improving concordance. Children and young people report that it is easier to remember to take one tablet per day than several, and this is also easier to manage for schools who often have concerns about health and safety in relation to managing and storing medication in schools. Whilst the effects of sustained-release preparations last up to 12 hours, some children and young people continue to report rebound effects.

Methylphenidate

There is an extensive evidence base supporting the use of stimulant medication for ADHD (Swanson *et al.* 1998). This is to address the core symptoms of hyperactivity, impulsivity and inattention, and in terms of improvements in some of the functional domains of psychosocial functioning (Wolraich *et al.* 2001). The most commonly used stimulant is methylphenidate hydrochloride (Ritalin, Equasym, Equasym XL, Concerta XL and Medicanet XL) and almost half of all children with hyperkinetic disorder take this drug (Swanson *et al.* 1995; Green *et al.* 2005).

For children aged over six years the starting dose of immediate-release methylphenidate is usually 5 mg twice or three times daily, increasing the dose and frequency of administration by weekly increments of 5–20 mg per dose with a maximum of 60 mg in the total daily dose. Local protocols should be agreed with NHS trusts and drug and therapeutic governance frameworks about practice parameters and recommended regimes in relation to titration of medication. Doses of methylphenidate above 60 mg are not recommended (NICE 2008) and the total daily dose should be divided. An adequate trial is between four and eight weeks. The last dose of methylphenidate should generally be given no later than 4 pm as one of the most common side effects is insomnia. Parents and children should be aware that, if the dose is given later than this, there is a risk of sleep disturbance.

For older adolescents, the use of modified or slow-release methylphenidate (Concerta XL, Equasym XL, Medikinet XL) for trials and continued use is recommended (NICE 2006; Banaschewski *et al.* 2006; NICE 2008). Daily doses range from 18 mg to 54 mg depending upon the product used and the clinicians' understanding of the pharmacokinetic properties of the medication. Although doses of 72 mg have been used, there is no licence for use of methylphenidate at this dose. This enables the clinician to tailor pharmacological interventions according to the needs of individual children and young people, thus optimising the positive effects and outcomes of treatment (Banaschewski *et al.* 2006).

Certain groups of children and young people should not take methylphenidate or should only use it with caution. This includes those with a diagnosis or family history of vocal or motor tics, Tourette's syndrome or other movement disorders. This is because stimulants can trigger tics such as eye-blinking, shrugging and throat-clearing, or make tics worse if they already exist. For those with a history of high blood pressure or heart problems, hyperthyroidism or glaucoma, methylphenidate is contra-indicated. There have also been concerns that stimulant medication can slow growth and present cardiovascular risks (Spencer *et al.* 1996; Klein *et al.* 1998; Nissen 2006). Although methylphenidate is not licensed for use in adults or older people, it has been recommended as the initial treatment for adults with ADHD (NICE 2008).

Dexamphetamine

A more potent stimulant than methylphenidate, dexamphetamine sulphate (dexedrine) is licensed for use in children and young people over the age of three years and for refractory cases of ADHD. However, it is not widely used in the UK since methylphenidate is used much more widely in clinical practice, and because dexamphetamine carries a higher risk for misuse (NICE 2006a). Like methylphenidate, dexamphetamine is a fast-acting drug which is rapidly absorbed within one hour. Dexamphetamine is not currently licensed for use in adults.

Managing stimulant side effects

Although considered to be generally safe, stimulants sometimes have unwanted side effects which can often lead to difficulties with compliance and the discontinuation of treatment for some children and young people (Schacher *et al.* 1997). It is a matter of clinical judgement and the wishes of the child and their family about whether stimulant treatment is discontinued in the face of adverse side effects (Ryan 2006). Common side effects of stimulant treatment include difficulty falling asleep at bedtime, decreased appetite, nervousness, stomach aches and headaches. Less common side effects include nausea, weight loss, changes in blood pressure and skin rash. Nurses should always empower children and young people and their parents or carers to manage unwanted side effects through healthy lifestyle choices (Department of Health 2004a). For example, there is a well-established evidence base on 'sleep hygiene' which focuses on strategies to improve the quality of sleep that is essential for emotional health and wellbeing. Children with ADHD and those around them suffer from shortened and disrupted sleep patterns (Stein 1999), and sleep hygiene should always be considered as part of child and family treatment strategies, whether or not this includes the use of stimulant medication. Similarly, headaches can often be managed by using relaxation techniques such as breathing exercises and progressive muscle relaxation, which can easily be taught by nurses as part of their holistic approach to treatment.

Stimulants often result in appetite and weight loss (Rapport and Moffitt 2002). Despite this, most studies show that children and young people continue to grow while medicated and concerns that long-term stimulant use may lead to growth retardation have proved to be unfounded (Spencer *et al.* 1998; Kramer at al. 2000; Beiderman and Faraone 2005). However, since growth in height may be less than expected in some children and young people (Beiderman *et al.* 2003), nurses should ensure that all those who are taking stimulants should have their height and weight monitored regularly. After they become stabilised on medication, six-monthly reviews of height and weight are sufficient for stimulant monitoring (NICE 2008).

Drug holidays

Some clinicians advocate medication or so-called 'drug holidays' for children and young people who are taking methylphenidate. This is intended to improve the efficacy of medication, reduce side effects such as insomnia and appetite suppression and improve general tolerability (Spencer *et al.* 1996; Martins *et al.* 2004). The advantages of medication-free periods on non-school days are to reduce any long-term risks of toxicity and slowed growth and to encourage the child to develop alternative coping mechanisms. The disadvantages are that the child is likely to struggle equally in the home environment and that families do not benefit from the positive effects of medication seen in school. Parents and carers should be encouraged to keep a diary of behaviour to monitor the effects of medication-free periods. Drug holidays are an area of controversy among clinicians, parents and children and young people themselves. For this reason, the National Institute for Health and Clinical Excellence advocates the need to look for alternative evidence about what happens to the symptoms of children with ADHD when doses are accidentally missed or weekend doses are omitted (NICE 2008).

Non stimulants

Stimulant medications have limitations since they are not an acceptable treatment choice for some children and families and compliance with treatment plans affects effectiveness (Perring 1997). A significant number of children and young people fail to respond positively to stimulants or cannot tolerate their side effects (Fonagy *et al.* 2002; Coghill 2003). Although methylphenidate remains the first-line recommended treatment for ADHD (NICE 2008), an alternative non-stimulant treatment is now available in the form of atomoxetine.

Atomoxetine

Atomoxetine (Strattera) is a selective noradrenaline transport blocker indicated for the treatment of ADHD. It is licensed for use by children aged over six years and has been shown to be effective with both children and adults (Spencer *et al.* 2001; Michelson *et al.* 2001; Michelson *et al.* 2003). The pharmacological action of this drug is very different to that of stimulants. Atomoxetine is usually taken once in the morning and provides 24-hour relief from the symptoms of ADHD. This provides clear advantages in relation to the effects of medication not wearing off. However, some patients have reported benefits in dividing the dose across the day (Adler 2006). Atomoxetine should be used with caution with people who have high blood pressure, increased pulse and cardiovascular or cerebrovascular disease. There have also been documented concerns about the risks of liver damage (Lim *et al.* 2006) and an increase in suicidal thoughts in children and young people taking atomoxetine (Rosack 2005). Monitoring of children and young people who are taking atomoxetine is crucial and should involve height and weight, blood pressure, pulse and mood.

After methylphenidate, atomoxetine is generally accepted as an alternative treatment for children and young people with ADHD. However, it may be considered as a first-line treatment where the child has comorbid tics or Tourette's syndrome, an anxiety disorder, or where there is coexistent substance misuse (NICE 2008). The effectiveness of atomoxetine for children and adolescents with ADHD is currently being reviewed as part of the Cochrane Collaboration.

Non-licensed medications

Methylphenidate and dexamphetamine are licensed for use by children and young people with ADHD in most European countries (Taylor *et al.* 2004). However, many medications used by children and young people do not have a product licence (Royal College of Paediatrics and Child Health 2000; Johnson and Clarke 2001). This is not unusual practice since many medications are not trialled on children and are used for reasons other than their licensed intention. Nonetheless, they can still have a positive effect on symptom reduction. The evidence for the effectiveness of non-licensed treatments is limited and has been reviewed by Biederman and Spencer (2000) and Taylor *et al.* (2004). Non-licensed medications that are used in the treatment of ADHD but do not have a product licence include clonidine, bupropion, modafinil, imipramine, risperidone, and nicotine patches. Tricyclic antidepressants are the most extensively researched non-stimulant medications and are occasionally prescribed off label for children and young people who do not respond to licensed medications (Findling and Dogin 1998). The use of tricyclics by children and young people with ADHD is currently being reviewed by the international Cochrane Collaboration.

Both licensed and unlicensed medications for ADHD have side effects and some carry special warnings which identify which groups of people should not be given the drug. Most have contra-indications for use, which means that certain groups of people are at higher risk, either through an existing medical condition or interaction with a medication they are already taking. Medication should only be prescribed by those with appropriate training and experience, and only after completing a comprehensive assessment including a full medical history (NICE 2008). Monitoring response to medication is a crucial part of the treatment process and this is a key part of the nursing role. Before a child starts treatment with medication, it is crucial to take a baseline measure of height, weight, pulse and blood pressure. This information should be plotted on centile charts so that progress over time can be monitored and reviewed. Nurses and other professionals have developed pre-treatment questionnaires, patient information leaflets and side effect checklists to assist with monitoring of methylphenidate and atomoxetine (Hill and Taylor 2001; Ryan 2007).

Involving children, young people and parents in decisions about medication

An important part of good clinical practice is involving service users in treatment decisions. This is not only a very clear message from service users (Mental Health Foundation 2001; Leon 2001), but involving families in treatment decisions including those related to ADHD medication use is also likely to lead to better outcomes. This is because improved knowledge about medication is directly linked to greater concordance and compliance (Liu *et al.* 1991; Bennett *et al.* 1996). Therefore, children and young people and their parents or carers should always be encouraged to ask questions about medication, and the Royal College of Psychiatrists have highlighted some of the important issues for children and young people and their parents or carers to discuss with clinicians. Recommended questions to ask include:

- What are the effects and side effects?
- What dose will be used?
- Will any monitoring be conducted whilst my child is on medication?
- Will there be collaboration with school?
- What should I do if I miss a dose?
- What should I do if my child takes too much?
- How long will they need to take medication for?

Continuation and discontinuation of medication

Little is known about the safety and efficacy of long-term medication use for ADHD. Following an adequate treatment response, children and young people who are taking medication for their ADHD should be reviewed at least once per year. This is to assess whether the medication is still effective, whether the dose is optimal and if side effects are causing impairment in day-to-day functioning in school and at home. When reviewing the need for continued treatment, it is important to consider what the effects of missed doses and planned medication-free periods have been and the views of the child and their parents or carers in relation to the relative costs and benefits of medication. Because many children and young people choose to stop taking medication (Marcus *et al.* 2005), it is important for nurses to continue education about ADHD, its challenges and effective self-management strategies, even after stimulant medications have been stopped (Meaux *et al.* 2006). Discontinuation of medication is always recommended in situations where there is concern about unwanted side effects which are detrimental to psychological and physical wellbeing, or when medication is no longer thought to be effective. However, complete discontinuation of medication should always be done in collaboration with clinicians who have knowledge and expertise about ADHD.

Stuart, a seven-year-old boy with ADHD and a simple motor tic was prescribed atomoxetine (Strattera). A routine health screening interview was conducted with Stuart and his parents and the contraindications for using atomoxetine were discussed. According to the BNF regimes, doses of the drug are determined by body weight; therefore, the phases of the trial were as follows:

0.5 mg atomoxetine per kg of body weight
0.5 mg × 25 kg = 12.5 mg = atomoxetine 10 mg for 7 days
1.2 mg atomoxetine per kg of body weight
1.2 mg × 25 kg = 30 mg = 30 mg atomoxetine for 35 days

Unfortunately, after several weeks the trial of atomoxetine treatment was unsuccessful in terms of reducing Stuart's hyperactivity, impulsivity and inattention. A trial of stimulant (methylphenidate) was therefore discussed with parents as the next treatment option. After discussion with Stuart and parents it was agreed that the positive benefits from stimulants outweighed the potential side effects of exacerbating the facial motor tic. The treatment regime agreed was:

Methylphenidate 2.5 mg three times a day for seven days
Methylphenidate 5 mg three times a day for seven days
Methylphenidate 7.5 mg three times a day for seven days
Methylphenidate 10 mg three times a day for seven days

The trial was reviewed at school with Stuart, his parents, the

SENCO, Stuart's class teacher and the behaviour support assistant. Conners questionnaires and both parental and teacher verbal reports demonstrated a decrease in hyperactivity, increase in concentration and reduction in impulsivity. It was reported that Stuart had produced more work of a better quality as the doses of treatment increased, and there was no evidence of an increase in facial motor tics. The higher dose of methylphenidate 10 mg three times a day produced significant loss of appetite and sleep disturbance without any greater treatment effect. Therefore, it was agreed that Stuart should continue on methylphenidate 7.5 mg three times a day with review in four weeks' time in the hyperkinesis nurse-led clinic.

Stuart continues with methylphenidate without any side effects. He is growing and gaining weight appropriately. His parents have been pleased with his progress in school. His concentration is better and his academic performance has improved. Stuart is more sociable, more included by his peer group and is making and keeping more friends. Parents have also made changes to their parenting style and feel more consistent in their approach and can be positive with Stuart on a regular basis.

Psychosocial interventions

Pharmacological treatments for ADHD may not always be the first choice of treatment for children and young people and their families or carers who may express a preference to try other interventions before medication. There have been many concerns expressed by service users that there is too little focus on their psychological and social needs and too much focus on symptoms and medication (Department of Health 2006; Department of Health 2008). Some parents hold the belief that the key to solving problems lies less in their child and more in their social networks or school (Poduska 2000; Taylor *et al.* 2004). They are often aware that there are limitations to the effectiveness of pharmacological treatments, particularly in terms of the effects of improvements in symptoms when medication is wearing off. This is supported by research findings which show that many of the benefits of stimulant medication are state-dependent. This means that their effects may only last for as long as the child or young person is receiving the medication and may not generalise to situations where medication treatment is absent (Whalen and Henker 1991).

For some children and young people medication is undoubtedly helpful in improving the core symptoms of hyperactivity, inattention and impulsivity, but for others medication may not be helpful (Swanson *et al.* 1995; Safren *et al.* 2005). Regardless of whether medication is effective, there are many other difficulties that children and young people face which pharmacological treatments will not directly address. These include interventions to address defiant and oppositional behaviour, strategies to enable children and young people to develop prosocial behaviour, and low self-esteem. In these circumstances, psychosocial interventions will be required alongside medication to address the core symptoms of ADHD.

Perhaps not surprisingly, the way in which families function, communicate and behave together impacts on outcomes. Families in which communications are hostile, critical or negative produce poorer outcomes (Baguley and Baguley 1999). Children's major support systems are through the family, and large population surveys have shown that families of children with hyperkinetic disorder are twice as likely as other children to live in families classified as having unhealthy functioning (Green *et al.* 2005). Psychosocial interventions are used to help children and young people and their families cope with the difficulties associated with ADHD. They are generally intended to improve individual, family, social and academic functioning and overall quality of life. This can be achieved through individual and group parenting programmes, social skills training and positive self-instruction. For some children and young people whose impairment caused by symptoms of ADHD is mild, improvements in psychological and social functioning can be facilitated by psychological interventions and parent skills training as first-line interventions (NICE 2008). However, there is no evidence that the use of psychosocial interventions alone to address the core symptoms of severe hyperactivity, impulsivity and inattention is effective.

Parenting programmes

It is not only the child or young person with ADHD that needs support. Parenting or caring for a child with this disorder can be a challenging task, and nurses should always consider family support needs as part of any assessment, treatment and management strategy. The last decade has witnessed a growing interest in early prevention programmes to interrupt the developmental trajectories that lead to poor outcomes for children and families with disorders such as ADHD. There is now a rapidly expanding evidence base showing that strategies to promote, prevent and intervene during childhood can offset the development of further problems and disorders in adolescence and adulthood (Fryers 2007). Working with parents and carers is the key to prevention and early intervention. 'Parenting programmes' is an overarching term that encapsulates parent support, parent education and parent training (Utting *et al.* 2006).

Originating in the US, there was tremendous growth in parent training programmes in the 1970s. Programmes such as the Parent Effectiveness Training (PET) reached 250,000 families and produced over 1000 trained instructors (Gordon 1975). Since then, a range of programmes have been designed to assist parents to manage their child's ADHD (Cousins and Weiss 1993; Zimmerman *et al.* 1996). In recent years there has been a move away from general or universal parent education and training towards 'third generation' or targeted programmes (Long 1997). In the US, this has partly been due to the increasing demand for specific interventions as managed-care companies exclude or restrict mental health services for children with behaviour problems including ADHD (Long 1997). In the UK, a number of studies have shown that parent-based therapies can be effective in producing positive behaviour change in pre-school children (Sonuga-Barke *et al.* 2001) and those with conduct disorder (NICE 2006b). However, parenting programmes for ADHD are broadly similar in both the UK and US.

How do parenting programmes work?

Rather than directly addressing the core symptoms of hyperactivity, impulsivity and inattention, parenting programmes are intended to help parents develop optimum strategies to cope with their child's behaviour (Anastopoulos *et al.* 1991; Anastopoulos *et al.* 1993). This is achieved through learning skills to cope with or compensate for ongoing difficulties. It has been suggested that caring for a young person with ADHD poses particular challenges and there is a need for consistency (Pentecost 2000). Most programmes include contingency management as well as standard behavioural techniques. Parents are taught the principles of behaviour modification and are supported to manage their children with confidence, thus fostering positive family relationships.

Parent training programmes in the UK have gained in popularity in recent years and this has partly been the result of media interest. The National Institute for Clinical Excellence (NICE) has undertaken a technology appraisal of the effectiveness of programmes for parents of children with conduct disorder (NICE 2006b). This guidance can be generally applied to parenting children and young people with ADHD. This is due to the very high comorbidity of ADHD with conduct problems (Jensen *et al.* 1997), the high likelihood that children with ADHD will have been included in the studies of conduct disorder on which the recommendations were based and the general principles of behaviour management that apply to the parenting of children with conduct problems and ADHD. The NICE guidance states that:

- Group-based training and education programmes are recommended.
- Individual-based training and education are only recommended when there are particular difficulties engaging with parents or a family's needs are too complex to be met by group-based parent training and education programmes.
- Programmes should demonstrate proven effectiveness based on evidence from randomised controlled trials or other suitably rigorous evaluation methods undertaken independently.

In addition, the NICE guidance further states that all parent training programmes, whether group- or individual-based, should:

- be structured;
- include relationship-enhancing strategies such as play and praise, and effective discipline strategies;
- incorporate learning opportunities that reflect social learning theory such as skills rehearsal and role play, and watching recorded vignettes as triggers for discussion of alternative parenting strategies;
- offer a sufficient number of sessions, with an optimum of 8–12, to maximise the potential benefits for participants;
- not be didactic but enable parents to identify their own parenting objectives;
- identify homework to be undertaken between sessions, to achieve generalisation of newly rehearsed behaviours to the home situation;
- be delivered by appropriately trained and skilled facilitators who are supervised, have access to necessary ongoing professional development and are able to engage in a productive therapeutic alliance with parents.

Randomised controlled trials have shown that parent training and family-based behavioural interventions are effective (Pelham *et al.* 1998). One rigorous study of a parenting programme for families of pre-school children in the UK found that improvements in ADHD symptoms were sustained for up to four months after treatment (Purdie *et al.* 2002). The most widely recognised programmes to meet the criteria set out in NICE guidelines are the Webster-Stratton and Triple P parenting programmes. These can easily be adapted to provide a focus on ADHD and are widely used.

Webster-Stratton

The Incredible Years parenting programmes have been developed over 25 years by Carolyn Webster-Stratton and her colleagues in the US. They have been positively and rigorously evaluated in both North America and Europe including the UK (Webster-Stratton 1998; Webster-Stratton 2000; Reid *et al.* 2003). The programmes are based on videotape modelling and are intended to strengthen parenting, enhance the problem-solving ability of children and reduce behaviour problems at home and at school (Webster-Stratton 1981). Basic Webster-Stratton programmes enable parents to play with their child; give effective praise and encouragement; motivate the child; set limits and implement rules; and manage poor behaviour. Advanced programmes focus on adult relationships and the effects of family-based difficulties such as mental disorder, marital problems and poor parental anger management. The parent survival course is a 10–12 week programme for parents of 4–8 year olds. This aims to teach parents how to play with their child and use positive reinforcement, effective limit setting, problem-solving and non-violent discipline strategies. Following the programme, there is evidence that levels of disturbance are reduced, parental use of negative interactions decreases and overall child adjustment improves (Fonagy *et al.* 2002).

Triple P

Triple P is a multi-level, preventative, parenting and family support strategy developed in Australia (Sanders *et al*. 2003; Sanders *et al*. 2004). It aims to enhance the knowledge, skills and confidence of parents to increase their resourcefulness and self-sufficiency. Triple P has been used successfully with parents of children who have ADHD (Bor *et al*. 2002; Hoath and Sanders 2002).

Implementing parenting programmes

It is important for nurses to enable parents to recognise that help with managing their child with ADHD in no way indicates weakness or lack of success as a parent (Shattell *et al*. 2008). Some parents benefit from written material or self-instruction manuals based on positive parenting and behavioural instruction techniques (Long *et al*. 1993). Nurses have been instrumental in helping to develop information manuals which can facilitate positive change in the ways parents manage their children with ADHD (Weeks *et al*. 1999). Other parents find manualised, didactic approaches patronising and prefer interactive training such as video modelling. Here, the nurses' approach to supporting parents should be flexible, adaptive and creative. Generally, it is important for the nurse to establish what mode of psychoeducation the parents would find helpful or unhelpful. This is an essential part of the engagement process and a vital component given the reportedly high rates of drop-out from parent training courses (Pisterman *et al*. 1992). Some parents will have particular needs which need to be incorporated into the design of the parenting programme. For example, depressed parents or those with ADHD themselves will require targeted nursing interventions that accommodate their difficulties and needs (Tatano-Beck 1999).

Individual psychological treatments

There is evidence that psychological treatments help produce positive outcomes for individuals or groups of children and young people with ADHD (Sonuga-Barke *et al*. 2001), and these are usually provided as part of wider psychosocial interventions. There are many different forms of psychological therapy and treatment. Choosing which approach to use depends on the developmental status of the child, the evidence base for use and the specific wishes of the child or young person and their parents or carers (Woolley 2006). Three main types of psychological interventions for ADHD exist. These are cognitive behavioural interventions (CBT), family therapy and social skills training. However, access to psychological therapies for ADHD and other disorders of childhood and adolescence is not readily available in all areas of the UK. Access is variable in specialist child and adolescent mental health services (CAMHS), and is rarely available in paediatric health settings.

This is despite the growing evidence base for their effectiveness (Fonagy *et al.* 2002) and the increasing profile of psychological therapies in government policy and strategy (Department of Health 2007).

Behaviour therapy

Behavioural approaches are commonly used to manage the disruptive, rule-breaking or antisocial behaviour of children with ADHD. These have been reviewed by the American Academy of Child and Adolescent Psychiatry in their practice parameters on conduct disorders (AACAP 1997), oppositional defiant disorder (AACAP 2007a) and ADHD (AACAP 2007b). Like other psychosocial therapies, behaviour therapy is less effective than medication in reducing the primary symptoms of hyperactivity, impulsivity and inattention. In addition, the improvements may be short-lived and fail to generalise across a range of settings other than the environment in which they occurred (AACAP 1997; NICE 2008). However, behaviour therapy has been shown to be effective in supporting children and young people to develop social skills and improve academic performance (Carlson *et al.* 1992). This is through behaviour modification systems such as token economy, star charts, response costs (DuPaul *et al.* 1992) and [time out from] positive reinforcement. Behavioural strategies to help manage ADHD are reviewed in chapter 9 on school-based interventions.

Cognitive interventions

Behaviour, affect and cognition are part of the human condition. Being aware of our thinking allows us to understand feelings and behaviour and how they interact. Cognitive interventions are designed to change negative beliefs by gaining insight into how one's thoughts, feelings and behaviour are connected (Woolley 2006). Cognitive interventions for children and young people with ADHD include verbal instruction training, cognitive therapy and cognitive behavioural therapy (CBT). Self-instructional training is probably the most widely used cognitively-orientated therapeutic approach for individuals with ADHD. It comprises several different techniques including modelling, self-evaluation, self-reinforcement and response cost (Meichembaum and Goodman 1971; NICE 2008).

As its name suggests, CBT combines cognitive interventions with behavioural theory. What we do depends to some extent on how we feel, and how we feel depends to some extent on what we think. When used with children and young people who have ADHD, the aim of CBT is to interrupt this cycle and link thoughts, feelings and behaviour to improve overall day-to-day functioning. This is to develop a more reflective, systematic and solution-focused approach to problem-solving and task management. CBT builds on the principles of behaviour therapy as outlined above by aiming to enhance skills of self-control. Amongst other things, this is achieved through enabling children and young people to develop skills of reflection, self-regulation, positive self-reinforcement and self-evaluation.

The ability to use cognitive interventions may be easier said than done with children who experience difficulties with information processing and who struggle to stop, look, listen and think. They require the child or young person to pay attention to and process social cues, to think about a situation, consider a range of options and to plan a response (Kendall *et al.* 1995). The principles of CBT have been translated into a number of practical strategies for use by children and young people with ADHD. These are often used in the school setting and have evolved from the 'Think Aloud' programme which originated in the US (Camp and Bash 1981). Other task-based strategies have been developed with the aim of improving functioning in specific areas such as relationships, recreation and leisure and school performance (Kendall 1978; Kendall 1982).

By focusing on more positive and effective ways of thinking, children and young people are better able to cope in situations which may generate negative thoughts and appraisals. When used specifically to support children and young people with ADHD, CBT may be helpful in reducing motor activity, improving planning skills and regulating impulsivity and behaviour control. However, as with behaviour therapy, there can be a problem with teaching children and young people to generalise the problem-solving strategies they have mastered to different settings and in using them spontaneously (Fonagy *et al.* 2002). Although research has shown that CBT is effective for symptoms of ADHD (Pelham and Waschbusch 1999), there is no evidence that it is more effective than medication (Abikoff 1991; AACAP 1997; NICE 2008).

Group therapy

Like many other psychological interventions for ADHD, very little literature reviews the effectiveness of group interventions. Several papers have been published in the US and UK, but studies have been small and conclusions should be interpreted with caution. The majority of group interventions for children with ADHD occur in school settings as part of the wider personal, health and social education (PHSE) curriculum. This is to address social skills-building and identity formation (DuPaul and Eckert 1997; Cantor 2000). Group interventions for children and young people with ADHD can have positive and negative implications. They can provide opportunities for peer support, role modelling and interpersonal skills-building. However, for young people who are shy or lack confidence, they can be intimidating and perpetuate difficulties associated with socialisation. Group interventions are also cost-effective, both in terms of time and resources (Dwivedi 1993; Horstmann and Steer 2007).

Family therapy

Living with the persistent intrusive and challenging behaviours often associated with ADHD can be physically and emotionally exhausting. These can generate a range of emotions such as fear, sadness, anger and guilt (Concannon and Tang 2005; Bull and Whelan 2006). Whilst family members play an invaluable role in the treatment and management of ADHD, the unfamiliar territory that comes with ADHD can often feel overwhelming. Like any chronic or persistent childhood disorder, the development of ADHD in the early years can extend the caregiving role (Jones *et al.* 2006).

It is not unusual for parents to feel impotent in terms of their child's difficulties associated with ADHD. In some cases, the assessment of a child with ADHD will have suggested that family factors are playing an unhelpful role in maintaining or exacerbating their difficulties. Here, it is essential to provide an intervention that aims to alter unhelpful patterns of family interaction. Family-based difficulties are closely associated with ADHD and family-based interventions have been extensively researched and systematically reviewed (Bjornstad and Montgomery 2005). The term 'family therapy' refers to a range of systemic, structural, behavioural, strategic and brief focused interventions and the various types of family therapy have been evaluated for use with children and young people who have ADHD (Carr 2000a; Carr 2000b). All appear to share the common objective of improving family functioning, interpersonal relationships and facilitating positive outcomes.

There has been a lack of robust studies to evaluate the effectiveness of family therapy for ADHD. Despite this, family interventions are used widely. A recent large five-year follow-up study of children and young people with ADHD indicated that two-thirds had received some family-orientated therapy guidance in the previous 12 months from mental health services (Ford *et al.* 2007). This is typically focused on psychoeducational packages, reducing tensions within the family through goal-setting, problem-solving and stress management and the improvement of communication patterns between family members. Nurses in specialist CAMHS often have a dual qualification and training in family therapy and support children and families who are living with ADHD.

At the time of writing this book, there are no randomised controlled trials (RCTs) that allow comparisons between family therapy interventions for ADHD and controls to be made (NICE 2008). However, a lack of RCT evidence does not necessarily mean that family interventions are ineffective. Indeed, it is generally agreed that using a systemic approach to understand the impact of ADHD on impairment and functioning can be useful and is promoted as part of day-to-day management of ADHD (Bernier and Siegel 1994). Furthermore, a systemic approach to the assessment, planning, implementation and evaluation of care and treatment interventions is also considered to be good practice (Department of Health 2004b). Further research is required to evaluate the effectiveness of family therapy for children and young people with ADHD (Bjornstad and Montgomery 2005).

The Multimodal Treatment Study of Children with ADHD (MTA)

Generic therapies and treatment orientations that focus exclusively on the child are declining. In their place, specialist strategies or multimodal treatment manuals represent a move towards systemic and contextual explanations of childhood mental disorder (Woolley 2006). Multimodal or combined treatment programmes aim to address multifaceted problems by including several therapeutic strategies and are generally more effective than single treatment interventions, particularly for ADHD (Kidd *et al.* 2000; Crystal *et al.* 2001; Stevens 2005; Vlam 2006). Steer (2005) suggests that the cornerstones of long-term multimodal management are:

- psychoeducation comprising information, explanation and counselling about ADHD for children, parents and carers;
- psychological and behavioural strategies;
- social support such as parent support groups, financial assistance and respite care;
- appropriate educational strategies and support in school, including help for children with coordination difficulties;
- discussion and consideration of pharmacotherapy.

However, multimodal treatments are not readily available, and reports from both the US and UK suggest that too often children and young people with ADHD receive little more than minimal psychological assessment and stimulant medication (Kidd 2000; NICE 2008). The MTA study (MTA Cooperative group 1999) is one of the most influential research studies in the field of ADHD to date. This was a large randomised controlled trial in the US involving the use of medication and psychosocial interventions for over 500 children aged 7–9 with a diagnosis of ADHD. The five-year study explored the effectiveness of treatments in the following ways:

1   Medication management involving highly specialised initiation of medication (methylphenidate) and review of efficacy with monthly follow-up appointments to evaluate and change medication regimes.
2   Highly structured behaviour modification which included 35 parent training sessions; an eight-week summer treatment programme to provide direct intervention with the child in playground and classroom settings; 12 weeks of support for teachers to deliver behavioural interventions; and teacher consultation to sustain the use of behavioural interventions in the school setting.

3   Combined medication management and behavioural management which included all the interventions in 1 and 2.
4   Routine care described as care that was routinely available in clinical settings.

The outcomes of the MTA study at 14 months suggested that high-quality medication management was most effective in treating symptoms. The use of behaviour modification was not found to add more benefits to medication, but influenced the amount of medication needed to be effective. When the MTA data was re-evaluated using the ICD-10 diagnostic criteria in order to represent the UK population more accurately than DSM-IV, evidence was found for the effectiveness of stimulant medication (methylphenidate) for the treatment of hyperkinetic disorder (Santosh *et al*. 2005). Further follow-up of the original cohort at 36 months showed that medication use changed significantly after the initial 14-month research algorithm. Young people who had not previously taken medication were starting, and those who had started medication at the outset of the study were stopping (Jensen *et al*. 2007). This was partly explained by participants reverting to 'treatment as usual' because the specialist intervention was no longer available to them at the end of the 14-month research study. However, the research team were struck by improvements made by participants in all groups from baseline to 36 months in the domains of overall functioning, global impairment and social skills (Jensen *et al*. 2007).

Complementary and alternative treatments

Understandably, many parents of children and young people are concerned about the immediate and long-term effects of taking medication and often ask nurses about alternative therapies. Little is known about the effectiveness of complementary and alternative medication for ADHD yet its use is reported to be widespread (Harrison *et al*. 2004). Just as the use of psychopharmacological treatments for ADHD has increased dramatically in recent years, so too has the market for herbal, natural, complementary and other alternative diagnostics and remedies for ADHD flourished (Stead *et al*. 2007). Some parents seek alternative therapies due to concerns about the physiological and psychological effects of pharmacological treatments on their children (Rice and Richmond 1997; Bjornstad and Montgomery 2005). Others object to their children taking medication on ethical grounds (Perring 1997; Singh 2005). Various alternative therapies for ADHD are described in the research literature and popular media including yoga, massage and acupuncture. One of the most widely researched strategies is meditation and this has been the subject of various studies and systematic reviews. However, there have been no controlled trials and the reviews on which some conclusions have been based have been unpublished. Another alternative treatment for ADHD is homeopathy, which has been the subject of a Cochrane systematic review.

This concluded that there is at present insufficient evidence to recommend the use of homeopathy for children and young people diagnosed with ADHD (Coulter and Dean 2007).

Relaxation training is widely used with children and young people who have ADHD. Although techniques vary, most involve the sequential tensing and relaxing of muscle groups and are intended to improve self-control and reduce anxiety and tension. Electroencephalography (EEG) biofeedback has been used since the 1970s with children and young people who have ADHD (NICE 2008). Proponents of this method suggest that people with ADHD can be trained to increase their beta activity which is associated with alertness and attention and decrease their theta rhythm, or slow wave brain activity, which is associated with feeling drowsy (Linden *et al.* 1996; Satterfield *et al.* 1973).

Psychoeducational interventions

A key part of the nurses' role is assisting young people towards recovery (Department of Health 2005; Till 2007). Rather than attempting to 'cure' people, nurses who apply the principles of recovery to their practice enable children and young people with ADHD to live and cope with their symptoms and maintain optimal psychological, social and educational functioning. Recovery is not something that is done to young people; rather it is a way of thinking about the therapeutic relationship and remaining hopeful and optimistic that children and families are capable of positive change and can be empowered to improve their lives. It has been suggested that the principles of recovery should underpin all that nurses do. Recovery should be reflected in all that we write in care plans, all that we say to service users and colleagues and in every intervention we offer (Till 2007). Education and advice about ADHD should therefore be at the heart of any treatment and management strategy. Psychoeducation involves informing the child and parents or carers about ADHD, helping families anticipate difficult developmental challenges and providing general advice to help improve the child's overall functioning. It is common practice for nurses to provide education about the illness or disorder as part of the recovery process. However, psychoeducation should commence at the point of diagnosis and continue throughout the treatment process (Jackson and Farrugia 1997).

In order to help children and young people adopt self-care strategies to help manage their ADHD education about the symptoms of hyperactivity, impulsivity and inattention is essential. Psychoeducational interventions can be provided by nurses in many forms, including verbal discussion, written information or through signposting the child and their parents or carers to self-help groups, web-based resources and voluntary sector services. Deciding which medium to use depends on a range of factors including beliefs about health and illness, attributions about causal and control mechanisms and of course service user choice. Specialist ADHD nurses have developed video-based resources for parents, teachers and other professionals (Thompson and Laver-Bradbury 1999a; Thompson and Laver-Bradbury 1999b). However, the nurse should always point out that there is a vast amount of information about ADHD in the public domain, and not all is underpinned by evidence or good practice. In order to assist parents to make informed choices, nurses should therefore offer to discuss any literature or other information that parents wish to discuss about ADHD. A range of information leaflets and booklets for young people are available such as those provided by YoungMinds, a national charity committed to improving the mental health of children and young people.

Summary

There is no 'one size fits all' approach to successfully treating and helping children and young people with ADHD. No single treatment is effective across all the domains of psychological, social and academic functioning in the child and in meeting the needs of parents or carers in supporting and managing their child. This illustrates the need for a multidisciplinary, multimodal approach which combines the evidence from a range of treatments to produce an individualised plan of intervention for the young person and their family or carers. Nurses are in key roles to help ensure that the treatment and management of ADHD becomes more holistic and focused on outcomes.

Although multimodal treatment strategies are heralded as the winning combination, all too often children with ADHD and their families or carers receive little more than stimulant medication. Along with a range of psychological and social interventions, psychopharmacological treatments are one of the major therapeutic options available to help children and young people with ADHD. They are undoubtedly helpful in reducing the core symptoms of hyperactivity, impulsiveness and inattention. However, access to pharmacological treatment is not always readily available. This can be due to a number of factors including lack of access to specialist services and a lack of appropriately trained clinicians willing or able to prescribe medication for ADHD. It is recommended that medication should only be used as part of a wider multimodal treatment strategy and alongside psychosocial interventions including individual and group parenting programmes, social skills training and self-instruction.

Despite a large evidence base that parenting programmes are effective in managing unwanted behaviours associated with ADHD, less than half of parents are offered such programmes as part of the treatment of their children (ADDISS 2006). Parents of pre-school children with a diagnosis of ADHD should be offered a parent training programme as a first-line intervention. Group-based parent training and education programmes are recommended in the management of children and young people with ADHD. These appear to be effective both in terms of generating behavioural compliance in children and by improving the coping strategies and self-esteem of parents. Nurses should be aware that some parents may be isolated or difficult to engage. Here, it is important to offer appointments in various locations and at flexible times.

Individual psychosocial interventions may be effective in helping children and young people develop improved social skills and academic performance in school. However, despite government strategies to improve access to psychological therapies, these are not always accessible, with long waiting times in some areas of the UK. Further research is required to evaluate the effectiveness of a range of treatments for children and young people with ADHD. It is important that nurses consider the support needs of parents and carers in their assessment, treatment and management of children and young people with ADHD. Parent support groups, self-help groups and access to ADHD organisations can provide parents with a network of support, information and advice. Nurses should be aware that not all information about ADHD which is available in the public domain is valid and reliable. For this reason, it is good practice to signpost parents and carers to reputable resources such as YoungMinds and the National Attention Deficit Disorder Information and Support Service (ADDISS) which provide resources and information about ADHD.

8 Service provision and care pathways

Key points

- The tiered model of service delivery is a framework to organise the commissioning, management and delivery for children and young people with mental health problems and disorders.
- As with all disorders of childhood and adolescence, intervention should be earlier rather than later and should occur in primary settings such as schools. Service provision should involve professionals who are trained to assess, treat, monitor and support children and young people with ADHD over long periods.
- The way in which children and young people are referred for assessment and treatment of ADHD varies widely across the UK. Many children face what has been referred to as a 'treatment lottery', where care pathways are arbitrary and the availability of specialist assessment and treatment services depends on their postcode.
- Increasingly, local protocols exist which define integrated care pathways and models of best practice for the assessment, diagnosis and management of ADHD. Stepped care models comprise several components including the identification of children with ADHD; management by parents and teachers; training and support for primary care and school based professionals; and care pathways to access specialist treatment.
- Healthcare providers of ADHD services should be commissioned to offer a wide range of interventions not only to address ADHD symptoms but also to manage the associated difficulties that accompany them.
- Signposting parents to local support groups can often be helpful. This helps provide a network of advice and advocacy which parents or carers often find supportive. Local groups can be an opportunity for parents or carers to seek and provide peer support, and many provide advice on stress management and the day-to-day management of children and young people with ADHD.

Introduction

Despite ADHD being a relatively common disorder of childhood, comprehensive assessment and treatment services are not routinely available in all areas of the UK. Although many areas of the UK have access to dedicated ADHD services, this varies from county to county and region to region. Lead responsibility for service provision varies, and paediatric services probably see more children and young people than specialist mental health services. Some ADHD services are hospital-based and are located in paediatric services, whilst others are hosted by specialist CAMHS teams (NHS Quality Improvement Scotland 2007). A number are commissioned and delivered in partnership between both these services and involve shared care arrangements (NICE 2008). Several specialist ADHD teams have developed to support a multi-agency approach to the assessment and treatment of children with ADHD. Often this is part of a wider service that also focuses on autistic spectrum disorders and other developmental disorders (Horstmann and Steer 2007). Most ADHD services in the UK cover a small catchment area and provide assessment and treatment services for local children and families. However, services that cover a wider area such as an NHS health board in Scotland or Wales or subregion in England also exist. The multidisciplinary composition of these services also varies, with some but not all having specialist ADHD nursing input.

How do children get referred to specialist services?

Parental or professional concerns about a child or young person's health, general development, behaviour or education can lead to referral to any one of a number of services or agencies (Sayal *et al.* 2002; Salmon *et al.* 2006). The way in which children and young people are referred for assessment and treatment of ADHD varies widely across the UK. Many children face what has been referred to as a 'treatment lottery', where the availability of specialist assessment and treatment services depends on their postcode (Audit Commission 1999). Children with mental health problems and disorders, including those with ADHD, often pass through a series of gates or filters before reaching specialist mental health services (Wolpert and Fredman 1994; McDougall and Crocker 2001). This means that for many families the journey from assessment can be long and arduous (Pryjmachuk 1999; NICE 2008) and care pathways can often be arbitrary. Guidelines recently published by the National Institute for Health and Clinical Excellence (NICE) aim to improve this by setting standards for good practice and defining models for referral within a 'stepped care' framework (NICE 2008).

Stepped care

Stepped care is a way of organising resources to enable efficiency and appropriate levels of service delivery matched to clinical need. Implementation of the diagnostic and treatment process for ADHD should be within the framework of such a structured and stepped pathway (NICE 2008). At present, service provision for children and families in the UK is compartmentalised and fragmented (Salmon *et al*. 2006). However, examples of good practice do exist. These are usually underpinned by robust management protocols which streamline referral processes by setting standards for specific referral to specialist ADHD services (Hill and Taylor 2001).

Shared care guidelines

It has been suggested that many specialist ADHD services are close to saturation point, and that referrals are on the increase (Salmon 2005). Many children and young people with ADHD require long-term prescribing and medication monitoring. As new ways of working are evolving for nurses and other professionals, this presents opportunities to develop new services and improve access. Indeed, in many areas of the UK this is already happening with shared care arrangements in place between GPs and specialist ADHD services and nurse prescribing as part of nurse-led ADHD clinics (Ryan 2007a; Ryan 2007b). However, in other areas shared care has been difficult to implement and general practitioners remain reluctant to refer to or become involved in joint management (Steer 2005). This is partly because some primary care professionals report that they do not feel adequately trained or experienced to work with children and young people with ADHD (Klasen and Goodman 2000; Thapar and Thapar 2002; Sayal *et al*. 2002).

The tiered model of service delivery

The child and adolescent mental health services (CAMHS) tiered model of service delivery (Health Advisory Service 1995) is a framework to organise the commissioning, management and delivery of mental health services for children and young people with metal health problems and disorders. This framework is currently the preferred model for planning and delivering child mental health services which often include ADHD services, and is now common currency across all children's services agencies (see Figure 8.1 on p. 129).

Tier 1

Parents and frontline professionals in primary services are usually the first to recognise the symptoms of ADHD. These include GPs, teachers, health visitors and school nurses. Sometimes referred to as universal, frontline or primary services, Tier 1 services are those in which children receive day-to-day care, education or healthcare interventions (Health Advisory Service 1995). Such services include those provided in schools, GP practices and children's homes, and professionals in these settings should have a basic understanding of ADHD and know how to refer a child for specialist assessment. Here, symptom checklists such as the Conners Rating Scale (Conners 1997) or Strengths and Difficulties Questionnaire (Goodman 1997) may be useful in identifying which children may need referral for a specialist assessment of ADHD. Parental advice is the most common intervention for children and young people with ADHD and is often delivered by health visitors or nurse specialists (NICE 2008). This may sometimes be combined with a parenting programme on an individual family or group basis and is often delivered by nurses and other professionals in child mental health or paediatric services.

Tier 2

Tier 2 services are provided by professionals with additional training or expertise in child and adolescent mental health. This includes community and hospital paediatricians, nurse practitioners with a special interest in ADHD, or nurse specialists in Youth Offending Services who may be concerned that a young person in contact with the criminal justice system has unmet mental health needs. Other Tier 2 CAMHS professionals who may be involved in the care, treatment or education of a child or young person with ADHD include educational psychologists, speech and language therapists or occupational therapists. The role of a Tier 2 professional is to provide direct assessment or treatment interventions for individual children and young people with less complex problems, and to provide support, guidance and training for Tier 1 professionals providing frontline services. Professionals working in services at Tiers 1 and 2 must be able to access specialist CAMHS. This is where they have concerns that a child or young person they are working with may require a full multidisciplinary assessment or specialist treatment for ADHD.

Tier 3

Tier 3 services are dedicated multidisciplinary teams providing comprehensive assessment, treatment and consultation services for children and young people with complex, persistent or severe mental health needs and disorders. Many referrals to Tier 3 CAMHS are of children and young people with ADHD (McDougall and Crocker 2001). Tier 3 teams usually comprise nurses, psychiatrists, psychologists, family therapists, social workers and therapists. Specialist Tier 3 ADHD assessment and treatment services are not routinely available in the UK. Over two-thirds of parents in a large survey stated that they had no access to a specialist ADHD clinic (ADDISS 2006). NICE guidelines recommend that mental health trusts and children's trusts that provide mental health services for children should consider developing specialist multidisciplinary teams with specific expertise in the assessment, diagnosis and management of ADHD (NICE 2008). Such teams should:

- provide diagnostic, treatment and consultation services;
- develop protocols, care pathways and transition arrangements;
- collaborate with primary care providers to develop shared care protocols;
- ensure children and young people with ADHD have access to psychological therapies.

This multidisciplinary, multi-agency approach to the assessment, treatment and management of children with ADHD should be based on a seamless care pathway (Keen *et al.* 1997). However, this is often not available due to a lack of cooperation among professionals, an absence of teamwork and a deficit of specialist resources (Cohen 2006). The use of protocols and integrated care pathways is a way of standardising care and will help ensure that nurses can deliver high-quality care and treatment services as advised in the NICE guidelines on ADHD.

Tier 4

Sometimes young people have very complex or debilitating mental disorders. Tier 4 CAMHS are highly specialised tertiary CAMHS and include in-patient child and adolescent units, specialised eating disorders services and forensic CAMHS, as well as multi-agency services such as home treatment services, community support teams and crisis teams. For children and young people with ADHD who have not responded to overall treatment in primary care and continue to experience significant impairments, referral to Tier 4 CAMHS may be indicated. However, admission to hospital would not usually be for ADHD per se but for additional comorbidity and an associated degree of risk to self or others (see Figure 8.1).

What is the role of practice parameters and clinical guidelines?

Clinical guidelines are systematic statements about best practice and are intended to assist clinicians and service users to make informed decisions about appropriate treatment options for specific conditions (Mann 1996; Kendall *et al.* 2005). A rapid increase in the number of clinical guidelines within health services means that clinicians are becoming increasingly guided by evidence of effectiveness. Protocols for ADHD focus on clinical interventions and care pathways and set standards for assessment, care and treatment. The majority of ADHD protocols summarise referral criteria, define the role and responsibilities of ADHD specialists and set out expectations of GPs, teachers and parents or carers (Hill and Taylor 2001). Most protocols

Tier 1
Services at primary level by professionals providing non-specialist CAMHS in health, education, social services and youth justice settings. This involves mental health promotion, early identification of mental health problems and, in some cases, treatment for less severe mental health problems, e.g. sleep, temper tantrums, behaviour problems at home/school and bereavement

Professionals
Health visitors, Portage Practice nurses, School nurses, Sure Start worker GPs, Voluntary sector workers, Youth workers, Teachers, Healthy Schools Project workers, Social workers, Family support workers

Tier 2
Individual professionals working relatively independently from other services, but relating to each other through a network. They provide training and consultation to Tier 1 workers, outreach to identify complex, severe or persistent mental disorders and signpost children and young people to specialist CAMHS at Tiers 2 or 3

Professionals
Clinical psychologist, Educational psychologist, Child and adolescent psychiatrist, YOT health nurse specialist, Primary mental health worker, Community paediatrician, Hospital paediatrician

Most children with mental health problems will be seen at Tiers 1 and 2

Tier 3
Specialist multidisciplinary child and adolescent teams

Professionals
Psychiatrists, Mental health nurses, Psychologists, Social workers, Family therapists and others providing assessment and treatment for children and young people with complex, persistent or severe mental disorders. Assessment for referrals to Tier 4
Provision of support and training for Tier 2; offer consultation to Tier 1 professionals

Tier 4
Specialist multidisciplinary child and adolescent teams

In-patient child and adolescent units may also have support from occupational therapists, speech and language therapists and creative therapists who specialise in art, music, drama or play therapy.

In-patient child and adolescent units Day units	Intensive home-based treatment services/crisis outreach teams	Out-patient services for eating disorders; neuropsychiatric problems; sexual abuse; OCD etc

Figure 8.1 NHS Health Advisory Service tiered model of service delivery (1995).

for ADHD are multi-agency agreements. They identify a single point of referral or entry, planned assessment and treatment interventions and set thresholds for where referral on to another agency may be required due to complexity or severity.

In both the UK and US, guidelines, parameters and protocols for good practice have had a profound impact on clinical practice (Hill and Taylor 2001; American Academy of Pediatrics 2000; American Academy of Child and Adolescent Psychiatry 2002). These have been developed from empirical evidence and the clinical consensus of experts, and set standards or principles in relation to best practice based on the available evidence. However, our knowledge about childhood mental disorder is in a process of evolution. Whilst the cause, effect and outcome of some disorders is partially understood, our knowledge of what works for other disorders is limited (Skuse 2003). Many research findings have not been evaluated. This is rapidly developing as clinical guidelines, practice parameters, systematic reviews and evidence-based briefings are published.

Following concern about the increasing use of medication for ADHD, and the wide variation in assessment and treatment protocols used in clinical settings, UK clinical guidelines have been developed to assist clinicians in assessing, treating and managing children, young people and adults with ADHD. Clinical and service recommendations are made based on the strength of empirical and clinical consensus, and all are intended to improve standards of care, reduce variations in quality of care and ensure that children and young people with ADHD receive services that meet their needs (NICE 2008). General guidelines for ADHD include those published in the US (Dulcan *et al.* 1997); New Zealand (Ministry of Health 2001); Scotland (Barton *et al.* 2001; Scottish Intercollegiate Guidelines Network 2001), and England and Wales (NICE 2008), as well as specific guidance on the use of stimulant medication including methylphenidate (NICE 2001; American Academy of Child and Adolescent Psychiatry 2002). However, a national study from the US found that only half of children and young people with ADHD receive care that corresponds to practice parameters on ADHD issued by the American Academy of Child and Adolescent Psychiatry (Hoagwood *et al.* 2000). This illustrates the need to ensure that guidelines are part of everyday clinical practice and service governance. Nurses and other professionals should be clear that ADHD guidelines are not a substitute for professional knowledge, experience or expertise. Rather, they complement professional practice and, like all guidelines, have their limitations.

Managing transitions

Later in this book we will hear that some young people with ADHD continue to experience symptoms of hyperactivity, impulsivity and inattention in adulthood and may require support from specialist ADHD or adult mental health services. However, the provision of adult ADHD services is limited in the UK and most adults are unable to access appropriate specialist services (Asherson 2005; Nutt *et al*. 2007). This may be due to the comorbid presentation of the ADHD with adult assessment and treatment services prioritising other aspects of the presentation such as personality difficulties, substance misuse and depression or anxiety. Where adult services do exist, the evidence from young people is that the transition process is not usually a positive event and is associated with significant concerns and anxieties (Willoughby *et al*. 2003; Beresford 2004). Various reports have confirmed that transitional arrangements for young people with ADHD are often poor, lack strategy and are frequently managed on a case-to-case basis (NHS Quality Improvement Scotland 2007).

It is not only transitions from children's to adult's services that young people with ADHD may require support with. There is well-documented evidence that the transitions from junior school to secondary school, or the process of leaving college to start employment can be stressful events for many children and young people (Litner 2003; Ward *et al*. 2003; While *et al*. 2004; Horstmann and Steer 2007). For children and young people, one-to-one teacher support decreases and the demands placed by a bigger peer group increase. For those with ADHD, the challenges may be greater due to deficits in skills of organising, planning and memory which are essential to manage this transition smoothly. It is therefore essential that nurses and other professionals assist young people with ADHD to navigate transitions successfully. School nurses and Connexions workers are well placed to support young people through periods of vulnerability by helping bridge the gaps between leaving school and starting vocational, training or employment activities (Department for Education and Skills 2001).

Care planning

Earlier in the book we heard that children and young people with ADHD require integrated care from multi-agency services. However, like many child and adolescent disorders, ADHD transgresses a multitude of agencies and services and integrated care is not easy to achieve. Where comorbidity exists children and young people with ADHD may be in contact with paediatric health services, specialist CAMHS and learning disability services. Where there are school-based difficulties they may require services from educational psychologists, speech and language therapists and behaviour support teams. Young people with ADHD whose behaviour problems are associated with antisocial or criminal behaviour may come into contact with social services, youth offending teams or the police.

With such a wide multi-agency array of professionals and services there exists real potential for inconsistency and poor communication. Here, the role of the nurse can be vital in coordinating interventions so that care and treatment programmes are seamless and delivered efficiently. It is vital that all services for children and families with ADHD are coordinated and integrated through seamless care packages. Where multi-agency arrangements for ADHD have been developed, these appear to be more successful than single-agency planning (Horstmann and Steer 2007). The role of the nurse in helping achieve interagency cooperation involves giving, receiving and seeking advice and consultation, co-working and networking with multi-agency colleagues and being creative and innovative in how they assess, plan and manage the multi-agency care plan.

What is the role of ADHD support groups?

In many European countries ADHD support groups have ambitious goals, both in relation to the support of individual children and families, and in public campaigning. For many, their credibility and rejection of factionalism or professional parochialism are important in persuading society of the importance of recognising and supporting children and young people with ADHD (Taylor *et al.* 2004). Nationally recognised ADHD information services such as the Attention Deficit Disorder Information and Support Service (ADDISS) or reputable charities such as YoungMinds often collaborate with local support groups to help ensure that children, young people and families are provided with consistent and accurate information about all aspects of ADHD.

Signposting parents to local support groups can often be helpful as part of the overall care package. This helps provide a network of advice and advocacy which parents or carers often find supportive (NICE 2008). Local groups can be an opportunity for parents or carers to seek and provide peer support, and many provide advice on stress management and the day-to-day management of children and young people with ADHD. Putting families in touch with local support groups or even national organisations can be supportive; these support groups can vary but most offer meetings for parents and can act as advocates for parents and young people, provide information and resources and offer direct input to young people. Whilst support groups may be helpful to some families, it is important to be aware that not all parents will like this approach. Here, nurses will need to consider whether another supportive intervention would be more appropriate and they should be flexible and creative.

Summary

Wherever possible, models for care and treatment should be based on evidence and established best practice guidelines. Various guidelines exist to guide clinicians, commissioners and managers on how best to plan, deliver and evaluate ADHD services. Yet all too often the services that children and families receive do not reflect best practice. The process of assessment and diagnosis for young people and families can often be frustrating and lengthy and care pathways are often arbitrary. The need for a consistent approach to the assessment of ADHD is required in order to improve care pathways and models of intervention. In the UK, guidelines published by the National Institute for Health and Clinical Excellence describe evidence-based interventions and models of service provision which are known to produce positive outcomes. Nurses should consult these best practice guidelines at every stage of the assessment and treatment process.

9　School-based interventions for ADHD

Key points

- Due to difficulties primarily with inattention, children and young people with ADHD experience academic underachievement, often fall behind their peers and have poor educational outcomes.
- School-based professionals including teachers and school nurses are frequently the first to recognise the symptoms of ADHD and are in key positions to support parents and refer the child for specialist assessment.
- Children with ADHD need school-based support in order that their educational, social and psychological needs can be met and they can reach their fullest potential.
- Pupils with ADHD are likely to benefit from a structured, consistent and predictable classroom environment where their ADHD is understood and supported by teachers and other school-based staff.
- Strategies for supporting children with ADHD in school can be used for individual children, in the classroom setting and through a 'whole school approach'. Behavioural strategies include paying positive attention to appropriate behaviour and compliance, providing clear and achievable instructions and using appropriate negative consequences for problem behaviour.
- Since the behaviour of children and young people with ADHD can often be oppositional and challenging to manage, teachers and other school-based professionals may benefit from guidance on behaviour management strategies from specialist ADHD nurses.

Introduction

It has been estimated that as many as 1% of school-age children in England and Wales have severe ADHD. In addition, as many as 5% experience symptoms which fulfil the criteria for ADHD as defined by ICD-10 (NICE 2008). This equates to around 69,000 children in England being severely affected, and approximately 345,000 mildly to moderately affected (Hill 2005). The symptoms of hyperactivity, impulsivity and inattention frequently manifest as overt behaviours which are disruptive in the classroom and school environment (DuPaul and Eckert 1997a). Almost two-thirds of children with hyperkinetic disorder are behind in their overall scholastic ability, and almost three-quarters have officially recognised special educational needs (Green *et al.* 2005). Population studies show that children with ADHD are more likely to be 'school refusers', or to have been absent from school for long periods at a time than other children (Green *et al.* 2005). The oppositional behaviour of between one-quarter and one-third of children and young people with ADHD will lead to their exclusion from school (Tannock 1999; Green *et al.* 2005; Barbaresi *et al.* 2007).

Research has shown a clear link between ADHD and impairment in overall academic functioning (Frazier *et al.* 2007; Barbaresi *et al.* 2007). Children and young people with ADHD have higher rates of specific and generalised learning problems (NICE 2008), poor reading skills (McGee *et al.* 1992; Swanson *et al.* 1999; Ford *et al.* 2004) and more speech and language difficulties (Hinshaw 2002). As many as half will have learning problems in reading, writing, spelling, mathematics and language and traditional teaching and learning systems may present many difficulties for pupils with ADHD (Green *et al.* 2005). Not surprisingly, the costs of education are high for this group of children and young people (Agency for Health Care Policy and Research 1999).

The behavioural difficulties that children and young people with ADHD show in school partly arise from their symptoms of hyperactivity, impulsivity and inattention, and the inability to meet demands for academic and social performance. As the school curriculum progresses, these demands may escalate, leading to a breakdown in the relationship between the child, school or college and family (McArdle 2005). Despite a vast international literature on the medical and behavioural management of children and young people with ADHD, there has been a lack of longitudinal studies and well-designed studies of direct relevance to the class or school setting (Merrell and Tymms 2004).

School-based mental health services

To date, much of the learning about school-based mental health services has come from the US where various models of intervention exist. These include support from school-based professionals including nurses; training for educational staff and school nurses; consultation for teachers and other school-based professionals and outreach from specialist child and adolescent mental health services (CAMHS) (Rones and Hoagwood 2000; Leighton 2006). Social skills programmes and student mediated conflict resolution programmes have been effective for some children and young people with ADHD in schools (Rhodes and Ajmal 1995; Wells *et al.* 2000), and nurse-led, school-based services have been successful in supporting children with ADHD develop positive self-esteem (Frame *et al.* 2003). However, the way in which school-based services for pupils with ADHD are provided differs between the US and UK. In the US, education systems operate under several legal mandates applicable to children with ADHD. Pupils with additional needs including ADHD may qualify for special educational services under the Individuals with Disabilities Education Act (IDEA) (Bussing *et al.* 2003).

Very few schools in the UK offer ADHD-specific interventions. However, many offer individual support and group programmes for social skills development which are often run by special educational needs coordinators (SENCOs) and teachers with a special interest in ADHD. These can be helpful in reducing aggressive or bullying behaviours which may be a consequence of or associated with ADHD (Rigby 2002). School nurses are ideally placed to assist in the provision of mental health services within schools as they work across education, health and social care boundaries (Frame *et al.* 2003; Leighton 2006). However, in both the US and the UK, the role of the school nurse with children and young people is not clearly defined.

Although school-based mental health services in the UK are not comprehensively available, recent investment in the emotional development of school-aged children is likely to make this an area of rapid growth (Department for Children, Families and Schools 2008). This is long overdue given the government's policy commitments to the mental health and psychological wellbeing and substantial investment in child and adolescent mental health services during the last decade (McDougall and Davren 2006). School nurses in particular have the potential to improve both educational and health outcomes for all school-age children including those with ADHD (Department for Education and Skills 2006).

How can schools and teachers help?

It has been posited that the origins of many of the difficulties that young people face lie less in themselves and more within the environment in which they live (Thomas 2004). This suggests that the key for positive change may be in the contexts in which children and young people with ADHD find themselves. Therefore, rather than change the child, changing the environment might be the intervention that is most helpful (Poduska 2000; Wood and Hughes 2005). Schools play a vital role in helping children develop emotional health and wellbeing and children and adolescents spend longer in school than in any other environment (WHO 1997). For this reason, schools have been identified as an ideal place to prevent and address child and adolescent mental health problems (DfES 2001; Leighton 2006).

A range of school-based professionals including school nurses, educational psychologists, SENCOs, speech and language therapists, learning mentors, classroom support assistants, pastoral staff and school counsellors play a key role in supporting children with ADHD achieve their potential. However, more than any other professional, teachers are the most commonly identified source of support for parents of children with ADHD (Sayal *et al*. 2006a). In the UK, two-thirds of parents of children with ADHD have consulted and discussed their concerns with their child's teacher (Sayal *et al*. 2006b). The proportion of children and young people observed by their teacher to be displaying ADHD symptoms is high (Gaub and Carlson 1997; Merrell and Tymms 2001). In addition, a large-scale survey of children in Great Britain found that it is often teachers who first recognise overactivity, impulsiveness and poor attention as this may impact on the academic performance and behaviour of children in their class (Green *et al*. 2005). Studies in the US have also shown that it is most often teachers who first notice the symptoms of ADHD (Kidd 2000). For these reasons, teachers are well placed to help improve outcomes for children by fostering the protective factors and resilience necessary for them to live with their ADHD (Sandberg 2002).

Despite government policy to improve child mental health training for frontline professionals (Department of Health 2004), and the very high level of contact teachers have with children who have ADHD, training about ADHD and mental health problems in general for teachers has been lacking (Gowers *et al*. 2004). Similar trends have been observed in the US (Snider *et al*. 2003), and there has been little in the way of research examining the knowledge, skills and competencies required by teachers to teach and manage children with ADHD. A small number of questionnaires and surveys from North America and Australia have focused on the training needs of elementary school teachers in relation to ADHD but these have not been widespread (Jerome *et al*. 1994; West *et al*. 2005). The provision of education for teachers has been reported to raise awareness and improve recognition of pupils with possible ADHD (Sayal *et al*. 2006a), but the impact of teacher awareness on the outcomes of children and young people with ADHD is yet to be determined.

Guidance for teachers and school-based staff

A range of policy and good practice guidance exists to help schools improve outcomes for children with ADHD. *Promoting Children's Mental Health Within Early Years and Schools Settings* (Department for Education and Skills 2001a) provides guidance for local education authorities, pre-school settings, schools and specialist child and adolescent mental health services. It offers pointers to and examples of good practice in terms of the early identification of mental health problems in children and young people in pre-school and school settings. There is a specific section on supporting children with ADHD which includes guidance on teaching and learning strategies.

NICE guidelines

As part of its public health programme, the National Institute for Health and Clinical Excellence (NICE) has produced guidance on social and emotional wellbeing in primary education (NICE 2008a). Through the development of comprehensive programmes, universal approaches and targeted interventions, local authority commissioners and professionals in schools are encouraged to focus on the development of social and emotional wellbeing and skills in all areas of the curriculum. The suggested areas for investment include problem-solving, coping, conflict resolution and understanding feelings. As part of targeted approaches addressing the needs of pupils with emotional and behavioural difficulties, the guidance makes a number of important recommendations for education commissioners, teachers and practitioners such as school nurses. These are intended to improve outcomes for all children who have social or behavioural problems including those with ADHD:

- Teachers and practitioners should be trained to identify and assess the early signs of anxiety, emotional distress and behavioural problems among schoolchildren.
- Teachers and practitioners should be able to assess when a specialist should be involved and make an appropriate referral.
- Children who are exposed to difficult situations such as bullying or racism, or who are coping with socially disadvantaged circumstances, are at higher risk and need additional support.
- Teachers and practitioners should be able to discuss the options for tackling these problems with the child and their parents or carers. They should also be able to agree an action plan, as the first stage of a 'stepped care' approach (as defined in NICE clinical guidance on ADHD).

Both the NICE guidelines on ADHD (2008b) and good practice guidance for schools and early years settings (Department for Educational and Skills 2001) recognise that transitions can be periods of vulnerability for all children, and particularly those with additional needs such as ADHD. There is a large body of research that shows that the transition from nursery to primary school, from primary to secondary school and from secondary school to higher education or employment can be highly stressful for children and young people with ADHD (Galton *et al.* 1999; Morris 1999; Barber and Olsen 2003). Although careful planning is advocated by a number of specialist agencies including the National Attention Deficit Disorder Information and Support Service (ADDISS), this does not always happen in practice (Horstmann and Steer 2007). It is therefore crucial that school nurses, teachers and other professionals help pupils with ADHD navigate transitions successfully by anticipating periods of difficulty and helping ensure that children and young people and their parents and carers are adequately prepared.

ADHD or something else?

Teachers and other school-based staff should be aware that there are many potential explanations for hyperactivity, impulsivity and inattention which do not include ADHD. For example, the inattentive child may have a sensory problem such as hearing loss or visual impairment. This may mean that they fail to read instructions on the board, or may miss what has been said by the teacher. Children with sensory impairments can also appear noisy and appear 'off task' as they cannot hear properly or attend to visual instructions. In addition, those with social communication disorders can also appear to be 'off task' when they are not engaged in a group social activity but attending to their own script, which they can focus and concentrate well on. Children and young people with learning disabilities or low cognitive abilities can experience inattention and frustration in the classroom, and this may masquerade as ADHD (Furman 2005). It is therefore important that teachers seek advice from health professionals such as school nurses if they are concerned that a child in their class may have unmet health or communication needs.

Inattention in school

Many of the difficulties that pupils with ADHD face in school are associated with inattention. Normal attention can be seen on a continuum from, on the one hand, highly attentive to, on the other, very easily distracted (Reid 2007). Inattention in a pupil with ADHD is considered to be beyond the realms of normal attention and manifests in a number of ways. They often struggle to focus, are easily distracted and may appear to be daydreaming. This is because children with ADHD seek additional stimulation when low levels of stimulation are present (Antrop *et al.* 2000). In a busy and highly stimulating environment such as the classroom setting, pupils with ADHD may be highly aroused. As a result, they have difficulty paying attention and may appear not to listen to the teacher. They may struggle to stay on task for more than a few minutes at a time, and disrupt other children's attempts to work or concentrate. ADHD is not due to a lack of knowledge or ability, but is a problem with sustaining attention, effort and motivation. This means that ADHD is a disorder of performing what one knows, rather than one of not knowing what to do.

Pupils with ADHD can be supported to improve their attention. Keeping stimuli to a minimum in the classroom setting is supported by research showing that distractions in the environment result in decreases in time spent on task (Whalen *et al.* 1979). Sitting an inattentive child at the front of the class can have a positive impact. Here, the child becomes less distracted by visual stimuli and is better able to concentrate on the task in hand. The teacher is more able to encourage, motivate and keep the child with ADHD on track and the rest of the class benefits from minimal disruption to their learning. Similarly, using worksheets, role play and exercises can help pupils with ADHD maintain attention and motivation, and helps reduce impulsivity.

Executive functioning

Psychologists and other professionals often refer to 'executive functioning' by which they mean the cognitive system which controls cognitive activities. These include planning, choosing appropriate actions and inhibiting inappropriate actions, and selecting relevant sensory information. Research shows that children and young people with ADHD have difficulties with executive functioning and their working memory (Barkley 1997a; Klingberg *et al.* 2002; Sergeant *et al.* 2002; Bitsakou *et al.* 2008). Our working memory allows us to retain, manipulate and filter information during a short period of time. Planning involves the ability to look ahead and work through a sequence of intermediary steps. Due to difficulties with executive functioning, the way in which children and young people process information, plan, make decisions and take actions may be impaired. This may make them forgetful and poorly organised, and they may find it difficult to manage time or follow complex instructions. Here, the use of class-based memory aides such as 'green for go' and 'red for stop' visual cues can be helpful (O'Regan 2006).

Due to difficulties with executive thinking, it is helpful if classroom-based tasks can be broken down to be concise, time-limited and simple to achieve. Complex tasks can easily be forgotten or the child with ADHD may become quickly bored. This is because children and young people with attention difficulties find it difficult to pace the progress of work and may tire easily, or finish a task prematurely (Zentall 1993; Levine 1997). Classroom projects should therefore be short in duration and longer assignments should be broken down into short attainable tasks that are promptly rewarded if they are completed satisfactorily. Children with ADHD can be forgetful, and may sometimes miss their medication, books or other equipment needed in school. Here, it may be helpful to use visual prompts to assist recall.

Concentration

Rushing to finish a piece of work can often mean that attention to detail is missed and careless mistakes can be made. It is not clear from research whether inaccuracy alone or a fast inaccurate response time is characteristic of children with ADHD (Fonagy *et al.* 2002). Sustained attention is the ability to maintain a consistent focus on a continuous activity. Selective attention is the ability to focus on relevant stimuli and ignore competing stimuli. This distractibility or inability to 'screen out' unwanted stimuli can place competing demands for attention and cause numerous distractions. Due to difficulties with attention span and concentration, pupils with ADHD may start off a task with great enthusiasm and vigour, but quickly lose pace and find it increasingly difficult to sustain attention. This can mean that work remains unfinished whilst other tasks get started. It is easy to see how the characteristics of inattention and impulsivity can be misinterpreted as a lack of interest and a wilful choice to avoid tasks (Leroux and Levitt-Perlman 2000). It is therefore important that the teacher helps the child pace themselves and plans small, sequential steps to complete pieces of classwork. Here, it is important to emphasise the quality or the child's work rather than the quantity they produce. In order to compensate for difficulties with stimulus control, children and young people with ADHD should receive more prompts, cues and reinforcements than those without ADHD will require. Children with ADHD will often require feedback on a regular basis to let them know if what they are doing is consistent with the task at hand. Computer-assisted learning is beneficial to children with ADHD. This is because the constant visual stimuli motivate and reward the child and the information processing that is required is suitable for a child who has difficulties with concentration and attention.

Hyperactivity in school

Hyperactivity in the classroom manifests in a number of ways. A pupil with ADHD will often stand out as being fidgety, overactive and generally restless. In a classroom setting where it is commonplace for children to sit still for long periods, children with ADHD may struggle to do so and this can be difficult for teachers to cope with. For those with the most severe form of hyperkinetic disorder, overactivity may be extreme with the child constantly wriggling, running and climbing. This group of children are often described by parents or teachers as being driven by a motor (Selikowitz 2006). In order to help manage the hyperactive pupil, classroom rules should be clear, simple and achievable. For example, it is no use teachers insisting that the child with ADHD should sit still for the whole lesson. This will simply not be possible and will set the child up to fail. Instead, it is helpful to describe how pupils are expected to behave during the lesson, and be clear about when children can move about the classroom and when it is discouraged.

Due to poorly developed gross and fine motor control, handwriting may be untidy. For this reason teachers should not insist on neatness and on children redoing untidy work. This is likely to be counterproductive and may further alienate the pupil with ADHD (O'Regan 2006). Instead, the specialist input of a speech and language therapist or occupational therapist may be helpful in developing strategies that can be applied in the classroom. These professionals can help pupils with ADHD develop the fine visual and motor skills needed for handwriting, along with help in visual perception, neurological and postural control, and the planning and organisation of tasks (O'Regan 2006). Not only does hyperactivity impact negatively on the individual child's academic performance but it also has the potential to disrupt the learning and behaviour of others around them. Here, careful consideration of seating arrangements can be productive. Simple, practical intervention such as sitting a child who is hyperactive next to a child who is calm and not easily provoked or distracted can be helpful.

Teachers should be forgiven for believing that channelling the hyperactive behaviour of pupils with ADHD into PE or games will solve problems. It has been suggested that as many as half of all children with ADHD have motor problems (Hartsough and Lambert 1985; Pitcher *et al*. 1987). Whilst some children with ADHD are excellent athletes, most are poorly coordinated and struggle with competitive sports. For example, catching a ball is difficult due to poor hand–eye coordination, and many have low muscle tone which may result in a poorly coordinated running style (Selikowitz 2006). This is not to say pupils with ADHD should not be encouraged to participate in physical education. On the contrary, joining in sports and games promotes opportunities to improve social interaction, turn-taking and good physical health.

Impulsivity in school

Impulsivity can be defined as difficulty with being able to think before acting (Selikowitz 2006). People who are impulsive often act and then think, rather than think and then act. Impulsivity by children with ADHD in school manifests at a cognitive and behavioural level. Due to difficulties with impulse control, children with ADHD often struggle to inhibit inappropriate verbal and physical responses. Cognitive impulsivity involves a tendency to blurt out answers to questions before the question is finished, interrupting others and struggling to take turns (Clark *et al*. 1999). Behavioural impulsivity may involve a disregard for the negative consequences of an action or the need for immediate gratification.

Deferred or delayed gratification is the ability to wait in order to obtain something that one wants. Children with ADHD often struggle in this area because they require instant gratification and suffer from poor impulse control. The so called 'Marshmallow experiments' and 'gift delay' impulse control studies in the 1960s illustrate this process nicely. In the first study a group of four-year-old children were tested by being given a marshmallow, and were promised another only if they could wait 20 minutes before eating the first one. Not surprisingly, some children could wait and others could not. In the second experiment, children were shown a gift-wrapped present but told they could only open it if they completed a puzzle. Researchers calculated a delay score based on how long the children could wait. Follow-up studies found that boys who had not delayed were irritable whereas those who had been patient were attentive.

Whilst most children without ADHD will learn to organise tasks and develop social competence in relation to turn-taking and listening, children with ADHD often struggle with these developmental tasks. 'Circle Time' as part of the PHSE curriculum may provide an appropriate forum to help children develop skills of turn-taking, listening to others and understanding social rules. Shouting out and talking out of turn can make pupils with

ADHD unpopular with peers who grow to resent the intrusiveness, and experience the child with ADHD as 'pushing in'. It can sometimes be helpful to encourage the child to practise a structured routine prior to answering a question. A three-step approach which encourages pupils to 'listen', 'think' and 'answer' can be effective. However, for children with ADHD, simply teaching the child the consequences of an action does not solve the problem. They lack the reflective and behavioural inhibition mechanisms needed to apply such teaching to everyday situations (Selkowitz 2006).

Tests and rating scales

Several psychometric tests have been developed to assess cognitive impulsivity and both sustained and selective attention. These include the Conners Continuous Performance Test (CPT) (Conners *et al.* 2000) and the Matching Familiar Figures Test (MFFT) (Kagan 1965). The CPT is often used by educational or clinical psychologists as part of a wider battery of tests to assess executive functioning and to support a diagnosis of ADHD. The MFFT is designed to measure reflection and impulsivity by requiring children to select repeatedly from several alternative figures the one that matches a standard. Children who are impulsive are likely to choose more quickly and make more errors than their non-ADHD peers who may be more reflective. Neither test is diagnostic, and both should only be used as part of a wider assessment strategy. Studies show that teacher-rated scales tend to provide a more accurate overview of a child's behaviour than do parent-rating scales (Taylor *et al.* 1996). A number of rating tools can be used by teachers to assist the diagnosis and monitoring of children with ADHD. In the US, clinical practice guidance suggests that teachers should be directly involved in the process of diagnosing ADHD by completing rating scales and providing information about behaviour in the school setting (American Academy of Child and Adolescent Psychiatry 2007). In the UK, the involvement of teachers in understanding how the child or young person functions in their learning environment is a crucial part of the overall assessment process but is not in itself diagnostic.

The most common rating scales used in school are the Conners Teacher Rating Scale (CTRS) (Connors 1989; Connors *et al.* 1998); the Strengths and Difficulties Questionnaire (SDQ) teacher version (Goodman 1999); the SNAP (IV) Rating Scale (Swanson 2001); and the Disruptive Behaviour Disorders Checklist (DBDC) (Pelham *et al.* 1992). These tools can be useful in helping teachers to distinguish ADHD from conduct disorder and other potential explanations for inattention and hyperactivity. Many other rating scales have been adapted for use in school, and these include the ADHD Rating Scale School Version (DuPaul 1998). This has separate scoring profiles for boys and girls and can be completed by teachers as well as parents.

Teaching strategies and lesson planning

All pupils have the right to a school experience which provides a broad, balanced and relevant curriculum including the National Curriculum, which is appropriately differentiated according to their needs (Department for Education and Skills 2001b). This is often referred to as 'mainstreaming' and includes pupils with and without ADHD. Although there is a statutory requirement to provide appropriate education for all children, including pupils with ADHD, practice within local education authorities varies (NICE 2008b). For children with ADHD it is important to understand their learning styles and the way they process information in order to help them achieve positive outcomes in the classroom. It has been suggested that children and young people struggle both in the normal school environment and in classes for children with special educational needs (Hjorne 2007). This makes supporting them appropriately a challenge for teachers and schools. Increasingly, curriculum design is drawn up to accommodate the needs of children with special educational needs within a mainstream setting and many schools will have an inclusion policy. However, many children with special educational needs, including those with ADHD, have experienced difficulties with inclusion and not all classroom staff, head teachers or local authorities have been able to meet their needs (Davis and Watson 2000).

Additional classroom support

Many children and young people with ADHD will often require additional classroom-based support from specialist services. They do not usually ask for this support themselves. This is because people with ADHD are poor at monitoring and regulating their behaviour (Barkley 1997b). It is therefore important that teachers and other classroom support staff recognise the need for additional support in their teaching strategies and lesson delivery. Some schools provide mentors to support pupils with additional needs in the classroom setting. Those with ADHD often have deficits with organising and planning their work, and mentors can assist them to stay 'on track'.

Additional support can include teaching services provided through behaviour and learning support teams, teaching assistants, educational psychologists and specialist CAMHS professionals. Identification of pupils with special educational needs, including ADHD, begins with 'School Action', the process whereby teachers, parents, SENCOs and other professionals monitor a child's progress. Some children with ADHD will need an individual education plan (IEP) to assist learning and/ or an individual behaviour plan (IBP) to identify specific behaviour difficulties, set targets and include intervention strategies. Others will require a full statement of special educational needs from the local education authority. This describes the type of assistance which may be required by particular pupils, including those with ADHD (Department for Education and Skills 2001). However, the process of 'statementing' can often be bureaucratic and time-consuming. This can result in local education authorities failing to provide pupils with ADHD with individualised school intervention programmes (Brown 2003).

Functional analysis

Functional assessment or functional analysis is a useful way of understanding the classroom-based behaviour of pupils with ADHD. This is a process sometimes used by educational or clinical psychologists to link behaviours with interventions and involves the following characteristics (Ervin *et al.* 1998):

- carefully defining the target behaviour in question so that the teacher is able to reliably monitor this behaviour;
- identifying antecedents and consequences to this behaviour in the classroom environment;
- generating hypotheses about the function of this target behaviour in terms of the antecedent factors that set the context for the behaviour and/ or consequences that maintain it;
- systematically manipulating antecedents and consequences to test hypotheses about their relationship to the target behaviour;
- implementing interventions that alter the functional antecedents or consequences so that the problem behaviour is replaced with appropriate behaviour.

Creating structure and consistency

With limited resources it is not easy to teach and manage a child with ADHD in a busy classroom environment. However, the tolerance and ability of teachers and other school-based professionals to cope with a child who has ADHD contributes to whether their ADHD is seen as problematic. Those who are child-centred, strong-minded and patient are likely to cope best with pupils who have ADHD (O'Regan 2006). There are several simple strategies that can be employed consistently and which may benefit a wide range of pupils including those with ADHD. A structure of consistent and predictable routines, rules and guidelines forms the basis of all teaching systems, and its importance is even greater for the pupil with ADHD (O'Regan 2006). This is because children and young people with ADHD often lack stimulus control, and the first step in any process of intervention is to create an orderly, well-structured environment (van der Krol *et al.* 1998). In addition, many people with ADHD are motivated to satisfy a need for immediate gratification (Young and Bramham 2007). It is therefore important to structure the learning experience to include reward systems. A fast-paced structure will be beneficial to pupils with ADHD who have a high intolerance and low boredom threshold, and who are sensitive to reward delay (Tripp and Alsop 2001).

Behavioural strategies

The development of human behaviour is an undoubtedly complex process. However, much of our behaviour is determined by the positive and negative consequences we receive from our interactions with others. Through a process of socialisation, children learn that positive behaviour is rewarded and that negative behaviour is either ignored or punished. Theoretical behavioural models include classical conditioning (Pavlov 1955), social learning theory (Bandura 1977) and operant learning (Skinner 1974). Behavioural interventions for children and young people with ADHD are intended to extinguish antisocial or disruptive behaviour and replace this with desirable, prosocial behaviour (Abramowitz *et al.* 1987). Teachers and other school-based professionals should remember that they are not only focusing on problem behaviour. In the absence of opportunities to develop prosocial behaviour, pupils will invariably replace one problem behaviour with another. Behavioural strategies for pupils with ADHD include paying positive attention to appropriate behaviour, verbally reinforcing compliance, providing clear and achievable instructions and using appropriate negative consequences for antisocial behaviour.

The behaviour problems of pupils with ADHD place an increased demand on the teacher who is charged with meeting the educational and social developmental needs of all children, including those with ADHD. Behavioural strategies for supporting children with ADHD in school can be used for individual children in the classroom setting and through a 'whole school approach'. Behavioural interventions are known to be effective in reducing hyperactivity and promoting social adjustment in pre-school, primary and secondary school populations (DuPaul and Eckert 1997b). School-based interventions should include both proactive and reactive strategies in order to maximise behaviour change. The most common school-based interventions for pupils with ADHD involve behaviour reinforcement strategies (Mulligan 2001). These are used to manage the associated behavioural disturbance that pupils with ADHD often bring into the classroom.

Positive reinforcement

Pupils with ADHD need to be rewarded or disciplined immediately. Long-term goal targets such as gaining a good end-of-term report will not motivate them. Instead, immediate, consistent, tangible results such as a sticker, certificate or points are required if a behavioural system is to work (O'Regan 2006). The most simple positive social reward is praise, and this is a powerful reinforcer for children with ADHD who require motivation to remain engaged in a task and believe in their abilities to succeed in that task. The pride achieved by accomplishing a task well, and the supportive approval from significant adults, siblings and peers adds to the pupil's self-esteem and positive self-image.

Children and young people with ADHD are often artistic and creative, and it is important to provide them with opportunities to be rewarded for their positive achievements. Many are also good at expressing themselves, are quick to put what they learn into practice and are enthusiastic to learn. Positive praise from teachers can be a powerful reinforcer, for like parents teachers are often significant adults in the eyes of a child. Practical rewards can also be helpful when supporting children to develop prosocial behaviour. Ideal rewards are immediate, practical, tangible, consistent, in proportion to achievement and administered in small amounts (Gelfand and Hartmann 1984). For younger children, the use of star charts can motivate them, whereas for adolescents or teenagers working towards extra leisure or recreational activities can be rewarding. In the school setting, the use of practical rewards must be managed with sensitivity, since there are financial, moral and equity issues for teachers and schools to consider. Positive behavioural change does not happen overnight and teachers should expect that progress may sometimes be slow. It is not just successes that should be rewarded. Rewarding effort is just as important, particularly for children who have been entrenched in negative behaviour cycles for a long time.

Discipline

Wherever possible, it is important to make the distinction between antisocial behaviour and behaviour problems that arise from hyperactivity, impulsivity and inattention. This is not always straightforward. We have heard that pupils with ADHD are generally more impulsive than others, have difficulty delaying gratification, have a lower frustration tolerance and have difficulty monitoring their own behaviours (Kendall 1999). As Barkley (1997b) points out, children and young people with ADHD do not usually lack knowledge about appropriate behaviour; they lack the ability to act on what they know.

We are also aware that many pupils with ADHD have coexisting conduct disorder and many are on developmental trajectories towards antisocial behaviour (Biederman *et al.* 1991; Jensen *et al.* 1997). Here, children and young people need to learn that there are social consequences for inappropriate, defiant or antisocial behaviour. Whilst teachers and parents are generally encouraged to reward good behaviour rather than punish poor behaviour, fair and consistent rules, boundaries and consequences are important external controls that enable young people with behaviour problems to develop internal controls and learn socially appropriate behaviour. The most common negative consequence for hyperactive or impulsive behaviour which is disruptive to others is verbal reprimands. However, verbal interventions may sometimes be ineffective, particularly those which are inconsistent.

Time out

It has been suggested that hyperactive children cannot be managed by logic, explanation and sweet reasonableness (Drabman *et al.* 1973). For children with ADHD whose behaviour is more challenging and disruptive, teachers may need to apply a range of distraction techniques. This includes the targeting of additional resources such as support from a learning mentor or teaching assistant. Occasionally, the use of behavioural strategies such as time out from positive reinforcement, often called 'time out' for short, may be effective. This involves the child or young person being placed away from the situation that is maintaining problematic behaviour for a short period of time. During this time they are expected to be quiet and comply with requests from the teacher. The rationale for using time out is that if there is no reward for a behaviour it will decrease and eventually become extinct. Ignoring undesired behaviour is therefore very effective if its function is to gain social attention (Wood and Hughes 2005). The way in which time out is used is also important. When asking children to temporarily leave the classroom, a non-verbal system such as a hand signal, note or other gesture may be more effective and 'face-saving' than telling them to do so in front of their peers (O'Regan 2006). Time out should only be used when other less potentially stigmatising interventions have failed. Repeated use of time out also reduces the impact of this intervention, particularly if the conditions and length of the intervention vary. It is also important that time out is used in conjunction with positive strategies to increase prosocial behaviour.

Whereas they are generally successful, behavioural interventions only work whilst they are being implemented. Even then, they require constant monitoring over time to help ensure continuing success and maximal effectiveness. In order to assist teachers and other school-based staff manage pupils with ADHD in the school setting, Pfiffner *et al.* (2006) suggest that the principles of behaviour management for pupils with ADHD outlined in Table 9.1 may be helpful.

Medication in school

There is strong evidence that stimulants produce beneficial effects on levels of the core symptoms of hyperactivity, impulsivity and inattention. In the school setting this manifests as a reduction in motor hyperactivity, longer attention span for repetitive tasks and a general improvement in behaviour problems. This is in terms of interference with peers, time spent off the chair, non-compliance with requests from the teacher, aggression and motor control (Abikoff and Gittelman 1985; DuPaul and Rapport 1993). Whether or not stimulants directly improve academic performance is an area of debate. There is a popular view among experts that these medications do not improve learning per se but lead to improvements in academic performance on tasks requiring repetition and concentration (Barkley and Cunningham 1978;

Table 9.1 Principles of effective behaviour management for pupils with ADHD

- Rules and instructions provided to pupils with ADHD must be clear, brief and often delivered through more visible and external modes of presentation than is required for the management of normal children.
- Consequences used to manage the behaviour of ADHD children must be delivered swiftly and more immediately than is needed for normal children.
- Consequences must be delivered more frequently, not just more immediately, to children with ADHD in view of their motivational deficits.
- The type of consequences used with pupils who have ADHD must often be of a higher magnitude, or more powerful, than those needed to manage the behaviour of normal children.
- An appropriate and often richer degree of incentives must be provided within a setting or task to reinforce appropriate behaviour before punishment can be implemented.
- Those reinforcers or particular rewards which are employed must be changed or rotated more frequently with pupils who have ADHD than normal children.
- Anticipation is the key to teaching and managing children with ADHD.
- Children with ADHD must be held more publicly accountable for their behaviour and goal attainment than other children.

Source: Pfiffner *et al.* 2006

Douglas *et al.* 1986). The diagnosis of ADHD should not be used to justify the use of stimulants for the sole purpose of improving academic performance, and in the absence of significant impairments (NICE 2008). Further studies are required to better understand the role of stimulants in children's learning and ability (Weber *et al.* 1992; Rapport *et al.* 1994).

The Department for Education and Skills and Department of Health have issued guidance on the management of medicines in schools (2005). This advises that teachers, school nurses and other members of staff can administer medication including controlled drug (CD) medication for children and young people with ADHD. This must be done using a healthcare plan and in accordance with the prescriber's instructions. The medication should be kept in a locked non-portable container and only named staff who have received training should have access. Schools are encouraged to keep written records for audit and safety purposes. Before school-based health professionals can administer medication for ADHD, there needs to be appropriate written consent from those who hold parental responsibility for the child concerned. Since research has shown that teachers understand very little about pharmacological treatments for ADHD (Snider *et al.* 2003), it is good practice for those who have prescribed medication for ADHD to liaise with the school. This is to discuss what the medication is for, how it is expected to help and how the school might be expected to support the child in achieving the treatment objectives. This information is usually contained in a pupil support plan which sets out who the medication is for, the required dosage, how and when the medication should be taken and any side effects that may occur. Taking medication can sometimes be a stigmatising experience for children and young people. It is therefore essential that school-based protocols for dispensing medication are discreet and recognise the child's right to privacy, dignity and confidentiality.

Social skills building

School-based professionals have a key role to play in supporting children to develop psychological health and wellbeing (Department of Health 2004). This involves helping pupils develop emotional literacy and positive social skills, and is increasingly promoted as part of the personal, health and social education (PHSE) curriculum (Department for Education and Skills 2003). Central to the development of emotional literacy is the development of social competence which can be defined as the behaviours and skills necessary to engage in developing and maintaining positive social relationships (Compas *et al.* 2002). There is no doubt that pupils with ADHD have social skills deficits (Rucklidge and Tannock 2001; Fonagy *et al.* 2002). They experience difficulty in forming and maintaining peer friendships and are often unpopular with other children due to their disruptive behaviour. This is not just within schools. In many cases children with ADHD will be excluded from social gatherings such as birthday parties, and difficulties with siblings may compound relationship difficulties (O'Regan 2006).

Like many interventions for children and young people with ADHD, social skills training originated in the US in the 1970s. A number of strategies are thought to be effective and can be taught on an individual or small-group basis (Turpin and Titheridge 2001). Whilst school-based group activities rarely focus directly on ADHD and are more likely to focus on anti-bullying initiatives (Offler 2000; NICE 2008), they often aim to support pupils to improve self-control, anger management and problem-solving. However, developing skills and competencies in these areas of interpersonal and social functioning is undoubtedly of value for children and young people with ADHD. They allow them to join class or school-based activities with confidence, manage peer rejection or teasing, use negotiation techniques and manage confrontation with teachers and parents (Frankel *et al.* 1997; Cantor 2000; Compas *et al.* 2002; Gol and Jarus 2005). Group activities can be facilitated by nurses to help children and young people with ADHD discuss problems, identify with others and share strategies to resolve conflict and distress. Nurses should be aware that, whilst groups can be useful for children who require the approval of their peers, they can also provoke anxiety for children who are shy or lacking in confidence.

Liaison with specialist CAMHS

Like all primary services, schools and early-years settings share a responsibility for promoting the mental health and wellbeing of children and young people (Department for Education and Skills 2001; Department of Health 2004). However, managing children with mental health problems or developmental disorders such as ADHD is not their core business. This means that teachers, school nurses and other educational professionals will often require support from specialist CAMHS where pupils have mental health problems or developmental disorders. In some cases, the disruptive behaviour of children with ADHD may be beyond the skills and competencies of teachers and school-based staff to cope with. Here, it is vital that there are strong links between schools and specialist CAMHS. In the first instance, school-based professionals should seek advice and consultation from their own educational support teams. They function to provide support for pupils at risk of developing emotional and behavioural difficulties in schools. These teams should in turn liaise with specialist child and adolescent mental health services professionals if they are concerned that a child in school may have unmet mental health needs.

Many schools have developed referral pathways in conjunction with primary and secondary healthcare professionals. An example of one such pathway is reported in an excellent paper by Salmon *et al.* (2006) as shown below. The pathway was developed by a multi-agency team. This included psychiatrists, paediatric neurologists, community paediatricians and specialist ADHD nurses, as well as educational psychologists, special educational needs (SEN) advisors, specialist behaviour teachers, social workers and a voluntary sector organisation supporting parents whose children have special educational needs (see Figure 9.1).

Decision point A: The school protocol for children with suspected ADHD should be followed and a decision made whether or not to continue with current interventions in school, or to discuss the child with a specialist teacher and/or educational psychologist.

Decision point B: Following discussion it may be agreed that further intervention is necessary. If so, the format of the intervention and personnel to be involved will be agreed, and the school will refer to a community paediatrician for medical screening.

Decision point C: Following further review of progress, referral to specialist CAMHS by community paediatrician if concerns persist.

Joint working with schools

Liaison between specialist CAMHS and schools is a two-way process which is vitally important. However, this relationship can often be poor (Weare 1999; Mental Health Foundation 2003; Brown 2003). This may be partly because health and educational services may have different goals and utilise different criteria. This is not surprising when we consider that these two services have evolved from different institutional bases, employ professionals from different professional backgrounds and operate within different governance and performance frameworks. Sloan *et al.* (1999) suggest that health professionals

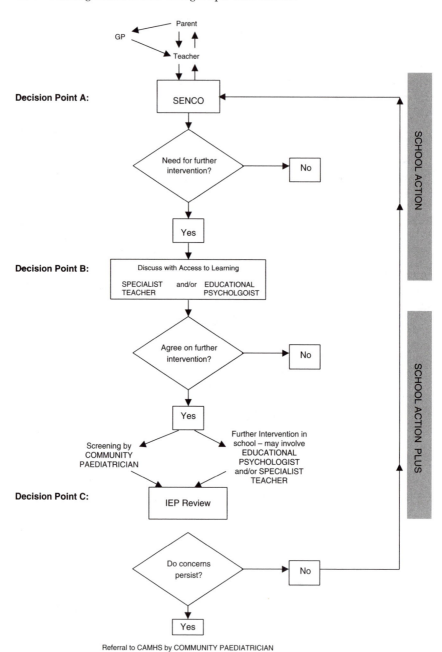

Figure 9.1 Assessment, treatment and follow-up of ADHD.
Source: Salmon *et al.* (2006)

tend to use internationally agreed criteria to confirm or rule out medical diagnoses around which to plan treatment. By comparison, teachers and other school-based professionals are more likely to focus less on labelling the problems and more on providing an educational plan (Sloan *et al.* 2003). Specialist ADHD nurses are in key positions to integrate these two perspectives, and support school-based staff including school nurses to effectively observe and manage a child with ADHD in the classroom. Specialist ADHD nurses should also be able to liaise with other professionals such as social workers, teachers, Connexion workers, school nurses and voluntary agencies. This is to enhance the understanding of the treatment options which are available and to support the young person throughout the treatment process (Porter 1988; Mitchell *et al.* 2004).

Teachers and classroom support staff often welcome feedback on how they are coping with a child with ADHD. This enables effective communication methods to be explored, and is an opportunity to discuss behaviour management strategies. Notwithstanding issues of consent, nurses or other health professionals should always liaise with the child's teacher. This is to advise them about the diagnosis, and to help establish whether special educational needs are likely to be present (NICE 2008). It is often helpful if a visit can take place in school where the child can be observed in the classroom and playground setting. Meeting the teachers and classroom support staff can provide valuable information about any positive or negative relationships the child may have formed, and is an opportunity to discuss classroom structure and task demands and to work through any specific problems the child may be experiencing. Local schools should have access to written information about ADHD. This should describe the symptoms, identify the support available to teachers and other school-based staff and highlight good practice guidance for the school-based management of pupils with ADHD.

Summary

Increasingly, schools are helping to improve social and emotional wellbeing in primary and secondary education through the social and emotional aspects of learning (SEAL) programme, the Healthy Schools agenda and other related school-based initiatives. Not surprisingly, children and young people with ADHD often feel different from their peers, and this can be reinforced by school-based approaches that emphasise difference. Being part of a special group requiring additional support can influence the ways in which a child forms their self-identity and the ways in which others view them. Balancing the need for additional support whilst at the same time promoting social inclusion and normalisation can be a difficult balance to achieve for teachers and other school-based professionals. School-based professionals including teachers, special educational needs coordinators and school nurses are in key positions to support children and young people with ADHD to improve psychological and social outcomes as well as reach their academic potential.

10 Adults with ADHD

Key points

- Having previously been thought to be exclusively a disorder of childhood and adolescence, there is now a growing recognition that ADHD persists into adulthood. However, access to specialist ADHD services for adults is variable and further research is needed to evaluate the adult outcomes of childhood ADHD.
- The majority of the research about ADHD comes from studies of children. Knowledge about the identification and recognition of ADHD in adults is less advanced, and the process of diagnosis and formulation is more complex.
- Many young people with ADHD make the transition from childhood to adulthood smoothly and do not develop serious mental health problems. However, adults with ADHD are at higher risk of developing mental health problems than their peers, and those with attention problems rather than hyperactivity or impulsivity are thought to have better outcomes.
- Adult ADHD is associated with high comorbidity and poor outcomes. Adults with ADHD use more healthcare services because of increased rates of accidents, and health problems associated with alcohol and substance misuse. Due to the demands placed on health, social care and criminal justice agencies there is a need for ongoing investigation, research and service evaluation.
- Due to relatively high prevalence rates of ADHD in adulthood, nurses and other professionals should be able to recognise the core symptoms of ADHD which are usually associated with inattention and manifest as difficulties in the areas of motivation, organisation and commitment.
- Since ADHD is a chronic disorder of childhood enduring into adulthood the risk of parents having this disorder themselves is high. This compounds the difficulties of living with and managing ADHD.
- Nurses working in specialist assessment, diagnosis and treatment services for adults should have a good understanding of neurobiology, psychopharmacology and multimodal assessment and treatment strategies.

Introduction

There is general consensus that ADHD is primarily a disorder of childhood and this is principally a book about children and young people. However, during the 1970s, Wood *et al.* (1976) reported initial findings related to 'minimal brain dysfunction' in adults. Follow-up studies of adults diagnosed as hyperactive as children led researchers to consider the possible persistence of ADHD into adulthood (Wood *et al.* 1976; Wender *et al.* 1981). During the mid 1990s there began to emerge a broader understanding that, for some young people, their symptoms persisted into adulthood (Hallowell and Ratey 1994). Subsequently, ADHD came to be reconceptualised as a life-span disorder and was no longer considered merely a condition of childhood (McGough and Barkley 2004; Barkley *et al.* 2007; NICE 2008). Since many children and young people with ADHD grow up to be adults with this disorder, and many health and care services in the UK provide 'cradle to grave' services, it therefore seems fitting to include a chapter about adult ADHD in this book.

How many adults have ADHD?

Population surveys estimate that 3–4% of adults have diagnosable ADHD (Faraone and Biederman 2005; Kessler *et al.* 2005a). In keeping with understanding ADHD as a developmental disorder, prevalence rates decline with age (Biederman *et al.* 2000). However, some studies suggest that as many as half of children with ADHD will continue to experience symptoms into adulthood (Spencer *et al.* 1998; Wender 2000). Of adults who were diagnosed as children, 15% continue to reach criteria for diagnosis in adulthood, and a further 65% have partial remission of their symptoms (Faraone and Biederman 2005; Faraone *et al.* 2006). It is important to acknowledge that the recognition of ADHD in children was rare before the mid-1990s. Retrospective studies show that many adults with ADHD have made numerous unsuccessful attempts to access help from health or social services as children or adolescents (Dalsgaard *et al.* 2002; Young *et al.* 2003a). It is likely that a large proportion of young people have therefore been left undiagnosed and untreated as children and present for the first time as adults (Keen *et al.* 2000; NICE 2008).

Service provision

Neither generic nor specialist assessment and diagnostic services for adults with ADHD are routinely available in the UK. For example, there are no dedicated teams for adults with ADHD in Scotland (NHS Quality Improvement Scotland 2007). The most common service model involves clinicians with a specialist interest in adult ADHD working as part of a generic team. In some areas, specialist neurodevelopmental services provide pharmacological and psychological interventions for adults with ADHD as well as a range of related conditions including autism. Like mental health services in general, there is a lack of defined care pathways for adolescents in transition to adult services (Asherson 2005; Nutt *et al.* 2007). As a result, young people, including those with ADHD, often fall through the gap (McDougall 2007). Generally speaking, adults with ADHD fall into three categories:

1   Those diagnosed as children or adolescents by paediatric services or child and adolescent mental health services (CAMHS) who require ongoing treatment or monitoring as adults.
2   Young people who have been diagnosed and treated in childhood but no longer require ongoing treatment or monitoring as adults.
3   Those who were undiagnosed as children or adolescents.

Children and young people diagnosed in childhood often require transition to adult mental health services. Adult mental health services provide assessment and treatment interventions for adults with a range of mental health problems. Many of these can appear similar to ADHD, particularly bipolar disorder, depression and personality disorders, and, to varying degrees, each of these disorders involves difficulties with activity, behaviour regulation, impulsiveness and inattention. Many adult mental health professionals will not have encountered ADHD and lack the knowledge skills and expertise to support an adult service user with ADHD. This makes the potential for misdiagnosis and inappropriate treatment high.

The National Institute for Health and Clinical Excellence (NICE) have considered the needs of adults within their guideline on the diagnosis and management of ADHD. Evidence suggests that outcomes for this age group are often poor and include negative work performance; mental ill health; difficulties with social functioning and relationships; and crime and antisocial behaviour (NICE 2008). Indeed, adults with ADHD may present for the first time to criminal justice services because of antisocial behaviour linked to their difficulties (Sayal 2008). This suggests that there is an important 'invest to save' principle for policy makers and service commissioners, and that early recognition, treatment and support is important.

How do symptoms of ADHD differ for adults?

To a large extent, our understanding of adult ADHD remains grounded in our conceptualisation of the disorder as it occurs in children (McGough and Barkley 2005). There is agreement that the symptoms of adult ADHD mirror the symptoms of ADHD in childhood (Weiss and Murray 2003). However, strict interpretation of ICD-10 or DSM-IV diagnostic criteria may be inadequate when we consider the needs of adults (NICE 2008). This is due to the developmental nature of ADHD, the changing nature of symptoms over time and because the ICD-10 and DSM-IV diagnostic criteria for ADHD were established with children and not adults in mind. For this reason it may be necessary to lower diagnostic thresholds and reframe symptoms in age-appropriate terms to understand day-to-day functioning and impairment in adults. For example, the symptoms of ADHD in adults do not manifest in the school setting but in the workplace. The number and severity of ADHD symptoms decline with age, thus reducing the prevalence of this disorder in adolescents and adults (Barkley 1997). It has been suggested that the intensity of hyperactivity also diminishes over time (Adler and Chua 2002). For those adults who continue to experience hyperactivity, this may be described as feelings of restlessness, lack of concentration and poor time management. Impulsivity may manifest through rapid, ill-considered decisions with little regard for consequences. Inattention may be exhibited as impatience and recklessness (Young and Bramham 2007) (see Table 10.1).

Although the symptoms of inattention, hyperactivity and impulsivity are the same in children and adults, the ways in which the core symptoms present vary according to age. Until research adequately defines developmentally appropriate symptoms, clinicians must use clinical judgement and flexibility in applying the ICD and DSM criteria for children to adults. Ongoing research and clinical involvement in defining the criteria for adult ADHD, including long-term follow-up studies of DSM-IV and ICD-10 diagnosed children and field trials of symptoms in adults, are crucial if the identification and management of adults with ADHD is to improve (McGough and Barkley 2005).

Inattention

The most prominent symptom of adult ADHD is reported to be inattention (Millstein *et al.* 1997; Wender 2000; Young and Bramham 2007). Because ADHD is characterised by difficulties with attention regulation and task organisation, adults with this disorder often report that they 'hyper-focus' on relatively unimportant details to the exclusion of more important issues. Inattention may become evident through a general lack of planning, poor task management, missing important deadlines and being late (Elliot 2002). This inability to plan, prioritise and sequence tasks can result in chaotic lifestyles that are difficult for others to tolerate. Procrastination refers to the mechanism for coping with anxiety associated with starting or completing any task or decision. Adults with ADHD often procrastinate and put off difficult tasks for significantly longer than other adults, and these tasks, once started with enthusiasm, frequently remain unfinished. Bills may be paid late and important letters may be forgotten. Many of the difficulties experienced by adults are associated with impaired executive functioning (Boonstra *et al.* 2005; Woods *et al.* 2002). These include poor organisation and task management, organisational skills and self-regulation. These are considered to be enduring traits from childhood that do not improve with medication or psychological intervention in adulthood.

Table 10.1 Comparison of core symptoms of ADHD in children and adults

Core symptom	Children	Adults
Hyperactivity	Restless	Feelings of inner restlessness
	Unable to sit still, especially in calm or quiet surroundings	Unable to relax
	Constantly fidgeting	Unhappy or discontented when inactive
	Unable to settle to tasks	Persistent motor hyperactivity
	Excessive physical movement	
Inattention	Short attention span, unable to concentrate	Interrupts frequently
	Easily distracted	Impatient and reckless
	Inability to stick at tasks that are tedious or time-consuming	Makes snap decisions
	Constantly changing activity or task	Feeling 'down' when bored or 'up' when excited or stimulated
		Difficulty following a conversation
		Awareness of other things going on around oneself despite trying to filter these out
		Difficulty reading or finishing a task
		Forgetfulness
		Procrastination
		Lateness with deadlines
Impulsivity	Unable to turn-take	Talking before thinking; interrupting conversation; impatience
	Rule-breaking	
	Poor sense of danger	Abruptly starting or stopping relationships; excessive involvement in pleasure-seeking activities without recognising potential consequences

Comorbidity

It is important to assess whether the overactivity, inattention or impulsivity of an adult can be explained in the context of one or more other psychiatric or psychosocial disorders. Chapter 5 outlines a range of mental disorders that can coexist in children and young people with ADHD, and comorbidity also exists with adults. It has been estimated that up to three-quarters of adult mental health service users have ADHD with one other comorbid problem, and one-third will have two or more mental health or psychosocial disorders (Asherson 2005). Personality disorders and ADHD both involve mood instability, impulsivity and anger outbursts, and bipolar disorder and ADHD also share many symptoms. There is evidence of increased alcohol and substance misuse in adults with ADHD, and this can partly be explained by risk-seeking behaviours, self-medication and poorer social skills in people with ADHD (Ingram *et al.* 1999; Barkley *et al.* 1996; Fergusson and Boden 2007). Oppositional behaviour, defiance and conduct disorder are often associated with children and young people who have ADHD (Taylor 1996), and this may evolve into antisocial personality disorder and criminal behaviour in adulthood (Rutter 1989; Wexler 1996; Fryers 2007). Indeed, research has suggested that a high proportion of the young adult male prison population would have met the criteria for ADHD as children, and the residual effects of their impulsive behaviour continue to manifest into their adult life as antisocial or criminal behaviour (Weiss and Hecthman 1993; Young *et al.* 2003b; Rosler *et al.* 2004; Gunter *et al.* 2008). For these reasons, it is essential that nurses working in criminal justice settings are aware of the causes and symptoms of ADHD and promote emotional health and wellbeing for this client group.

ADHD and relationship difficulties

Very few studies have investigated the impact of adult ADHD on family relationships. However, one of the most common complaints of adult service users in the clinical setting is marital and relationship problems (Eakin *et al.* 2004). Adults with ADHD report significantly higher rates of adjustment and higher rates of separation and divorce than normal controls (Eakin *et al.* 2004). There are several reasons why ADHD makes sustaining a positive personal relationship difficult. Adults with ADHD have a low frustration tolerance (Wilens *et al.* 1995). Often described as having a 'short fuse', they can be impatient or irritable when others do not follow their train of thought or reasoning. A tendency to overreact to minor frustrations can have a negative impact on family life, friendships and relationships at work. This trait of impatience in adults is equivalent to the child with ADHD who is unable to wait. Low frustration tolerance can make the child with ADHD unpopular with their peers and therefore the adult with ADHD frequently falls out with partners, friends and work colleagues.

Difficulty 'switching off' is often reported by adults with ADHD. They are unable to filter a barrage of cognitions and report feeling overwhelmed by a constant stream of thoughts which makes it difficult to rest and relax. Adults with ADHD often report mood-related difficulties such as depression (Rapport *et al.* 2002). Notwithstanding the strong comorbidity with bipolar disorder and ADHD (Faraone *et al.* 1997), adults without cyclical mood disorders report changes in mood without any apparent trigger. They may feel depressed when inactive, and low mood may be associated with a poor self-image, underachievement from poor task management and difficulties in personal relationships arising from ADHD. Thrill-seeking behaviour is a common feature of adult ADHD. This serves to satisfy the need for immediate gratification and excitement. High-risk behaviours such as extreme sports, substance misuse and irresponsible sexual activity are often associated with impulsivity and a lack of concern for consequences.

ADHD and parenting

Since ADHD is a chronic disorder of childhood enduring into adulthood the risk of parents having this disorder themselves is high. This compounds the difficulties of living with and managing ADHD and can lead to a cycle of difficulties, especially as the success of parenting programmes for parents of children with ADHD is highly influenced by the presence of parental ADHD (Sonuga-Barke *et al.* 2002; Harpin 2005). It has been reported that parents with ADHD have more difficulty monitoring their child's behaviour and struggle to set effective limits (Murray and Johnston 2006).

Diagnosis

There has been an increased public focus on ADHD in recent years, and many adults seek assessment or treatment for undiagnosed ADHD after recognising their symptoms during the assessment or treatment of ADHD involving their children. Others seek help following encouragement or advice from family members or professionals. Frequently there is a concern that ADHD may underlie other behavioural or mental health problems, and some adults may have previously been misdiagnosed with a different disorder or problem. Much has been written about the validity of ADHD diagnosis in childhood and controversy and scepticism does not end in adulthood. This arises from the difficulties of obtaining verifiable information from adults about their childhood, the relatively undeveloped evidence base for treatments in adulthood and concerns about substance misuse with controlled drugs.

The diagnosis of ADHD in adults can be a challenging process since it includes making judgments based on clinical interviews, rating scale results, informant ratings and objective supporting evidence (Murphy and Adler 2004). Due to high levels of comorbidity, the potential for misdiagnosis is high. Borderline and antisocial personality disorder, bipolar disorder and, to a lesser extent, psychotic disorders can each be experienced by adults with ADHD. Comprehensive assessment and diagnostic services should be available in order to fully evaluate the core symptoms of ADHD in the context of other mental health problems experienced by adults. Chapter 2 outlines the diagnostic systems used to classify ADHD, and the skills required to make an accurate diagnosis of adult ADHD are broadly the same as those needed to diagnose a child or adolescent. However, adults are often better able than children to sustain their attention and suppress their behaviour during the course of assessment. This illustrates the need to supplement observation with other assessment methods, and the need to explore functioning over a longer period of time (Asherson *et al.* 2005). Various recognised interview schedules exist, but these can be time-consuming to use in clinical practice and are mostly used in research. In order to help assess and diagnose ADHD in adults the British Association for Psychopharmacology (Nutt *et al.* 2007) suggests that the following traits and characteristics may be indicative of ADHD:

* lack of attention to detail or carelessness;
* inattention in tasks or activities the person finds tedious;
* difficulty listening;
* failure to follow instructions;
* starting many tasks but finishing few;
* poor organisational skills;
* avoidance or dislike of tasks that require sustained mental effort;
* losing or misplacing things;
* distractibility;
* forgetfulness;
* fidgeting;
* restlessness or inability to sit still in low-stimulus situations;
* inappropriate or excessive activity;
* difficulty keeping quiet and talking out of turn;
* unfocused mental activity with difficulty turning thoughts off;
* blurting out responses with poor social timing;
* trouble waiting if there is nothing to do;
* interrupting or intruding on others;
* irritability, impatience or frustration;
* labile mood or hot temper;
* stress intolerance;
* impulsive or risk taking activities.

What are the implications of being diagnosed as an adult?

Due to a lack of specialist adult ADHD services, the process of diagnosis is often long and difficult for service users. Just as the diagnosis of a child or adolescent should be addressed with sensitivity and support, so too does the diagnosis of adults need to be managed with care and compassion. The ways in which adults react to receiving a diagnosis of ADHD will differ, and the psychological supports they may require to adjust and cope may be different to those that children find helpful. Psychoeducation is as important with adults as it is with children, although this will require a different foundation and emphasis. It has been suggested that adults move through a 6-stage model of psychological acceptance during their diagnosis of ADHD (Young *et al.* 2008):

* relief and elation;

- confusion;
- anger;
- sadness and grief;
- anxiety;
- accommodation and acceptance.

Service user views suggest that some adults find that a diagnosis of ADHD explains their experiences and difficulties and provides hope through the option of treatment. To some service users, knowing they feel different to other people and having this validated can be a liberating experience. Understanding why simple everyday tasks are so difficult to manage may bring a sense of relief. Others find a diagnosis of ADHD less welcome. They may feel sad about having a recognised 'problem' or angry that their ADHD was not acknowledged or validated in childhood. Some adults with ADHD may resent what they consider to be lost opportunities at school and in employment. They may look back to their childhood, marriage or work history and remember being thought of as lazy or stupid by parents, teachers, partners or employers (Asherson 2005; Young and Bramham 2007). Due to the support needs that adults with ADHD have, nurses should ensure that service users are given appropriate information about local and national support groups, voluntary organisations for adults with ADHD and other sources of advice and advocacy (NICE 2008).

Assessment

The overall objective for a clinical assessment of ADHD in adults is to obtain an overview of the current difficulties, the background to these difficulties and the impact of symptoms on personal, family, social and occupational functioning (NICE 2008). In order to develop an understanding of the presenting difficulties, an adult ADHD assessment requires a comprehensive childhood history. This may sometimes be difficult to remember in detail, and, with the consent of the adult concerned, the use of third-party information may assist the process. Just as the degree and level of impairment in children affects diagnosis, so too is impairment central to the diagnosis of adults with ADHD. The assessment should therefore not only focus on current symptoms but on the impact of impairment on day-to-day functioning. This should include self reports and information provided by partners, other family members or carers.

Rating scales

A range of diagnostic checklists and rating scales may assist the process of assessment of adults. These include the World Health Organisation (WHO) Adult ADHS Self Report Scale (ASRS) (Kessler 2005b); and the Wender Utah Rating Scale (WURS) (Wender 1981). The former focuses on DSM-IV symptoms of ADHD and includes a short-form version used for screening. The latter aids the retrospective diagnosis of childhood ADHD and addresses retrospective symptoms in childhood and current functioning within the domains of hyperactivity and inattention (Ward *et al*. 1993). The WURS has been shown to be valid in differentiating adults with and without ADHD, but has not been standardised on a UK population (Young and Braham 2007). The Conners Adult ADHD Rating Scale (CAARS) (Conners *et al*. 1998; Conners *et al*. 1999) is also widely used. This can be rated using a self report version or completed by a professional. The long version has 66 items covering nine subscales of problem behaviour. The short version has abbreviated subscales, includes 26 items and can be used for screening purposes. The Brown Adult ADHD Rating Scale (BADDS) (Brown 1996) and the Copeland Symptom Checklist for Adult ADHD (Copeland 1991) may also be useful. However, the BADDS does not thoroughly assess impulse control and hyperactivity and is more useful for assessing deficits in executive functioning associated with ADHD (Young and Bramham 2007).

Like all ratings scales, those used to assess ADHD in adults have limitations. Used in isolation, they are insufficient to make a diagnosis and should therefore only be used in conjunction with a full developmental history, substance misuse history and clinical interview. A medical or neurological examination may often be necessary to help rule out other causes of poor concentration and inattention. Gathering information which is reliable is often difficult when assessing adult ADHD. Children do not always reliably report their ADHD symptoms and this is no different for adults (Young and Bramham 2007). They may be aware of inattention, hyperactivity or impulsivity, but may not readily associate these with impairment or dysfunction in their day-to-day life. Like assessment during childhood, it is therefore important to explore the accuracy and validity of information provided about ADHD in adulthood from several sources.

Treatment

Treatments for ADHD in adults comprise medication, psychosocial interventions such as cognitive behavioural therapy and coaching, and self-help strategies such as positive self instruction.

Pharmacological treatments

Many young people whose ADHD persists into adulthood develop coping mechanisms which effectively compensate for their ADHD symptoms without the need for pharmacological interventions. For others, core symptoms may return rapidly when psychostimulants are discontinued, and treatment with medication may be required over a longer term (NHS Quality Improvement Scotland 2007). As with children and adolescents, pharmacological interventions address the core symptoms of ADHD. However, the range of treatment options is limited since methylphenidate is not licensed for use in adults. Despite this, methylphenidate has been recommended as the firstline medication for this age group (NICE 2008). Similarly, atomoxetine is only licensed for use in adults if it has been started in childhood, but is again recommended for the treatment of ADHD in adulthood (NICE 2008). The monitoring of side effects is an important part of pharmacological treatment. Although concerns about the impact of stimulants on growth diminish in adulthood, regular monitoring of blood pressure, pulse and overall wellbeing should be part of any ongoing pharmacological treatment for an adult with ADHD. This can be carried out by nurses and other professionals with appropriate training.

Psychological interventions

Psychological treatments for ADHD in adults can be helpful, and there is some evidence that cognitive behavioural therapy (CBT) is effective (Safren *et al*. 2005a; Rostain and Ramsay 2006). Cognitive interventions include positive self-talk, repetition and rehearsal, problem-solving, anger management and strategies to improve self-esteem (Young and Bramham 2007). Motivational interviewing can assist the process of assessing impairment rather than the core symptoms of ADHD (Safren *et al*. 2005b). However, research with adults who have ADHD has lagged behind the rapid growth of research into the use of CBT with children and adolescents, and this is largely due to the underrecognition of ADHD in adults (Ramsay and Rostain 2003). Furthermore, when treating adults with ADHD, current practice in the UK does not routinely include the provision of psychological interventions (NICE 2008). This is an area which requires future investment. As many young people with ADHD mature into adulthood and their symptoms remit, treatment with medication may no longer be recommended. The need for psychological treatment may continue, if not arise, to address low self-esteem and feelings of hopelessness (NICE 2008).

Furthermore, some adults with ADHD will not want to take medication even if this is recommended, or stimulant medication may be ineffective or intolerable (Wilens *et al*. 2002). There are also concerns about substance misuse by adults (Wilens *et al*. 2006). In such cases, alternative treatments should be available. Where psychological interventions can be provided, adults with ADHD should be offered a course of individual or group CBT to address functional impairment as a key priority. This should be tailored to the needs of each individual. In planning treatment sessions, it is important for nurses to consider factors such as attention span, working memory and time management when considering psychological interventions. Practical strategies such as the use of diaries, lists and the use of alarm clocks are simple ways in which adults with ADHD can assist memory and task organisation.

Summary

Whilst once thought to be exclusively a condition of childhood, it is now understood that ADHD is a lifespan disorder and that symptoms persist over time. Nurses are in unique positions to recognise symptoms in service users of all ages and provide holistic care and treatment interventions to facilitate optimal outcomes and enhance quality of life. Adult behaviours linked to ADHD are associated with the childhood symptoms of hyperactivity, attention deficit, unfocused thinking, disorganisation and impulsivity. This can have a negative effect on interpersonal, social and occupational functioning, and adult ADHD is associated with high comorbidity and a range of poor outcomes. Adults with ADHD are more likely to misuse substances, attempt suicide and have problematic personal and social relationships. Due to high levels of unmet need and the demands placed on health, social care and criminal justice agencies there is a need for ongoing investigation, research and service evaluation. Adult mental health professionals including psychiatrists and nurses should receive basic awareness training to assist identification of ADHD in adults. Skills and competencies should also be available within teams to diagnose and provide pharmacological and psychological treatments for adults with ADHD.

11 Nurse prescribing and ADHD

Key points

- There has been more research into the use of medication for ADHD than in any other area of child and adolescent psychopharmacology.
- Nurses can facilitate access to medication for children and young people with ADHD through the rapidly-expanding area of independent and supplementary prescribing.
- In order to have the competence, skills and knowledge to be a supplementary prescriber, nurses are required to undertake independent, extended and supplementary prescribing training.
- Nurses should only practise within the sphere of their competence, knowledge and skills, and this applies equally to nurse prescribing.
- Nurses are well placed to offer holistic care to children and young people with ADHD and their families or carers.

Introduction

In the UK, nurses make up a quarter of the specialist child and adolescent mental health (CAMHS) professional workforce (Audit Commission 1999). New ways of working in mental health services (Department of Health 2007) and the development of non-medical prescribing are service innovations that will enhance young people's access to medication interventions for ADHD. Nurses have traditionally delivered nursing assessments for ADHD as well as psychosocial interventions. These have included parenting skills training groups, social skills training groups and individual behaviour management and psychoeducation to young people and their families about ADHD. Non-medical prescribing is part of a new ways of working programme to produce a capable and flexible workforce. Nurse prescribing supports children and young people with ADHD, and enhances the contribution that nurses have to make to modern holistic care and treatment interventions.

Background to nurse prescribing

In recent years, nursing has become increasing professional, with higher academic requirements and a growing evidence base which underpins our practice. This had led to an increased emphasis on nurses gaining additional therapeutic and technical skills such as psychosocial interventions and nurse prescribing (Till 2007). Nurse prescribing is one of the most radical and controversial developments in the history of nursing (O'Dowd 2007; Barlow *et al.* 2008) The practice of non-medical prescribing in mental health comes primarily from the US, where nurse prescribing has occurred for nearly 40 years, and this extended role for nurses is now part of everyday practice (Nolan *et al.* 2001). Nurse prescribing in the UK has been slower to develop, and has only really evolved in recent years after a series of legislative changes. This has been frustrating for some nurses who are keen to embrace the opportunities that non-medical prescribing will bring patients and the nursing profession. However, the pace of change has recently increased, and the future development of non-medical prescribing is likely to have a dramatic effect on the role of the nurse in treating children and young people with ADHD.

The concept of nurse prescribing was first considered in 1986 with the introduction of *The Cumberledge Report*, the product of a community nursing review commissioned by Baroness Cumberledge (Department of Health 1986). This set out the Government's intentions to allow rapid access to appropriate treatments and was followed by two Crown reports (Department of Health 1989; Department of Health 1999). Primary legislation permitting nurses to prescribe was passed in 1992. Prior to this, only doctors had been able to prescribe medication. Disappointingly, the introduction of non-medical prescribing in adult mental health services has been less enthusiastically taken up than in other areas of health service provision. Some mental health nurses have expressed fear that the therapeutic relationship they cherish with patients will be altered (Nolan and Badger 2000). Others have embraced this extended role for nurses, and foresee many benefits for service users and the nursing profession as a whole (Turner 2007; McDougall and Ryan 2008).

As legislation has continued to change to enable access to medicines for patients, there has also been a move away form the restrictive framework originally introduced alongside nurse prescribing. Nurses have now been given independent prescribing rights and can now prescribe any licensed medicine, including controlled drugs, for any medical condition (Department of Health 2006). The legislation continues to evolve and one anticipated update will allow nurses to prescribe controlled drugs independently. There are currently two types of non-medical prescribing available for nurses to utilise:

1. Independent prescribing

Independent prescribing is defined as 'the prescriber takes responsibility for the clinical assessment of the patient, establishing a diagnosis and the clinical management required, as well as for prescribing where necessary and the appropriateness of any prescription' (Department of Health 2003).

2. Supplementary prescribing

Supplementary prescribing is defined as 'a voluntary prescribing partnership between an independent prescriber (IP) (doctor) and a supplementary pre-scriber (SP) (nurse or pharmacist), to implement an agreed patient-specific CMP with the patient's agreement' (Department of Health 2003).

Clinical management plans (CMPs)

The efficacy and safety of medicines trialled with adults cannot automatically be assumed in children and adolescents. Indeed, the large majority of medi-cines used to treat children and adolescents in the UK are only licensed for use in people over 18 years of age. They are tested for safety and efficacy with adult populations and children and adolescents are excluded from the trials. Therefore, medicines that do not have a licence for use with children and young people can only currently be prescribed by nurses using supplementary prescribing and a clinical management plan. The exception to this is atomox-etine (Strattera) a licensed medicine for ADHD which has been trialled with children, and one that can be prescribed independently by nurses without the need for a clinical management plan. The CMP identifies clear parameters in relation to the medicines which can be prescribed, identifies the range of dosage, and sets safety and review procedures. It states which treatments can be started, stopped or titrated by the nurse (see Figure 11.1).

Training, skills and knowledge

Through their basic training, nurses develop skills and knowledge in psy-chopharmacology, physical health and mental health. This provides the bed-rock upon which to provide holistic assessments for ADHD and then go on to deliver medication treatment. However, the amount of education that nurses receive about medicines varies, and there have been mixed views about whether pharmacology should even be included in the curriculum (Morrison-Griffiths *et al.* 2002).

Within the UK, training for non-medical prescribing is robust and the Nursing and Midwifery Council (NMC) has sought to protect the public by ensuring that nurses can demonstrate the knowledge, skills and competence to practise safely. Nurse prescribing training is delivered within a higher education institution (HEI) as a 'dual qualification' course (Bradley and Nolan 2005). During the training, each nurse is assigned to a medical practitioner who acts as their prescribing mentor for the duration of their course. Examin-ations are undertaken to demonstrate skills and competence within the domains of assessment, history-taking and diagnostic and communication

Patient Name: ID number, date of birth, ID sticker Nicola Gorman	Patient medication sensitivities/allergies: None
Independent Prescriber(s): Drs Brown and Smith	**Supplementary Prescriber:** Joanne Collins
Condition(s) to be treated ADHD	**Aim of treatment** To improve concentration, reduce hyperactivity and impulsivity

Medicines that may be prescribed by SP:

Preparation	Indication	Dose schedule	Specific indications for referral back to the IP
1. Methylphenidate IR 2. Methylphenidate MR 3. Dexamphetamine	To improve concentration, reduce hyperactivity and impulsivity	1. 2.5 mg to 20 mg tds 2. 10 mg to 72 mg daily 3. 2.5 mg to 30 mg bd	Failure to respond to treatment Adverse drug reactions

Guidelines or protocols supporting clinical management plan:

Departmental protocols

BNF for Children guidelines, section 4.4 CNS stimulants and other drugs used for ADHD

Frequency of review and monitoring by:

Supplementary Prescriber One month after trial of medication Then each school term	**Supplementary Prescriber and Independent Prescriber** Annual review joint review
Process for reporting ADRs: Yellow card system. Verbal and written report by SP to IP	**Shared record to be used by IP and SP:** CAMHS case notes

Agreed by Independent Prescriber(s)	Date	Agreed by Supplementary Prescriber(s)	Date	Date agreed with patient/carer

Figure 11.1 Example of clinical management plan.

Source: Ryan 2007

skills. Final written examinations are required before nurses can act as independent or supplementary nurse prescribers. All nurses who prescribe are professionally obliged to engage in ongoing personal development planning, and keep their practice up to date. The Knowledge Skills Framework (KSF) and their professional portfolio can assist them to do this systematically (Department of Health 2004a). Guidance issued by the NMC sets out the standards and proficiencies for programmes of preparation for nurse prescribers, as well as outlining standards of conduct that nurses, midwives and specialist community public health nurses are required to meet in their practice as registered nurse prescribers (NMC 2006a; NMC 2006b).

In their guidance on ADHD, the National Institute for Health and Clinical Excellence (NICE 2008) specifically states that practitioners who are treating children and young people should have a good knowledge base in relation to the different drugs used for ADHD and the immediate release and modified release preparations that are available. The pharmacokinetic and pharmacodynamic effects of each drug used for ADHD should be fully understood by the nurse. This refers to the process by which the medicine is absorbed, distributed, metabolised and eliminated from the body, and what action the drug has on the brain. A sophisticated understanding of drug action is essential in order to tailor each medication regime to the individual child, to understand potential drug interactions and to reach optimum treatment outcomes. In order to have the competence, skills and knowledge to be a supplementary prescriber, nurses are required to undertake independent, extended and supplementary prescribing training. Supplementary prescribing is a collaborative process between the nurse, doctor, child and family (Shuttle 2004). With the extension of nurses' roles in supplementary prescribing and a move away from traditional nursing practice, clear frameworks to review the process of nurse prescribing need to be introduced within NHS Trust clinical governance structures (Jones and Harbone 2005).

Prescribing for children and young people

Along with psychological and psychosocial interventions, medication is one of the major therapeutic tools available to help people with mental health problems (Brimblecombe *et al.* 2005). Interest in non-medical prescribing in CAMHS and in particular ADHD services has been strong. Nurse prescribing offers new ways of working and changes the therapeutic relationship between the nurse, doctor and their patient. However, not all nurses will want or need to become nurse prescribers. Nurses who do choose to prescribe continue to be bound by their code of professional conduct when implementing nurse-prescribing decisions. They should involve children and young people in the process of obtaining consent to treatment, provide information accurately, truthfully and clearly and work within their knowledge, skills and competence (Nursing & Midwifery Council 2008). The use of pharmacological treatments for children and adolescents with mental health problems has a relatively well-developed evidence base. Health technology appraisals and clinical guidelines which have included children in their scope have reviewed the use of medication for depression (NICE 2005), obsessive compulsive disorder (NICE 2005), ADHD (NICE 2006 and 2008) and bipolar disorder (NICE 2006).

It has been recognised that there are special considerations to make when prescribing medications for children and young people (Sutcliffe 1999; Department of Health 2004b; BNF 2008). The British National Formulary (BNF) for children acknowledges this concern and is an important reference document for nurses who prescribe and monitor medication in children and young people who have ADHD. There has been more research into the use of medication for ADHD than in any other area of child and adolescent psychopharmacology (Coghill 2003). In particular, methylphenidate has been used for over 50 years for the treatment of ADHD. NICE have reviewed the evidence base for the use of licensed medications for ADHD, which included methylphenidate, dexamphetamine and atomoxetine. All these treatments were found to be effective for ADHD (NICE 2006).

Prescribing for ADHD

When working with children and young people and their families or carers it is important to ensure that there is collaboration when considering prescribing for ADHD. As discussed in chapter 7, medication is only one part of a comprehensive package of care and wider treatment strategy. NICE have set parameters for the use of medication depending upon the age of the child and the severity of their symptoms and associated impairment (NICE 2008). Nurses need to be able to make a comprehensive assessment of the young person and their family, taking into account developmental considerations and the needs of families. This has been discussed earlier in chapter 3. Only when a diagnosis of ADHD has been made and there has been careful consideration of other comorbid difficulties should the decision to prescribe medication be taken. The National Prescribing Centre (NPC) have developed a framework of prescribing competencies that can be interpreted in the context of nursing practice and the scope of professional practice. This prescribing pyramid can be helpful to nurses in signposting prescribing decisions. Each step should be considered before the next step is approached (see Figure 11.2). The NPC guidance encourages nurses to consider whether writing a prescription is the most appropriate course of action, or whether there are alternative interventions that may be more effective (NPC 1999).

As we have heard, psychopharmacology is used to relieve the core symptoms of inattention, hyperactivity and impulsivity and there have been many trials of effectiveness (Heyman and Santosh 2002). Parents and young people's choice will be a further factor in the decision-making process. When a diagnosis has been made it is important to liaise with the child, family and school to discuss the implications of the diagnosis and the treatment options

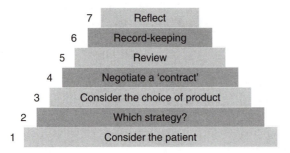

Figure 11.2 The prescribing pyramid.

that are available. Information should be made available to parents and carers and teachers, and this should also be provided for children and young people in a form that is suited to their age and developmental understanding.

Pre-medication screening

Before any medication is prescribed a number of standard assessments should be undertaken (Ryan 2006; NICE 2006; NICE 2008). As discussed, ADHD is often associated with other problems and disorders and the pre-medication screening process enables the nurse to take these into account. The side effects of prescribed and non-prescribed medications can have unwanted effects such as irritability, cognitive difficulties, anxiety and agitation and motor restlessness. These can appear to be symptoms of ADHD. During the assessment process it is therefore essential that the nurse asks about any prescribed, over-the-counter and illegal substances the child or young person may have been taking. It may often be appropriate to liaise with other colleagues to gather as much information as possible about the following factors:

- learning disability;
- autistic spectrum disorder;
- anxiety and depression;
- developmental problems;
- epilepsy;
- tics and Tourette's syndrome;
- substance misuse.

The following information should be reviewed and recorded in the clinical notes:

- pre-medication screening checklists for all medications used for ADHD, with specific relevance to each medication (see Figure 11.3);
- physical monitoring of height and weight (recorded on centile chart), blood pressure and pulse (centile recorded);

- enquiry about any family history of cardiac disease and further investigation where indicated (e.g. electrocardiograph);
- baseline monitoring of ADHD symptoms, comorbidity and side effects of treatment prior to any treatment implementation;
- verbal and written information about the medication, how it works, benefits and side effects of treatment for parents and also age-appropriate information for children.

Name		
DoB		
Consultant		
	Child	**Family**
Anxiety		
Epilepsy		
Psychosis		
Drug/alcohol dependency		
Tic/Tourette's		
Thyroid disorder		
Angina		
Glaucoma		
Expresses suicidal ideas		
Low mood or depression		
High or low blood pressure		
Irregular heart beat/arrhythmia		
Kidney problems		
Liver problems		
Drug allergies		
Other medicines prescribed, over-the-counter or herbal remedies		
Dose calculation		
Clinical examination		
Height	Centile	
Weight	Centile	
BP	Centile	**Pulse**
Signed		**Date**

Figure 11.3 ADHD medication checklist.

Medication trials

Medication for ADHD should be conducted on a trial basis in order to assess side effects and efficacy of treatment. It is important to explain the process of the trial of medication to the child, parents or carers and their teachers. Medication should not be used in pre-school children (NICE 2008), and licensed medications are used from six years onwards. The exception to this is dexamphetamine which can be used from three years and is licensed for refractory cases of ADHD. During the early stages of treatment, nurses should meet regularly with children and young people and their parents or carers as well as provide support over the telephone. This is to discuss response to treatment and any concerns the family may have about side effects.

To assist with the process of monitoring during the medication trial, a range of questionnaires have been produced (Hill and Taylor 2001). These should be used alongside general measures of change such as the Conners questionnaire which can be rated by the young person where appropriate (Conners 1989a), by parents (Conners 1989b) and by teachers (Conners 1989c). These measures are used to assess the severity of ADHD symptoms and provide evidence of change in response to medication and other treatments. Gathering information in the form of questionnaires and verbal information during the review of the trial will assist the nurse in understanding whether there have been any positive or negative treatment effects. In summary, the medication trial review should include the following:

- review at school with parents, teachers and young person;
- review of questionnaires and verbal reports;
- continued prescribing decision or not;
- commencement of treatment;
- offer other psychosocial intervention;
- review in one month by nurse in a nurse-led clinic;
- review each term thereafter when established on treatment.

Titration of medication

The decision about which medication should be used will be determined by many factors. These include choice by young people and parents or carers, safety issues and contraindications of using a particular treatment (Hill and Taylor 2001; Taylor *et al.* 2004; NICE 2006; NICE 2008). With the exception of atomoxetine (Strattera), the majority of medicines have not been adequately tested with children and young people. There is widespread acceptance within the research literature about the use of methylphenidate (Ritalin, Concerta XL, Equasym XL and Medikinet XL) and dexamphetamine (Dexedrine). The medications used for ADHD are licensed for use in children and young people; however, methylphenidate and dexamphetamine are controlled drugs and can currently only be prescribed on a supplementary basis by nurses. However, atomoxetine can be prescribed independently by nurses without the use of a clinical management plan.

Methylphenidate hydrochloride

Methylphenidate is used to increase attention and reduce hyperactivity and is licensed for use in the UK for children aged six years and over. Methylphenidate comes in immediate release (IR) and modified release (MR) preparations and is known by the trade names Ritalin, Equasym, Equasym XL, Concerta XL and Medikinet XL. NICE (2008) recommends that methylphenidate should be used as the initial treatment for ADHD and that this should be conducted as a trial. Stimulants have limitations since they are not an acceptable treatment choice for some families and concordance with treatment plans impacts upon effectiveness. There have been concerns expressed about young people taking methylphenidate with cannabis and/or alcohol but there are no contra-indications of using methylphenidate with cannabis and/or alcohol. However, if there is a family history or past personal history of psychosis or cannabis use, methylphenidate use should be very carefully monitored (NICE 2008).

Mechanism of action

The mechanism of methylphenidate is not fully understood. It is thought that methylphenidate promotes the release of dopamine from the presynaptic vesicles and then blocks the reuptake of dopamine back to the presynaptic nerve endings (Scahill *et al*. 2004). Dopamine is now recognised as playing a central role in mediating many brain pathways necessary to human behaviour. Treatment with methylphenidate usually commences at a low dose and is gradually increased over a period of weeks until there is a positive treatment response or unwanted side effects appear. Dosages are dependent upon the weight of the child and practitioners should always consult national and local guidelines and use their clinical judgement when considering treatment regimes. Careful titration of doses needs to be considered in order to improve positive response to treatment. Modified release (MR) preparations are used as a single dose in the morning and immediate release (IR) preparations are given in two or three divided doses. Stimulants are short-acting medications and some children metabolise these faster than reported in the literature (Greenhill 1995). Even when a positive response to medication has been achieved, it is therefore sometimes necessary for the nurse to adjust the timing of doses to avoid 'rebound effects'. These can occur when the medication is clearing the system and manifest as an increase in the core symptoms of hyperactivity, impulsivity and inattention (Swanson *et al*. 1998; Ludwikowski and DeValk 1998). Careful and detailed titration of dosage and timing is likely to lead to a positive response (MTA Cooperative Group 1999; Taylor *et al*. 2004).

Atomoxetine

Atomoxetine (Strattera) is a selective noradrenaline transport blocker indicated for the treatment of ADHD. This drug is newly licensed and therefore is a black triangle drug and any adverse effects need to be reported using the yellow card system. This is the system for reporting suspected adverse drug reactions run by the Medicines and Healthcare Products Regulatory Agency (MHRA). Atomoxetine is licensed for use in children over the age of six years. The advantages of this drug are that it provides all-day relief from symptoms and does not wear off like methylphenidate preparations. However, the data about the effectiveness of the drug is limited as atomoxetine has only recently been introduced in the UK and trials have been short in duration (Bailey 2003).

Mechanism of action

Atomoxetine was initially developed as an antidepressant and like tricyclic antidepressants is a noradrenaline reuptake inhibitor (Rains and Schahill 2006). Atomoxetine is well absorbed after oral administration and is minimally affected by food, therefore can be administered with or without food. Treatment with atomoxetine in children and young people up to a weight of 70 kg is commenced at the rate of 0.5 mg per kg for one week. After seven days the dose should increase to 1.2 mg per kg for at least another four weeks to assess efficacy. For children and adolescents over 70 kg in weight doses start at 40 mg a day for one week and the dose is increased dependent upon treatment response and tolerability to 80 mg. The maximum dose of atomoxetine is 100 mg per day for at least a further four weeks to assess efficacy.

Dexamphetamine

Dexamphetamine is used to increase attention and reduce hyperactivity and is licensed for use in the UK for children aged three years and over for refractory ADHD. NICE (2008) recommends that atomoxetine is used if there is no treatment response to methylphenidate which should be used as a firstline treatment.

Non-licensed preparations

Use of other non-licensed medications can be considered for the treatment of ADHD, but this is outside of the knowledge, skills and competence of the nurse prescriber (Department of Health 2007; Nursing & Midwifery Council 2007; Department of Health 2008). NICE (2008) has recommended that, if there is no treatment response to methylphenidate, atomoxetine or dexamphetamine then an opinion from a regional specialist unit should be sought.

Medications that have been previously used for ADHD without a product licence include:

- clonidine (antihypertensive);
- modafinil (CNS stimulant used for daytime sleepiness);
- tricyclic antidepressants (imipramine);
- selective serotonin reuptake inhibitors (SSRIs) (fluoxetine);
- serotonin noradrenaline reuptake inhibitors (SNRIs) (venlafaxine);
- bupropion (smoking cessation);
- atypical antipsychotic (risperidone) although these are not recommended for use in children and young people with ADHD (NICE).

Monitoring response to treatment

The nurse plays an important role in the baseline and continued monitoring assessment of height, weight, blood pressure and pulse, effectiveness of treatment and any adverse side effects. Following on from the trial review, a decision whether to continue with medication is made. If one medication proves to have intolerable side effects or is deemed not to be effective another medication can be trialled. Nurses are well placed to offer routine monitoring of medication and to provide other psychosocial interventions. Routine monitoring should focus on general mental health assessment at each appointment, particularly focusing on tics, depression, irritability, social withdrawal and lack of spontaneity. The potential for drug misuse or diversion should be considered by the nurse. However, reports of substance misuse and diversion are not common among young people with ADHD. The following physical factors should also be routinely monitored:

- blood pressure and pulse;
- height and weight;
- side effects of medication;
- positive and negative responses to treatment;
- progress at school.

Reviewing medication

Nurses who prescribe medicines for children and young people with ADHD should regularly review their effectiveness. Recently published guidance on good practice in medicines management (Department of Health 2008) suggests that the following issues should be discussed during the review:

- Are the medicines making a positive difference?
- What side effects are being experienced?
- What are the options for addressing these?
- What healthy-living options such as sleep hygiene might be appropriate?

• Is the young person having trouble remembering to take their medication?

Monitoring side effects

Medication used for the treatment of ADHD is a commonplace and can often be influential in treatment outcomes. Difficulties such as unwanted effects from medication including poor appetite, disrupted sleep and headaches are well documented and it is important to ensure that young people do not feel any worse whilst taking medication for ADHD. A key part of the nurse prescribing role is monitoring the positive and negative effects of pharmacological treatments through regular and ongoing review. The frequency of this review should be negotiated with the child or young person and their parents or carers. Treatment for ADHD is likely to be long-term and the development of the therapeutic relationship is important (Ryan 2007). Although considered to be generally safe, the drugs used to treat ADHD sometimes have unwanted side effects. In many cases, these subside after the first few weeks of commencing treatment. For some children and young people, however, ongoing side effects can lead to difficulties with compliance and the discontinuation of treatment. Nurses should be familiar with the properties of the medications that they prescribe and administer (Keogh and Doyle 2008). Side effects can often be ameliorated by adjusting the dose or timing of the dose (Ludwikowski and DeValk 1998). It is a matter of clinical judgement and the wishes of the child and their family about whether stimulant treatment is discontinued in the face of intolerable side effects. See Table 11.1 for the most common side effects of methylphenidate and atomoxetine and Table 11.2 for a side effects rating scale.

Nurses who prescribe medicines for children and young people can report unwanted side effects to the MHRA using the 'Yellow Card' system. The MHRA will be particularly interested to know about any suspected side

Table 11.1 Common side effects of methylphenidate and atomoxetine

Methyphenidate	Atomoxetine
Insomnia and difficulty falling asleep	Nausea and upset stomach
Decreased appetite	Decreased appetite
Weight loss	Tiredness
Nervousness and dysphoria	Dizziness
Nausea	Mood swings
Headaches	Suicidal thoughts
Changes in blood pressure	Liver toxicity
Skin rash	Skin rash
Tics	

Table 11.2 ADHD medication side effects questionnaire

Child's name:	Date:				
Children and young people may have unwanted effects of treatment as well as good effects. For each item, please tick in a box on each line how much that statement applies to you or your child over the last few days based on what you have seen. 0　　　is not at all 1　　　is a few occasions only 2　　　is about half the time 3　　　is most of the time 4　　　is all the time					
	0	1	2	3	4
Stares or daydreams a lot					
Talks less than usual with others					
Disinterested in other children					
Poor appetite					
Irritable					
Complains of stomach ache					
Complains of headache					
Drowsy, tired or sleepy					
Looks sad, miserable, low mood					
Crying spells					
Looks anxious or tense					
Seems unsteady or dizzy					
Excited					
Has trouble getting off to sleep					
Has nightmares					
Displays twitches (tics)					
Expresses suicidal ideas					
Constipation					
Dry mouth					
Is there anything else you would like to add?					

Source: adapted from Hill and Taylor 2001

effects that are not mentioned in the patient information leaflet that came with the medication, and/or a suspected side effect that has caused problems severe enough to interfere with everyday activities (Department of Health 2008).

Good practice in nurse prescribing

Nurses who prescribe medicines for children and young people with ADHD are bound by the NMC code of professional conduct and their own NHS trust guidelines regarding record-keeping and the issuing of prescriptions. They should always demonstrate the decision-making process in their prescribing practice by maintaining clear and contemporaneous records. Armstrong (2006) points out that clinical supervision helps ensure that clinical practice is safe and effective and nurses remain accountable and up to date. The use of reflective practice and clinical supervision provide opportunities for nurses who prescribe medicines to discuss any dilemmas related to medicines before making treatment decisions (Ryan 2007).

How can nurse prescribing add value?

Nurses are in an ideal position to integrate drug treatments with a wide range of non-pharmacological therapies, and to do so in a knowledgeable, safe and effective manner that is acceptable to service users (Nolan *et al.* 2004a; Jones *et al.* 2005). There is also evidence from the US that nurse prescribing is cheaper than medical prescribing and is equally safe and effective (Nolan *et al.* 2001; Nolan *et al.* 2004b). Due to a historical lack of resources, child and adolescent mental health services are notorious for having long waiting lists (Jones and Bhadrinath 1998). Prior to the development of nurse prescribing, medication management traditionally required a joint appointment for a child and their parents with a psychiatrist or paediatrician. This was often a time-consuming process which left young people and families waiting for treatment. It is well known that delays to treatment can threaten engagement and exacerbate young people's conditions (Terry 2003). It has been shown that nurses can complete episodes of care by competently prescribing medicines. This not only improves patient choice and access to medicines but also frees up psychiatrist or paediatrician resources to perform other interventions. This can be seen as a win-win-win situation where new ways of working can benefit service users and both nurses and psychiatrists alike.

Firstly nurse prescribing provides more timely commencement of treatment and routine follow-up for children and young people. Secondly, medication for ADHD is always initiated on a trial basis and the review would require the presence of a child psychiatrist or paediatrician. As an independent and supplementary prescriber nurses can complete this task autonomously. This again saves medical time and does not create delays in trying to arrange joint appointments for two busy clinicians. Thirdly, in the absence of nurse prescribing, any alteration to treatment regimes must be authorised by a child psychiatrist or paediatrician. This again can create an unnecessary delay in changes to treatment. Nurse prescribing enables decisions to be made by the supplementary nurse prescriber during ongoing appointments, this being more effective and timely for the child and family.

What are the risks of nurse prescribing?

Like all new ways of working and changes to clinical practice, there exist personal and organisational risks associated with non-medical prescribing. These have to be balanced against the potential benefits associated with nurse prescribing for children and young people with ADHD. An increase in the numbers of professionals prescribing medicines of course increases the overall risk of prescribing errors. Drug errors are a serious matter for the NHS, and can have severe direct and indirect effects on service users (National Patient Safety Agency 2002). However, there is no evidence that nurses are more likely to make prescribing errors than doctors who themselves do not always practise within national prescribing guidelines (Department of Health 2001; Nolan *et al*. 2001). Despite this, nurses who are supplementary or independent prescribers should ensure that they have professional indemnity insurance through membership of their professional body or trade union. A further risk for nurses and nursing is that of moving away from holistic care to a biomedical approach to practice (Bailey 1999). This has been referred to as the drift from caring to curing (Nolan and Bradley 2005). Other nurse commentators have cautioned against this too, suggesting that nurses must examine their relationships with the pharmaceutical industry and ensure their prescribing judgements are objective and ethical (Kersenich 2000; Lipley 2000; Ashmore and Carver 2001; Hemingway 2003).

Doctors' views of nurse prescribing

It is not only nurses who have been ambivalent about nurse prescribing. The prospect of nurse prescribing has triggered unease among many doctors. Although some doctors have welcomed nurse prescribing, others have felt anxious that nurses are not adequately trained or competent to prescribe (Horton 2002; Avery and Pringle 2005; Turner 2007). Yet others object because they perceive nurse prescribing as encroaching on their professional territory (Gunn 1990; Jones and Harborne 2005). Descriptions of nurses as 'pseudo-psychiatrists', 'medicine checkers' and 'physician extenders' have all received negative coverage in the UK and US nursing press. The motivation of nurses who wish to prescribe has been called into question by some commentators, believing this to be driven by a desire for autonomy and power rather than a wish to ensure that service users are given the best possible treatment as quickly as possible. In order that professional rivalry, perceived threat and conflict are avoided, teams must foster positive multidisciplinary working relationships (Shuttle 2004). This depends on strong nursing and medical leadership and is crucial if nurse prescribing is to be accepted, supported and successfully implemented for the benefit of children and families with ADHD.

Summary

The changes in prescribing regulations to allow nurses to practise as independent prescribers are aimed at improving patients' access to medicines. This is important as it enables patients to benefit from improved care, easier access to the medication they need and greater choice in the way they receive treatment. Nurse prescribing is conducted within a framework of ensuring patient safety, making better use of health professional skills and promoting multidisciplinary team-working. Some have argued that nurse prescribing is considerably quicker, much cheaper and more efficient than medical prescribing. Independent and supplementary nurse prescribing has undoubtedly enhanced patient care within specialist ADHD clinics and child and adolescent mental health services. The principles of nurse prescribing are not unique to ADHD and can be applied to the treatment of other mental disorders of childhood where medication is shown to be an effective part of the treatment package. This includes depression, anxiety and obsessive compulsive disorder where NICE guidelines have advocated more frequent review of medicines. Medications can be of significant value for children and young people with ADHD, but they can also cause harm if they are not used appropriately. It is essential that their management is as effective as possible, and nurses need to have appropriate supervision and guidance in prescribing psychotropic medication. Nurses will need to engage in continued professional development to keep their knowledge up to date, be aware of changes to the formulary and maintain their level of competency in nurse prescribing.

12 Good practice and the legal framework

Key points

- The close therapeutic relationship that evolves whilst assessing, treating and monitoring children and young people with ADHD can generate complex moral, ethical and legal dilemmas. It is therefore essential that nurses and other professionals are clear about the legal context in which they practise and their duties in relation to confidentiality and information sharing.
- Before embarking on assessment, treatment or management of a child or young person with ADHD, it is essential that consent is provided. In order for consent to be valid, the child or young person must be capable of consenting, the consent must be freely given and the child or young person involved must be given appropriate information.
- Nurses should ensure that children, young people and families are fully involved at every stage of the treatment process. They should be given verbal and written information in a form which is suited to their age, communication and developmental needs.
- There is very clear and consistent evidence that children and young people as well as their parents and carers want to be involved in decisions about their care and treatment. Whilst the principle of working in partnership with young people and families is straightforward, putting this into nursing practice when working with children and young people with ADHD can be a complex task. This is because the wishes and views of children, young people and their families or carers are often different and sometimes contradictory.
- Advocacy is a vitally important part of the nurses' role and is part of their code of professional conduct. Advocacy for children and young people and their parents or carers involves speaking on their behalf and promoting their best interests at a clinical and service-planning level.

Introduction

Legal, ethical and good practice issues are important in determining the care and treatment decisions made by nurses, doctors and other professionals. Foreman (2006) describes a model for routine ethical practice by doctors which can easily be applied to nursing children and young people with ADHD. This is based on three key assumptions that should guide ethical practice decisions:

1   Ethical practice is consistent with the four principles of beneficence, non-maleficence, justice and a respect for autonomy.
2   Ethical concerns lead to legal processes, which are intended to ensure ethical practice.
3   Decisions are based on the best interests of patients.

All nursing decisions that affect children and young people with ADHD must be underpinned by a legal and ethical framework which is consistent with the nurse's standard of conduct, performance and ethics (NMC 2008). To make accountable decisions, nurses must be able to defend their clinical practice decisions and to do so effectively they need to understand the legal and policy context in which they practise. The close therapeutic relationship that evolves whilst assessing, treating and monitoring children and young people with ADHD can generate complex moral, ethical and legal dilemmas. It is therefore essential that nurses and other professionals are clear about their duties in relation to consent, confidentiality and information sharing.

Policy

There are two overarching frameworks within which nurses provide care and treatment services for children and young people with ADHD. These are Every Child Matters, published by the former Government Department for Education and Skills (DFES 2003), and the National Service Framework for Children, Young People and Maternity Services, often referred to in short as the Children's NSF (Department of Health 2004).

Every Child Matters is a 10-year vision for the modernisation of children's services. This sets out the Government's plans to help ensure that each and every child is enabled to be healthy, stay safe, enjoy and achieve, make a positive contribution and achieve economic wellbeing (Department for Education and Skills 2003). England and Wales have separately published National Service Frameworks for Children, Young People and Maternity Services (Department of Health 2004; Welsh Assembly Government 2005). Closely linked to the Every Child Matters programme, they each set standards and define service models for children across all NHS and social care settings. There are five core standards in the NSF which focus on involving children and families, interagency working, competent commissioning and care pathways. In addition there are six specific standards which focus on children and young people with particular needs. These should be cross-referenced and read in conjunction with the core standards. Nurses are encouraged not to read any of the chapters in isolation (see Table 12.1).

Involving children and young people

Involving children and young people in decisions about the care and treatment they receive as well as in designing and evaluating service delivery has been a central plank of government policy for the last decade. Listening to the views of young people is at the heart of the NHS modernisation agenda and the principle of service user involvement is firmly embedded in Every Child Matters (Department for Education and Skills 2003), the National Service Framework for Children, Young People and Maternity Services (Department of Health 2004) and the Children's Plan (Department for Children, Schools and Families 2008). The NHS Plan emphasises the importance of placing service users at the centre of services (Department of Health 2000). However, systematically involving children and young people in service design and delivery can be a complex process. There are several reasons for this including a poor track record of user involvement in child and adolescent mental health services (CAMHS), stigma that may be associated with discussions about mental health and behaviour problems, and worries about overloading children who may already be vulnerable, under considerable stress and facing many changes and difficult choices (Street and Herts 2005).

In the field of health, it has been argued that too much emphasis has been placed on the views of parents and carers, and that this is at the expense of understanding the things that children and young people want to change about the services that they receive (Davis 2007). Children and young people are important users of health services and, although there has been a drive

Table 12.1 National Service Framework for Children, Young People and Maternity Services

---

Core standards
Standard 1: Promoting health and wellbeing, identifying needs and intervening early
Standard 2: Supporting parents
Standard 3: Child, young person and family-centred services
Standard 4: Growing up into adulthood
Standard 5: Safeguarding and promoting the welfare of children and young people

Specific standards
Standard 6: Children and young people who are ill
Standard 7: Children in hospital
Standard 8: Disabled children and young people and those with complex needs
Standard 9: Mental health and psychological wellbeing of children and young people
Standard 10: Medicines for children and young people
Standard 11: Maternity services

---

towards participation in health care by adults, children and young people are rarely directly included. There has historically been a view that parents can accurately represent their children's views. However, this cannot always be assumed to be the case, particularly as children mature and become more independent. Recent surveys of children and young people have very clearly demonstrated that they want to be directly involved in decisions about their care and treatment and influence the ways in which services are planned and delivered (Laws 1999; Department of Health 2002; OCC 2007; Pugh *et al.* 2006; Vasiliou-Theodore and Penketh 2008).

Involving parents and carers

Whilst the principle of working in partnership with young people and families is straightforward, putting this into nursing practice when working with children and young people with ADHD can be a complex task. This is because the wishes and views of children, young people and their families or carers are often different and sometimes contradictory. Parents and carers usually know their children better than doctors and nurses and bring expertise and knowledge to the therapeutic alliance with professionals. This partnership approach is the key to the successful treatment or management plan, and professionals should recognise that parents are crucial to completing assessment measures, implementing behaviour strategies and giving their children hope to live with and manage their ADHD. The perspectives of children and families can be measured using a range of evaluation tools such as section B of the Health of the Nation Outcome Scales for Children and Adolescents (HoNOSCA). This can be completed by nurses as well as young people themselves (Gowers *et al.* 2002; Gowers *et al.* 1998).

Providing age-appropriate information

The National Service Framework for Children, Young People and Maternity Services advocates that young people should participate in the decision-making process (Department of Health 2004). To do this effectively they require information which is valid, relevant, accurate, up to date and easily accessible. Children, young people and families should be given verbal and written information in a form which is suited to their age, communication and developmental needs at every stage of the assessment and treatment process. This should include information about the various psychological and pharmacological treatment options including no treatment, the relative risks and benefits of accepting or refusing the treatment, and side effects of any medication that is being considered. The expectations of treatment should be explored as fully as possible. Nurses who work with children and young people with ADHD should be committed to the provision of child-centred care and recognise that the needs of children are different to those of adults.

Children and their parents require information on which to base their decisions about treatment for ADHD.

ADHD and the legal framework

Human Rights

Along with nearly 100 other countries, the United Kingdom Government has ratified the United Nations Convention on the Rights of the Child (United Nations 1991). All articles have relevance to young people, but importantly where consent to treatment is concerned a number of articles are relevant. Article 3 states the right 'not to be subjected to torture or to inhuman or degrading treatment or punishment'. This can be related to helping nurses negotiate treatment decisions with young people who have ADHD. Article 12 makes clear that children and young people have the right 'to express their own views about matters that concern them, dependent upon their age and maturity', and article 13 states that 'information should be made freely available to children and young people, either orally, in print, in the form of art or by any other method the child wishes'. Article 14 determines a right to 'freedom from discrimination'. This is important when we consider that children with ADHD often experience social and educational exclusion.

Children Acts

The Children Act received Royal Assent in 1989 and was implemented in 1991. The principles of the Act are to support parents or carers in child care matters and to allow them to reinforce their position of autonomy in the care of children at the same time as protecting them from significant harm. The Children Act 2004 complements the 1989 act by requiring agencies to work more collaboratively together and promote the wellbeing of children and young people and to continue to safeguard young people.

Parental responsibility

The Children Act 1989 defines 'parental responsibility' as the duties, rights and authority which a parent has in respect of a child. Wherever the assessment or treatment of a child for ADHD is being considered, the person or persons with parental responsibility must be identified and their views taken into consideration. It is usually the child's parents who have parental responsibility, but shared or full parental responsibility may also be provided by the local authority if the child is 'looked after' by the local authority or the subject of a care order.

Consent to treatment

The National Service Framework for Children advocates that young people should participate in the decision-making process and that information provided should be valid, relevant, accurate, up to date, easily accessible and well presented and is appropriate to their level of understanding, before young people can decide whether to consent to, or refuse treatment (Department of Health 2004). Wherever the assessment or treatment of a child for ADHD is being considered, the person or persons with parental responsibility must be identified, and their views sought as appropriate. In addition, the views of the child should be sought, regardless of their age or understanding.

Providing consent for treatment decisions depends on age. When obtaining consent from parents it is only legally necessary to obtain consent from one parent who holds parental responsibility. However, if there is another parent who shares parental responsibility, it is good practice to obtain their consent too (Jones 2003). Even very young children have views about their treatment, and these should always be sought regardless of their age and understanding (Tan and Jones 2001). However, involvement in treatment decisions is not the same as consent for treatment decisions. The Department of Health has published guidance for children and young people on consent and what they have a right to expect from health service providers. Young people are given guidance about:

- how consent is asked for and given;
- what you need to know before giving consent;
- how old you should be to give consent on your own;
- when your parents can be involved;
- when other people can give consent for you;
- what to do if you're asked to help with research.

Nurses may find this useful in helping children and young people make informed decisions about ADHD assessment and treatment decisions (Department of Health 2001).

Confidentiality

The close therapeutic relationship that evolves whilst assessing, treating and monitoring children and young people with ADHD can generate complex moral, ethical and legal dilemmas. It is therefore essential that nurses and other professionals are clear about their duties in relation to confidentiality and information sharing. They should be aware of the rights of children and parents, national guidelines for best practice and local operational policies in relation to confidentiality and information sharing. Unless there are compelling reasons otherwise, children's rights to confidentiality should be strictly observed. Young people aged 16 and 17 are entitled to the same duty of confidentiality as adults. This means that unless failure to share information is likely to lead to harm to others, information about the child concerned cannot be shared without their explicit consent.

Guidance for nurses and other professionals about information sharing and consent is contained in *Working Together to Safeguard Children* (Department for Education and Skills 2006). Children under the age of 16 who have the capacity and understanding to take decisions about their own treatment are also entitled to make decisions about the use and disclosure of information they have provided in confidence. For example, they may be receiving treatment or counselling about which they do not want their parents to know. The nurse may try to persuade the child or young person to allow their parents to be informed about the treatment but they are not legally obliged to do so and nurses should be careful not to make the young person feel pressured.

Safeguarding vulnerable children

There are two situations when a child's confidentiality may need to be breached without necessarily obtaining their consent. The main indication is where there is information disclosed that suggests that the child may be at significant risk of harm or abuse. In these circumstances it is good practice for the nurse to support the child or young person to make the disclosure themselves. However, if the child is unable or unwilling to do this, the nurse is professionally obliged to report the disclosure on their behalf. In addition, where a competent young person or child is refusing treatment for a life-threatening condition, the duty of care would require confidentiality to be breached to the extent of informing those with parental responsibility for the child who might then be able to provide the necessary consent to the treatment. In both scenarios, nurses must have a clear understanding of their duties and have ready access to service policies on confidentiality and information sharing. NHS trusts usually have access to legal advice where there are complex legal or ethical dilemmas. For more routine advice about confidentiality, consent and information sharing, nurses should be able to access professional advice from within their organisation or professional body. For safeguarding children or child protection matters, nurses should have access to named and designated professionals who can assist them to make safe and competent decisions that may affect the welfare of a child. National guidance for nurses and other professionals related to safeguarding and protecting vulnerable children is also available (Department for Education and Skills 2006).

Advocacy

Advocacy is a vitally important part of the nurses' role and is in keeping with their code of professional conduct (Nursing & Midwifery Council 2008). Advocacy for children and young people and their parents or carers involves speaking on their behalf and promoting their best interests at a clinical and service-planning level. It involves helping children and young people to navigate the mental health system and to access independent and confidential information, culturally sensitive advice, representation and support (Valentine 2004). Advocacy by nurses on behalf of children and young people can occur at a range of different levels. This may be through representing the views of the child or young person at a review or case conference, informing them of their rights or making their voice heard throughout the care and treatment process. Nurses also share a responsibility to speak on behalf of children and young people at a strategic level. This may be in relation to CAMHS service planning or by representing their views and wishes to CAMHS service managers and commissioners. It is not always appropriate or possible for nurses to advocate on behalf of a particular child or adolescent. The young person may have a complaint that they do not want the nurse or service provider to know about. Independent advocacy services can also help children and young people to understand their rights, make complaints about their care, treatment or detention and provide confidential advice. In 2002, the Department of Health published national standards for the provision of children's advocacy services (Department of Health 2002).

Summary

Nurses should be committed to the provision of child-centred care and thus recognise that children's health needs are different from those of adults. Service commissioners and managers should take note of children's needs in terms of planning health, social and educational services. In addition, nurses should respect the views, wishes and experiences of parents in relation to their child. However, despite knowing their children better than professionals, parents and carers of children with ADHD sometimes feel excluded from treatment decisions. In a large survey, only half of parents had received written information about medical treatment options for ADHD when their child was first diagnosed (ADDISS 2006). It is therefore crucial for nurses to fully involve parents and carers at every stage of the assessment and treatment process.

Bibliography

Chapter 1 What is ADHD, and what is not?

Adler, L. and Chua, H. (2002). Management of ADHD in adults. *Journal of Clinical Psychiatry*, 63(12), 29–35.

Akhondzadeh, S., Mohammadi, M. and Khademi, M. (2004). Zinc sulphate as an adjunct to methylphenidate for the treatment of attention deficit hyperactivity disorder in children: a double blind and randomised trial. *BMC Psychiatry*, 8(4), 1–6.

American Psychiatric Association. (1994). *Diagnostic and Statistical Manual of Mental Disorders* (4th Edition). Washington: APA.

Amen, D. and Carmichael, B. (1997). High resolution brain SPECT imaging in ADHD. *Annals of Clinical Psychiatry*, 9(2), 10.1023/A:1026201218296.

Anderson, J. (1996). Is childhood hyperactivity the product of Western culture? *Lancet*, (348), 73–74.

Armstrong, T. (2006). Canaries in the coal mine: the symptoms of children labelled ADHD as biocultural feedback. In: Lloyd, D., Stead, J. and Cohen, D. (Eds). *Critical New Perspectives on ADHD*. London: Routledge.

Armstrong. (1995). *The Myth of the ADD Child*. New York: Dutton.

Arnold, E. (1996). Sex differences in ADHD: conference summary. *Journal of Abnormal Child Psychology*, (24), 555–569.

Arnold, E. and DiSilvestro, R. (2005). Zinc in attention deficit/hyperactivity disorder. *Journal of Child and Adolescent Psychopharmacology*, 15(4), 619–627.

Arnold, L., Votolato, N. and Kleycamp, D. (1990). Does hair zinc predict amphetamine improvement of ADD/hyperactivity? *International Journal of Neuroscience*, (50), 103–107.

Baldwin, S. and Anderson, R. (2000). The cult of methylphenidate: clinical update. *Critical Public Health*, (10), 81–86.

Baldwin, S. and Cooper, P. (2000). How should ADHD be treated? *The Psychologist*, (13), 598–602.

Banerjee, T., Middleton, F. and Faraone, S. (2007). Environmental risk factors for attention deficit hyperactivity disorder. *Acta Paediatrica*, (96), 1269–1274.

Barkley, R. (2002). Major life activity and health outcomes associated with attention deficit hyperactivity disorder. *Journal of Clinical Psychiatry*, 63(12), 10–15.

Barkley, R. (1996). Attention deficit hyperactivity disorder. In: Mash, E. and Barkley, R. (Eds). *Child Psychopathology*. New York: Guilford Press.

Barkley, R. (1990). *Attention Deficit Hyperactivity Disorder: A Handbook for Diagnosis and Treatment.* New York: Guilford Press.

Baughman, F. (2006). *The ADHD Fraud: How Psychiatry Makes Patients of Normal Children.* British Columbia: Trafford Publishing.

Baughman, F. (2001). Questioning the treatment for ADHD. *Science*, (291), 591.

Bhutta, A., Cleves, M., Casey, P., Cradock, M. and Anand, K. (2002). Cognitive and behavioral outcomes of school age children who were born preterm: a meta-analysis. *Journal of the American Medical Association*, (288), 728–737.

Biederman, J. and Faraone, S. (2005). Attention deficit hyperactivity disorder. *Lancet*, (366), 237–248.

Biederman, J., Faraone, S., Keenan, K., Benjamin, J., Krifcher, B. and Moore, C. (1992). Further evidence for familial-genetic risk factors in ADHD: patterns of comorbidity in probands and relatives in psychiatrically and paediatrically referred samples. *Archives of General Psychiatry*, (49) 728–738.

Biederman, J., Faraone, S. and Monuteaux, M. (2002b). Differential effect of environmental adversity by gender: Rutter's index of adversity in a group of boys and girls with and without ADHD. *American Journal of Psychiatry*, (158), 1556–1562.

Biederman, J., Mick, E., Faraone, S., Braaten, E., Doyle, A., Spencer, T., Wilens, T., Frazier, E. and Johnson, M. (2002a). Influences of gender on attention deficit hyperactivity disorder in children referred to a psychiatric clinic. *American Journal of Psychiatry*, (159), 36–42.

Brady, G. (2005). ADHD, diagnosis and identity. In: Newnes, C. and Radcliffe, N. (Eds). *Making and Breaking Children's Lives.* Ross on Wye: PCCS Books.

Breggin, P. (2001). *Talking Back to Ritalin: What doctors Aren't Telling You About Stimulants and ADHD* (rev ed). Cambridge MA: Perseus.

British Psychological Society. (2000). *Attention Deficit/Hyperactivity Disorder: Guidelines and Principles for Successful Multi-Agency Working: Report of a Working Party of the British Psychological Society.* Leicester: BPS.

Brown, R., Freeman, W. and Perrin, J. (2001). Prevalence and assessment of attention deficit/hyperactivity disorder in primary care settings. *Pediatrics*, (107), 43.

Brown, R., Madan-Swain, A. and Baldwin, K. (1991). Gender differences in a clinic referred sample of attention deficit disordered children. *Child Psychiatry and Human Development*, (22), 111–128.

Canon, M., McKenzie, K. and Sims, A. (2004). ADHD is best understood as a cultural construct. *British Journal of Psychiatry*, (184), 8–9.

Carey, W. and Diller, L. (2001). Concerns about Ritalin. *Journal of Pediatrics*, (139), 338–340.

Caspi, C., McClay, J., Moffitt, T., Mill, J., Martin, J., Craig, I., Taylor, A. and Poulton, R. (2002). Role of genotype in the cycle of violence in maltreated children. *Science*, (297), 851–854.

Castellanos, F., Lee, P., Sharp, W., Jeffries, N., and Greenstein, D. (2002). Developmental trajectories of brain volume abnormalities in children and adolescents with attention deficit/hyperactivity disorder. *Journal of the American Medical Association*, (9), 1740–1748.

Charatan, F. (2000). US parents sue psychiatrists for promoting Ritalin. *British Medical Journal*, (321), 723.

Cheon, K., Ryu, Y., Kim, Y., Namkoong, K., Kim, C. and Lee, J. (2003). Dopamine transporter density in the basal ganglia assessed with [I-123] IPT SPET in children with attention deficit hyperactivity disorder. *European Journal of Nuclear Medicine and Molecular Imaging*, (30), 306–311.

Cohen, D. (2006). Critiques of the ADHD enterprise. In: Lloyd, D., Stead, J. and Cohen, D. (Eds). *Critical New Perspectives on ADHD*. London: Routledge.

Conners, C., Goyette, C. and Southwick, D. (1976). Food additives and hyperkinesis: a controlled double-blind experiment. *Pediatrics*, (58), 154–166.

Connors, C. (1989). *Connors Teacher Rating Scales Manual*. New York: Multi-Health Systems.

Conrad, P. and Potter, D. (2000). From hyperactive children to ADHD adults: observations on the expansion of medical categories. *Social Problems*, 47(4), 559–583.

Cuffe, S., Moore, C. and McKeown, R. (2005). Prevalence and correlates of ADHD symptoms in the National Health Interview Survey. *Journal of Attention Disorders*, 9(2), 392–401.

Curran, S. and Taylor, E. (2000). Attention deficit hyperactivity disorder: biological causes and treatments. *Current Opinion in Psychiatry*, (13), 397–402.

Currie, J. and Stabile, M. (2006). Child mental health and human capital accumulation: the case of ADHD. *Journal of Health Economics*, 25(6), 1094–1118.

Davis, J. (2007). Disability, childhood studies and the construction of medical discourses. In: Lloyd, D., Stead, J. and Cohen, D. (Eds). *Critical New Perspectives on ADHD*. London: Routledge.

Dean, D. (2005). ADHD and its impact on family life. *Mental Health Practice*, 8(9), 20–23.

Department of Health. (2003). *Our Inheritance, Our Future: Realising the Potential of Genetics in the NHS*. London: HMSO.

Dobson, R. (2004). Could Fidgety Philip be proof that ADHD is not a modern phenomenon? *British Medical Journal*, (329), 643.

Dwivedi, K. and Banhatti, R. (2005). Attention deficit/hyperactivity disorder and ethnicity. *Archive of Diseases in Childhood*, 90(1), 10–12.

Dwivedi, K. and Sankar, S. (2004). Promotion of prosocial development and prevention of conduct disorders. In: Dwivedi, K. and Brinley-Harper, P. (Eds). *Promoting the Emotional Wellbeing of Children and Adolescents and Preventing their Mental Ill Health: a Handbook*. London: Jessica Kingsley.

Eiraldi, R., Mazzuca, L., Clarke, A. and Power, T. (2006). Service utilization among ethnic minority children with ADHD: a model of help-seeking behaviour. *Administration and Policy in Mental Health and Mental Health Services Research*. 10.1007/s10488–006–0076–9.

Faraone, S. (2005). The scientific foundation for understanding attention-deficit/ hyperactivity disorder as a valid psychiatric disorder. *European Child and Adolescent Psychiatry*, 14(1), 1–10.

Faraone, S., Doyle, A., Mick, E. and Biederman, J. (2001). Meta-Analysis of the association between the 7-repeat allele of the dopamine D4 receptor gene and attention deficit hyperactivity disorder. *American Journal of Psychiatry*, 158, 1052–1057.

Faraone, S., Perlis, R., Doyle, A., Smoller, J., Goralnick, J. and Holmgren, M. (2005). Molecular genetics of attention deficit/hyperactivity disorder. *Biological Psychiatry*, (57), 1313–1323.

Faraone, S., Sergeant, J., Gillberg, C. and Biederman, J. (2003). The worldwide prevalence of ADHD: is it an American condition? *Worldwide Psychiatry*, (2), 104–113.

Farrington, D. (2007). Childhood risk factors and risk-focused prevention. In:

McGuire, M., Morgan, R. and Reiner, R. (Eds). *The Oxford Handbook of Criminology* (4th Edition). Oxford: Oxford University Press.

Feingold, B. (1975). Hyperkinesis and learning difficulties linked to artificial food colors and flavors. *American Journal of Nursing*, (75), 797–803.

Fergusson, D., Horwood, L. and Lynskey, M. (1993). Prevalence and comorbidity of DSM-III-R diagnoses in a birth cohort of 15-year-olds. *Journal of the American Academy of Child and Adolescent Psychiatry*, 32, 1127–1134.

Fonagy, P, Target, M, Cottrell, D, Phillips, J. and Kurtz, Z. (2002). *What Works for Whom?: a Critical Review of Treatments for Children and Adolescents*. London: Guilford Press.

Ford, T., Sayal, K., Meltzer, H. and Goodman, R. (2005). Parental concerns about their child's emotions and behaviour and referral to specialist services: general population survey. *British Medical Journal*, (331), 1435–1436.

Furman, L. (2005). What is attention deficit hyperactivity disorder? *Journal of Child Neurology*, 20(12), 994–1002.

Gaub, M. and Carlson, C. (1997). Gender differences in ADHD: a meta-analysis and critical review. *Journal of the American Academy of Child and Adolescent Psychiatry*, (36), 1036–1045.

Gershon, J. (2002). A meta-analytical review of gender differences in ADHD. *Journal of Attention Disorders*, (5), 143–154.

Gill, M., Daly, G., Heron, S., Hawi, Z. and Fitzgerald, M. (1997). Confirmation of association between attention deficit hyperactivity disorder and a dopamine transporter polymorphism. *Molecular Psychiatry*, (2), 311–313.

Gingerich, K., Turrock, P. and Litfin, J. (1998). Diversity and attention deficit hyperactivity disorder. *Journal of Clinical Psychology*, (54), 415–426.

Gleeson, D. and Parker, D. (1989). Hyperactivity in a group of children referred to a Scottish Child Guidance Service: a significant problem. *British Journal of Educational Psychology*, (59), 262–265.

Goodman, R. (1997). The strengths and difficulties questionnaire: a research note. *Journal of Child Psychology and Psychiatry*, (38), 581–586.

Green, H., McGinnity, A., Meltzer, H., Ford, T. and Goodman, R. (2005). *Mental Health of Children and Young People in Great Britain*. London: ONS.

Greenhill, L. (1998). Diagnosing attention deficit/hyperactivity disorder in children. *Journal of Clinical Psychiatry*, (59), 31–41.

Harrison, L., Manocha, R. and Rubia, K. (2004). Sahaja yoga meditation as a family treatment programme for children with attention deficit hyperactivity disorder. *Clinical Child Psychology and Psychiatry*, 9(4), 479–497.

Hawkins. J., Herrenkohl, T., Farrington, D., Brewer, D., Catalano, R., Harachi, T. and Abbot, R. (1998). Understanding and preventing crime and violence: findings from the Seattle Social Development Project. In: Thornberry, T. and Krohn, M. (Eds). *Taking Stock of Delinquency: an Overview of Findings from Contemporary Longitudinal Studies*. New York: Kluwer/Plenum.

Hinshaw, S. (2002). Preadolescent girls with attention deficit/hyperactivity disorder: 1: background characteristics, comorbidity, cognitive and social functioning, and parenting practices. *Journal of Consulting and Clinical Psychology*, (70), 1086–1098.

Ho, T., Leung, P. and Luk, E. (1996). Establishing the constructs of childhood behavioural disturbance in a Chinese population: a questionnaire study. *Journal of Abnormal Child Psychology*, (24), 417–431.

Holmes, J., Payton, A., Barrett, J., Harrington, R., McGuffin, P., Owen, M., Ollier, W.,

Worthington, J., Gill, M., Kirley, A., Hawi, Z., Fitzgerald, M., Asherson, P., Curran, S., Mill, J., Gould, A., Taylor, E., Kent, L., Craddock, N. and Thapar, A. (2002). Association of DRD4 in children with ADHD and comorbid conduct problems. *American Journal of Medical Genetics*, 114(2), 150–153.

International Consensus Statement on ADHD. (2002). *Clinical Child and Family Psychology Review*, (5), 89–111.

Jackson-Brown, F. (2005). ADHD and the philosophy of science. In: Newnes, C. and Radcliffe, N. (Eds). *Making and Breaking Children's Lives*. PCCS Books: Ross on Wye.

Jensen, P., Kettle, L., Roper, M., Sloan, M., Dulcan, M., Hoven, C., Bird, H., Bauermeister, J. and Payne, J. (1999). Are stimulants overprescribed?: Treatment of ADHD in 4 US communities. *Journal of the American Academy of Child and Adolescent Psychiatry*, 38(7), 797–804.

Johnson, M. (1997). *Developmental Cognitive Neuroscience*. Oxford: Blackwell Publishing.

Jones, D. (2003). *Communicating with Vulnerable Children: a Guide for Practitioners*. London: Gaskell.

Kendall, J. (1999). Sibling accounts of attention deficit hyperactivity disorder (ADHD). *Family Process*, (38), 117–136.

Kent, L. (2005). Biological factors. In: Gowers, S. (Ed). *Seminars in Child and Adolescent Psychiatry* (2nd Edition). London: Gaskell.

Kidd, P. (2000). Attention deficit/hyperactivity disorder in children: rationale for its integrative management. *Alternative Medicine Review*, 5(5), 402–428.

Kirk, M., Tonkin, E., Skirton, H. and Carberry, A. (2006). Genetics in mental health nursing: is it part of your role? *Mental Health Practice*, 10(1), 15–18.

Kirley, A., Hawi, Z., Dly, G., McCarron, M., Mullins, C., Millar, N., Waldman, I. and Gill, M. (2002). Dopaminergic system genes in ADHD: towards a biological hypothesis. *Neuropsychopharmacology*, 27(4), 607–619.

Konofal, E., Lecendreux, M., Deron, J., Marchand, M., Cortese, S., Zaim, M., Mouren, M. and Arnulf, I. (2008). Effects of iron supplementation on attention deficit hyperactivity disorder in children. *Pediatric Neurology*, 38(1), 20–26.

Kozielec, T. and Starobrat-Hermelin, B. (1997). Assessment of magnesium levels in children with attention deficit hyperactivity disorder (ADHD). *Magnesium Research*, 10(2), 143–148.

Krause, K., Dresel, S., Krause, J., Kung, H. and Tatsch, K. (2000). Increased striatal dopamine transporter in adult patients with attention deficit hyperactivity disorder: effects of methylphenidate as measured by single photon emission computed tomography. *Neuroscience Letters*, (285), 107–110.

LaHoste, G., Swanson, J. and Wigal, S. (1996). Dopamine D4 receptor gene polymorphism is associated with attention deficit hyperactivity disorder. *Molecular Psychiatry*, (1), 121–124.

Lahti, J., Raikkonen, K., Kajantie, E., Heinonen, K., Personen, A. and Jarvenpaa, A. (2006). Small body size at birth and behavioural symptoms of ADHD in children aged five to six years. *Journal of Child Psychology and Psychiatry*, (47), 1167–1174.

Leo, J. and Cohen, D. (2003). Neuroimaging studies of ADHD: broken brains or flawed research? *Journal of Mind and Behavior*, (24), 29–56.

Li, D., Sham, P. and Owen, M. (2006). Meta-analysis shows significant association between dopamine system genes and attention deficit hyperactivity disorder (ADHD). *Human Molecular Genetics*, (15), 2276–2284.

Linnet, K., Dalsgaard, S. and Obel, C. (2003). Maternal lifestyle factors in pregnancy risk of attention deficit hyperactivity disorder and associated behaviors: a review of the current evidence. *American Journal of Psychiatry*, (160), 1028–1040.

Linnet, K., Wisborg, K., Agerbo, E., Secher, N., Thomsen, P. and Henriksen, T. (2006). Gestational age, birth weight, and the risk of hyperkinetic disorder. *Archives of Disease in Childhood*, (91), 655–660.

Lloyd, D. and Norris, C. (1999). Including ADHD? *Disability and Society*, (14), 505–517.

Lloyd, D., Stead, J. and Cohen, D. (2006). *Critical New Perspectives on ADHD*. London: Routledge.

McCann, D., Barrett, A., Cooper, A., Crumpler, D., Dalen, L., Grimshaw, K., Kitchin, E., Lok, K., Porteous, L., Prince, E., Sonuga-Barke, E., Warner, J. and Stevenson, J. (2007). Food additives and hyperactive behaviour in 3-year-old and 8/9-year-old children in the community: a randomised, double blinded, placebo controlled trial. *Lancet*. Published online September 6, 2007, 1–8 [DOI:10.1016/S0140–6736(07)61306–3].

McCubbin, M. and Cohen, D. (1997). Empirical, ethical and political perspectives on the use of methylphenidate. *Ethical Human Science*, (1), 81–101.

McGee, R. and Feehan, M. (2001). Are girls with problems of attention under-recognised? *Journal of Psychopathology and Behavioral Assessment*, (13), 187–198.

McLoyd, V., Cabello, R. and Mangelsdorf, S. (1997). The effects of poverty on children's socioemotional development. In: Noshpitz, J. (Ed). *Handbook of Child and Adolescent Psychiatry*. New York: Wiley.

Maniadaki, K., Sonuga-Barke, E. and Kakouros, E. (2006). Adults' self-efficacy beliefs and referral attitudes for boys and girls with ADHD. *European Journal of Child and Adolescent Psychiatry*, 15:132–140 DOI 10.1007/s00787–005–0514–3.

Mann, E., Ikeda, Y. and Mueller, C. (1992). Cross-cultural differences in rating hyperactive-disruptive behaviors in children. *American Journal of Psychiatry*, (149), 1539–1542.

Maras, P. and Cooper, P. (1999). Sex differences, gender issues and EBDs. In: Cooper, P. (Ed). *Understanding and Supporting Children with Emotional and Behavioural Difficulties*. London: Jessica Kingsley.

Mattes, J. and Gittelman, R. (1981). Effects of artificial food colourings in children with hyperactive symptoms. *Archives of General Psychiatry*, (38), 714–718.

Maughan, B., Brock, A. and Ladva, G. (2004). Chapter 12: mental health. In: Office for National Statistics. (Ed). *The Health of Children and Young People*. London: ONS.

Mellor, D., Storer, S. and Brown, J. (1996). Attention deficit hyperactivity disorder: perceptions, practice and politics. *Journal of Paediatrics and Child Health*, (32), 218–222.

Merrell, C. and Tymms, P. (2005). Rasch analysis of inattentive, hyperactive and impulsive behaviour in young children and the link with academic achievement. *Journal of Applied Measurement*, (6), 1–18.

Mill, J. and Petronis, A. (2008). Pre and peri-natal environmental risks for attention deficit hyperactivity disorder (ADHD): the potential role of epigenetic processes in mediating susceptibility. *Journal of Child Psychology and Psychiatry*, doi: 10.1111/j.1469–7610.2008.01909.x.

Naidermeyer, E. and Naidu, S. (1998). Rett syndrome, EEG and the motor cortex as a model for better understanding of attention deficit hyperactivity disorder (ADHD). *European Child and Adolescent Psychiatry*, 7(2), 69–72.

National Institute for Health and Clinical Excellence. (2008). *Attention Deficit Hyperactivity Disorder: Diagnosis and Management of ADHD in Children, Young People and Adults*. London: NCCMH.

Nigg, J. and Breslau, N. (2007). Prenatal smoking exposure, low birth weight and disruptive behaviour disorders. *Journal of the American Academy of Child and Adolescent Psychiatry*, (46), 362–369.

Oas, P. (2001). *Curing ADD/ADHD Children*. North Carolina. Pentland Press.

O'Connor, T., Dunn, J., Jenkins, J., Pickering, K. and Rasbash, J. (2001). Family settings and children's adjustment: differential adjustment within and across families. *British Journal of Psychiatry*, (179), 110–115.

Olfson, M., Gameroff, M., Marcus, S. and Jensen, P. (2002). National trends in the use of psychotropic medications by children. *American Journal of Psychiatry*, 160, 1071–1077.

Pastor, P. and Reuben, C. (2005). *Racial and Ethnic Differences in ADHD and LD in Young School-Age Children: Parental Reports in the National Health Interview Survey*. Public Health Reports, (120), 383–392.

Plizska, S., Carlson, C. and Swanson, J. (1999). *ADHD with Comorbid Disorders: Clinical Assessment and Management*. New York: Guilford Press.

Plomin, R. and Bergeman, C. (1991). The nature of nurture: genetic influences on environmental measures. *Behavioral and Brain Sciences*, 14(3), 373–427.

Polanczyk, G., Lima, M., Horta, B., Biederman, J. and Rohde, L. (2007). The world-wide prevalence of ADHD: a systematic review and metaregression analysis. *American Journal of Psychiatry*, (164), 942–948.

Rafalovich, A. (2001). The conceptual history of attention deficit hyperactivity disorder: idiocy, imbecility, encephalitis and the child deviant. *Deviant Behaviour*, 22(2), 93–115.

Ramchandani. P., Joughin, C. and Zwi, M. (2002). Attention deficit hyperactivity disorder in children. *Clinical Evidence*, (7), 262–271.

Reid, R., Hakendorf, P. and Prosser, B. (2002). Use of psychostimulant medication in South Australia. *Journal of the American Academy of Child and Adolescent Psychiatry*, 41(8), 906–913.

Reid, R., Riccio, C., Kessler, R., DuPaul, G., Power, T., Anastopoulos, A., Rogers-Adkinson, D. and Noll, M. (2000). Gender and ethnic differences in ADHD as assessed by behavior ratings. *Journal of Emotional and Behavioral Disorders*, 8(1), 38–48.

Richardson, A. (2004). Clinical trials of fatty acid treatment in ADHD, dyslexia, dyspraxia and the autistic spectrum. *Prostaglandins, Leukotrienes and Essential Fatty Acids*, (70), 383–390.

Richardson, A. and Montgomery, P. (2005). The Oxford-Durham study: a randomised controlled trial of dietary supplementation with fatty acids in children with developmental coordination disorder. *Pediatrics*, 115 (5), 1360–1366.

Richardson, A. and Puri, B. (2002). A randomised, double-blind, placebo-controlled study of the effects of supplementation with highly unsaturated fatty acids on ADHD-related symptoms in children with specific learning disabilities. *Progress in Neuro-psychopharmacology and Biological Psychiatry*, (26), 233–239.

Rowe, K. (1988). Synthetic food colourings and hyperactivity. *Australian Paediatric Journal*, 24(2), 143–147.

Rowe, K. and Rowe, K. (1994). Synthetic food coloring and behaviour: a dose response effect in a double-blind, placebo-controlled, repeated-measures study. *Journal of Pediatrics*, (125), 691–698.

Rubia, K., Overmeyer, S., Taylor, E., Brammer, M., Williams, S., Simmons, A., Andrew, C. and Bullmore, E. (1999). Hypofrontality in attention deficit hyperactivity disorder during higher order motor control: a study with FMRI. *American Journal of Psychiatry*, (156), 891–896.

Rubia, K., Smith, A., Brammer, M., Toone, B. and Taylor, E. (2005). Abnormal brain activation during inhibition and error detection in medication naïve adolescents with ADHD. *American Journal of Psychiatry*, (162), 1067–1075.

Rutter, M. (1988). *Studies of Psychosocial Risk: the Power of Longitudinal Data*. Cambridge: Cambridge University Press.

Rutter, M., Cox, A., Tupling, C., Berger, M. and Yule, W. Attainment and adjustment in two geographical areas: 1: the prevalence of psychiatric disorder. *British Journal of Psychiatry*, (126), 493–509.

Rutter, M., Giller, H. and Hagell, A. (1998). *Antisocial Behaviour by Young People*. Cambridge: Cambridge University Press.

Ruxton, C. (2004). Health benefits of omega-3 fatty acids. *Nursing Standard*, 18(48), 38–42.

Salmon, J. (2005). Hyperactive children. In: Williams, R. and Kerfoot, M. (Eds). *Child and Adolescent Mental Health Services: Strategy, Planning, Delivery and Evaluation*. Oxford: Oxford University Press.

Sayal, K. (2008). Attention deficit hyperactivity disorder. In: Jackson, C., Hill, K. and Lavis, P. (Eds). *Child and Adolescent Mental Health Today: a Handbook*. London: Pavilion.

Schacher, R. and Tannock, R. (2002). Syndromes of hyperactivity and attention deficit. In: Rutter, M. and Taylor, E. (Eds). *Child and Adolescent Psychiatry* (4th Edition). Oxford: Blackwell Publishing.

Searight, H. and McLaren, L. (1998). Attention deficit hyperactivity disorder: the medicalization of misbehaviour. *Journal of Clinical Psychology in Medical Settings*, 5(4), 467–495.

Sever, Y., Ashkenazi, A. and Tyano, S. (1997). Iron treatment in children with attention deficit hyperactivity disorder: a preliminary report. *Neuropsychobiology*, (35), 178–180.

Shannon, W. (1922). Neuropathic manifestations in infants and children as a result of anaphylactic reactions to foods contained in their dietary. *American Journal of Child Disabled Children*, (24), 89–94.

Shaw, P., Eckstrand, K., Sharp, W., Blumenthal, J., Lerch, J., Greenstein, D., Clasen, L., Evans, A., Giedd, J. and Rapoport, J. (2007). Attention deficit hyperactivity disorder is characterised by a delay in cortical maturation. *Biological Sciences/Psychology*, 104(49), 19649–19654.

Shrag, P. and Divoky, D. (1975). *The Myth of the Hyperactive Child*. New York: Pantheon.

Singh, I. (2004). Doing their jobs: mothering with Ritalin in a culture of mother-blame. *Social Science and Medicine*, (59), 1193–1205.

Singh, I. (2002). Bad boys, good mothers and the 'miracle' of Ritalin. *Science in Context*, 15(4), 577–603.

Sonuga, B. and Balding, J. (1993). British parents' beliefs about the causes of three forms of childhood psychological disturbance. *Journal of Abnormal Child Psychology*, (21), 367–376.

Sonuga-Barke, E. (1998). Categorical models in child psychopathology: a conceptual and empirical analysis. *Journal of Child Psychology and Psychiatry and Allied Disciplines*, (39), 115–133.

Spencer, T., Biederman, S., and Mick, E. (2007). Attention deficit hyperactivity disorder: diagnosis, lifespan, comorbidities and neurobiology. *Journal of Pediatric Psychology*, 32(6), 631–642.

Spender, Q., Salt, N., Dawkins, J., Kendrick, T. and Hill, P. (2001). *Child Mental Health in Primary Care*. Oxford: Radcliffe Medical Press.

Sprich, S., Bierderman, J., Crawford, M., Mundy, E. and Faraone, S. (2000). Adoptive and biological families of children and adolescents with ADHD. *Journal of the American Academy of Child and Adolescent Psychiatry*, (39), 1432–1437.

Starobrat-Hermelin, B. and Kozielec, T. (1997). The effects of magnesium physiological supplementation on hyperactivity in children with attention deficit hyperactivity disorder (ADHD): positive response to magnesium oral loading test. *Magnesium Research*, 10(2), 149–156.

Stevenson, J. and Williams, D. (2000). Parental investment, self-control and sex differences in the expression of ADHD. *Human Nature*, (11), 405–422.

Still, G. (1902). The Goulstonian lectures on some abnormal psychical conditions in childhood. *Lancet*, (1), 1008–1012.

Swanson, J., Sergeant, J., Taylor, E., Sonuga-Barke, E., Jensen, P. and Cantwell, D. (1998a). Attention deficit hyperactivity disorder and hyperkinetic disorder. *Lancet*, (351), 429–433.

Swanson, J., Sunohara, G., Kennedy, J., Regino, R., Fineberg, E., Wigal, T., Lerner, M., Williams, L., LaHoste, G. and Wigal, S. (1998b). Association of the dopamine receptor D4 (DRD4) gene with a refined phenotype of attention deficit hyperactivity disorder (ADHD): a family-based approach. *Molecular Psychiatry*, 3(1), 38–41.

Szatmari, P., Offord, D. and Boyle, M. (1989). Ontario Child Health Study: prevalence of attention deficit disorder with hyperactivity. *Journal of Child Psychology and Psychiatry and Allied Disciplines*, (30), 219–230.

Tannock, R. (1998). ADHD: Advances in cognitive neurobiological and genetic research. *Journal of Child Psychology and Psychiatry*, 39(1), 65.

Taylor, E., Dopfner, M., Sergeant, J., Asherson, P., Banaschewski, T., Rothenberger, A., Buitelaar, J., Coghill, D., Danckaerts, M., SonugaBarke, E., Steinhausen, H. and Zuddas, A. (2004). European clinical guidelines for hyperkinetic disorder: first upgrade. *European Child and Adolescent Psychiatry*, 13(1), 1–30.

Timimi, S. (2005). *Naughty Boys: Antisocial Behaviour, ADHD and the Role of Culture*. London: Palgrave Macmillan.

Timimi, S. (2004). Developing non-toxic approaches to helping children who could be diagnosed with ADHD and their families: reflections of a UK clinician. *Ethical Human Psychology and Psychiatry*, (6), 41–52.

Timimi, S. (2002). *Pathological Child Psychiatry and the Medicalisation of Childhood*. Hove: Brunner/Routledge.

Timimi, S. and Radcliffe, N. (2005). The rise and rise of ADHD. In: Newnes, C. and Radcliffe, N. (Eds). *Making and Breaking Children's Lives*. Ross-on-Wye: PCCS Books.

Timimi, S. and Taylor, E. (2004). ADHD is best understood as a cultural construct. *British Journal of Psychiatry*, (184), 8–9.

Thapar, A., Holmes, J., Poulton, K. and Harrington, R. (1999). Genetic basis of attention deficit and hyperactivity. *British Journal of Psychiatry*, 174, 105–111.

Thapar, A., Langley, K., Asherson. P. and Gill, M. (2007). Gene-environment interplay in attention-deficit hyperactivity disorder and the importance of a developmental perspective. *British Journal of Psychiatry*, 190, 1–3.

Thapar, A., O'Donovan, M. and Owen, M. (2005). The genetics of attention deficit hyperactivity disorder. *Human Molecular Genetics*, 14 (2), 275–282.

Tredgold, A. (1908). *Mental Deficiency (Amentia)* New York: W. Wood.

Utting, D., Bright, J. and Henricson, C. (1993). *Crime and the Family: Improving Child Rearing and Preventing Delinquency*. London: Family Policy Studies Centre.

Voeller, K. (2004). Attention deficit hyperactivity disorder (ADHD). *Journal of Child Neurology*, (19), 798–814.

Voigt, R., Llorente, A., Jensen, C., Fraley, J., Berretta, M. and Heird, W. (2001). A randomised, double-blind, placebo-controlled trial of docosahexaenoic acid supplementation in children with attention deficit/hyperactivity disorder, *Journal of Pediatrics*, 139(2), 189–196.

Volkow, N., Wang, G., Fowler, J., and Logan, J. (2002). Relationship between blockade of dopamine transporters by oral methylphenidate and the increases in extracellular dopamine: therapeutic implications. *Synapse*, (43), 181–187.

Wender, P. (1995). *Attention Deficit/Hyperactivity Disorder in Adults*. New York: Oxford University Press.

Wiesz, J. and Weiss, B. (1991). Studying the 'referability' of child clinical problems. *Journal of Counselling and Clinical Psychology*, (59), 266–273.

Williams, J. and Ross, L. (2007). Consequences of prenatal toxin exposure for mental health in children and adolescents: a systematic review. *European Child and Adolescent Psychiatry*, (16), 243–253.

Willoughby, M. (2003). Developmental course of ADHD symptomatology during the transition from childhood to adolescence: a review with recommendations. *Journal of Child Psychology and Psychiatry*, 44(1), 88–106.

Wolraich, M., Wilson, D. and White, J. (1995). The effect of sugar on behavior or cognition in children: a meta-analysis. *Journal of the American Medical Association*, (274), 1617–1621.

Zametkin, A., Liebenauer, L. and Fitzgerald, G. (1993). Brain metabolism in teenagers with attention deficit hyperactivity disorder. *Archives of General Psychiatry*, (50), 333–340.

Chapter 2 Diagnostic frameworks and ADHD

American Psychiatric Association. (1994). *Diagnostic and Statistical Manual of Mental Disorders* (4th Edition). Washington: APA.

Asherson, P. (2005). Clinical assessment and treatment of attention deficit hyperactivity disorder in adults. *Expert Review of Neurotherapeutics*, 5(4), 525–539.

Biederman, J. and Faraone, S. (2005). Attention deficit hyperactivity disorder. *Lancet*, (366), 237–248.

British Psychological Society. (2000). *Attention Deficit/Hyperactivity Disorder: Guidelines and Principles for Successful Multi-Agency Working: Report of a Working Party of the British Psychological Society*. Leicester: BPS.

Crowe, M. (2000). Psychiatric diagnosis: some implications for mental health nursing care. *Journal of Advanced Nursing*, 31(3), 583–589.

Ellis, D. (2003). The value of nursing diagnosis. In: Barker, P. (Ed) *Psychiatric and Mental Health Nursing: the Craft of Caring*. London: Arnold.

Faraone, S., Biederman, J. and Spencer, T. (2006). Diagnosing adult attention deficit hyperactivity disorder: are late onset and subthreshold diagnoses valid? *American Journal of Psychiatry*, (163), 1720–1729.

Frisch, N. and Kelley, J. (2002). Nursing diagnosis and nursing theory: exploration of factors inhibiting and supporting simultaneous use. *Nursing Diagnosis*, April–June 2002,

Gadow, K., Nolan, E. and Litcher, L. (2000). Comparison of attention deficit/hyperactivity disorder symptom subtypes in Ukrainian schoolchildren. *Journal of American Academy of Child and Adolescent Psychiatry*, (39), 1520–1527.

Gillberg, C. (2003) ADHD and DAMP: a general health perspective. *Child and Adolescent Mental Health*, 8(3), 106–113.

Gillberg, C. (1981). *Neuropsychiatric Aspects of Perceptual, Motor and Attentional Deficits in 7-Year-Old Swedish Children*. Unpublished thesis, Uppsala University. Acta Universitas Upsaliensis. No. 408.

Gordon, M., Antshel, K., Faraone, S., Barkley, R., Lewandowski, L., Hudziak, J., Biederman, J. and Cunningham, C. (2006). Symptoms versus impairment. *Journal of Attention Disorders*, 9(3), 465–475.

Gowers, S. and Glaze, R. (2005). Classification and epidemiology. In: Gowers, S. (Ed). *Seminars in Child and Adolescent Psychiatry* (2nd Edition). London: Gaskell.

Hill, P. and Taylor, E. (2001). An auditable protocol for treating attention deficit hyperactivity disorder. *Archives of Disease in Childhood*, (84), 404–409.

Hoyt, K. and Cajon, E. (1997). Validating nursing with NANDA, NIC and NOC. *Journal of Emergency Nursing*, 23(6), 507–509.

Institute of Medicine. (1989). *Research on Children and Adolescents with Mental, Behavioral and Developmental Disorders*: Washington DC: National Academy Press.

Kidd, P. (2000). Attention deficit/hyperactivity disorder in children: rationale for its integrative management. *Alternative Medicine Review*, 5(5), 402–428.

Landgraf, J., Rich, M. and Rappaport, L. (2002). Measuring quality of life in children with attention deficit hyperactivity disorders and their families: development and evaluation of a new tool. *Archives of Pediatric and Adolescent Medicine*, (156), 384–391.

Landgren, M., Kjellman, B. and Gillberg, C. (2000). Deficits in attention, motor control and perception (DAMP): a simplified school entry examination. *Acta Paediatrica*, (89), 302–309.

Lee, S., Schacher, R., Chen, S., Ornstein, T., Charach, A., Barr, C. and Ickowicz, A. (2008). Predictive validity of DSM-IV and ICD-10 criteria for ADHD and hyperkinetic disorder. *Journal of Child Psychology and Psychiatry*, 49(1), 70–78.

Maughan, B., Brock, A. and Ladva, G. (2004). Chapter 12: mental health. In: Office for National Statistics. (Ed). *The Health of Children and Young People*. London: ONS.

National Institute for Health and Clinical Excellence. (2008). *Attention Deficit Hyperactivity Disorder: Diagnosis and Management of ADHD in Children, Young People and Adults*. London: NCCMH.

Nolan, P. (1998). *A History of Mental Health Nursing*. London: Chapman and Hall.

Parsons, S. (2003). Classification and nursing. In: Barker Barker, P. (Ed). *Psychiatric and Mental Health Nursing: The Craft of Caring*. London: Arnold.

Pineda, D., Ardila, A. and Rosselli, M. (1999). Prevalence of attention deficit/hyperactivity disorder symptoms in 4- to 17-year-old children in the general population. *Journal of Abnormal Child Psychology*, (27), 455–462.

Rasmussen, P. (1982). *Neuropediatric Aspects of Seven-Year-Old Children with Perceptual, Motor and Attentional Deficits*. Unpublished thesis. University of Gothenburg.

Roberts, R., Attkinson, C. and Rosenblatt, A. (1998). Prevalence of psychopathology among children and adolescents. *American Journal of Psychiatry*, (155), 715–725.

Robins, E. and Guze, S. (1970). Establishment of diagnostic validity in psychiatric illness: its application to schizophrenia. *American Journal of Psychiatry*, (126), 983–987.

Ryan, N. (2007a). Non-medical prescribing in a child and adolescent mental health service. *Mental Health Practice*, 11(1), 40–44.

Ryan, N. (2007b). Nurse prescribing in child and adolescent mental health services. *Mental Health Practice*, 10(10), 35–37.

Rydelius, P. (2000). DAMP and MBD versus AD/HD and hyperkinetic disorders. *Acta Pediatrica*, (89), 266–268.

Schacher, R. and Tannock, R. (2002). Syndromes of hyperactivity and attention deficit. In: Rutter, M. and Taylor, E. (Eds). *Child and Adolescent Psychiatry* (4th Edition). Oxford: Blackwell Publishing.

Shaffer, D., Gould, M., and Brasic, J. (1983). A children's global assessment scale (CGAS). *Archives of General Psychiatry*, (40), 1228–1231.

Shoemaker, J. (1984). *NANDA Delphi Study*. Philadelphia: NANDA.

Spitzer, R. and Wakefield, J. (1999). DSM-IV diagnostic criterion for clinical significance: does it help the false positives problem? *American Journal of Psychiatry*, 156(12), 1856–1864.

Taylor, E., Dopfner, M., Sergeant, J., Asherson, P., Banaschewski, T., Rothenberger, A., Buitelaar, J., Coghill, D., Danckaerts, M., Sonuga-Barke, E., Steinhausen, H. and Zuddas, A. (2004). European clinical guidelines for hyperkinetic disorder: first upgrade. *European Child and Adolescent Psychiatry*, 13(1), 1–30.

Taylor, E., Sandberg, S., Thorley, G. and Giles, S. (1991). *The Epidemiology of Childhood Hyperactivity: Maudsley Monographs*. London: Oxford University Press.

Timimi, S. (2004). Developing non-toxic approaches to helping children who could be diagnosed with ADHD and their families: reflections of a UK clinician. *Ethical Human Psychology and Psychiatry*, (6), 41–52.

Vlam, S. (2006). Attention deficit/hyperactivity disorder: diagnostic assessment methods used by advanced practice registered nurses. *Pediatric Nursing* 32(1), 18–24.

Williams, R. and Salmon, G. (2002). Collaboration in commissioning and delivering child and adolescent mental health services. *Current Opinion in Psychiatry*, (15), 349–353.

World Health Organisation. (1993). *The ICD-10 Classification of Mental and Behavioural Disorders: Clinical Descriptions and Diagnostic Guidelines*. Geneva: WHO.

Chapter 3 Assessment and diagnosis

Achenbach, T. (1995). Diagnosis, assessment and comorbidity in psychosocial treatment research. *Journal of Abnormal Child Psychology*, (23), 45–65.

Achenbach, T. (1991). *Manual for the Child Behaviour Checklist 4–18 and 1991 Profile*. US Research Center for Children, Youth and Families/Achenbach System of Empirically Based Assessment (ASEBA).

American Academy of Child and Adolescent Psychiatry. (2007). Practice parameter for the assessment of the family. *Journal of the American Academy of Child and Adolescent Psychiatry*, 46(7), 922–937.

Armstrong, M. (2006). Young people, self-harm and nursing. In: McDougall, T. (Ed). *Child and Adolescent Mental Health Nursing*. London: Blackwell.

Baker, P. and Eversley, J. (2000). *Multilingual Capital*. London: Battlebridge.

Barker, P. (2003a). Person-centred care; the need for diversity. In: Barker, P. (Ed). *Psychiatric and Mental Health Nursing: the Craft of Caring*. London: Arnold.

Barker, P. (2003b). The value of nursing diagnosis. In: Barker, P. (Ed). *Psychiatric and Mental Health Nursing: the Craft of Caring*. London: Arnold.

Barker, P. (1997). *Assessment in Psychiatric and Mental Health Nursing: In Search of the Whole Person*. Cheltenham: JK Stanley Thornes.

Barkley, R. (1991). The ecological validity of laboratory and analogue assessment methods of ADHD symptoms. *Journal of Abnormal Child Psychology*, (19), 149–178.

Barkley, R. and Murphy, K. (1998). *Attention Deficit Hyperactivity Disorder: a Clinical Workbook* (2nd Edition). New York: Guilford Press.

Bird, S. and Emond, A. (2007). Attention deficit or lack of attention? *Archives of Disease in Child Education Practice*, (92), 76–81.

British Psychological Society. (2000). *Attention Deficit/Hyperactivity Disorder: Guidelines and Principles for Successful Multi-Agency Working: Report of a Working Party of the British Psychological Society*. Leicester: BPS.

Broderick, C. and Schrader, S. (1991). The history of professional marriage and family therapy. In: Gurman, A. and Kniskern, D. (Eds). *Handbook of Family Therapy*. New York: Brunner/Mazel.

Brown, G. (2003). Assessment of attention deficit hyperactivity disorder. *Nursing Times*, 99(25), 34–36.

Brown, G. and Bruce, K. (2004). A nurse-led ADHD service for children and adolescents. *Nursing Times*, 100(40), 36–38.

Brown, T. (1996). *Brown Attention Deficit Disorder Scales*. Texas: Psychological Corporation, Harcourt Brace and Company.

Brunette, E. (1995). Management of ADHD in the school setting: a case study. *Journal of School Nursing*, (11), 33–38.

Bussing, R., Gary, F., Mills, T. and Wilson-Garvan, C. (2003). Parental explanatory models of ADHD: gender and cultural variations. *Social Psychiatry and Psychiatric Epidemiology*, (38), 563–575.

Caldwell, C., Wasson, D., Anderson, M., Brighton, V. and Dixon, L. (2005). Development of the nursing outcome (NOC) label: hyperactivity level. *Journal of Child and Adolescent Psychiatric Nursing*, 18(3), 95–102.

Canino, I. and Inclan, J. (2001). Culture and family therapy. *Child and Adolescent Psychiatric Clinics of North America*, (10), 601–612.

Christner, R., Stewart, J. and Freeman, A. (2007). *Handbook of Cognitive-Behavior Group Therapy with Children and Adolescents*. London: Routledge.

Chu, S. (2003a). Attention deficit hyperactivity disorder (ADHD) part 1: a review of the literature. *International Journal of Therapy and Rehabilitation*, 10(5), 218–227.

Chu, S. (2003b). Attention deficit hyperactivity disorder (ADHD) part 2: evaluation and intervention. *International Journal of Therapy and Rehabilitation*, 10(6), 254–263.

Conners, C. (1998a). Rating scales in attention deficit/hyperactivity disorder: use in assessment and treatment monitoring. *Journal of Clinical Psychiatry*, (59), 24–30.

Conners, K., Sitarenios, G., Parker, J. and Epstein, J. (1998b). The revised Conners Parent Rating Scale (CPRS-R): factor structure, reliability and criterion. *Journal of Abnormal Child Psychology*, 26(4), 257–268.

Conners, K., Sitarenios, G., Parker, J. and Epstein, J. (1998c). Revision and restandardization of the Conners Teacher Rating Scale (CTRS-R): factor structure, reliability and criterion. *Journal of Abnormal Child Psychology*, 26(4), 279–291.

Conners, C. (1997a). *Conners' Rating Scales Revised Technical Manual*. New York: Multi Health Systems.

Conners, C. (1997b). A new self report scale for assessment of adolescent psychopathology: factor structure, reliability and diagnostic sensitivity. *Journal of Abnormal Child Psychology*, 25(6), 487–497.

Department of Health. (2007). *New Ways of Working for Everyone: Developing and Sustaining a Capable and Flexible Workforce*. London: HMSO.

Department of Health. (2006). *Improving Patients' Access to Medicines: a Guide to Implementing Nurse and Pharmacist Independent Prescribing in the NHS in England*. London: HMSO.

Department of Health. (2004). *The National Service Framework for Children, Young People and Maternity Services: Standard 9 – Mental Health and Psychological Wellbeing of Children and Young People*. London: HMSO.

DuPaul, G., Power, T., Anastopoulos, A. and Reid, R. (1998). *ADHD Rating Scale IV: Checklists, Norms and Clinical Interpretation*. New York: Guilford.

Flaskas, C. (1997). Engagement and the therapeutic relationship in systemic therapy. *Journal of Family Therapy*, (19), 263–282.

Furman, L. (2005). What is attention deficit hyperactivity disorder? *Journal of Child Neurology*, 20(12), 994–1002.

Garcia-Jimenez, M., Lopez-Pison, J. and Blasco-Arrelano, M. (2006). The primary care paediatrician in attention deficit hyperactivity disorder: an approach involving a population study. *Revista de Neurologia*, 41(2), 191–192.

Goodman, R. (1997). The strengths and difficulties questionnaire: a research note. *Journal of Child Psychology and Psychiatry*, (38), 581–586.

Goodman, R., Meltzer, H. and Bailey, V. (1998). The Strengths and Difficulties Questionnaire: a pilot study on the validity of the self report version. *European Child and Adolescent Psychiatry*, 7(3), 125–130.

Harborne, A., Wolpert, M. and Clare, L. (2004). Making sense of ADHD: a battle for understanding parents' views of their children being diagnosed with ADHD. *Clinical Child Psychology and Psychiatry*, 9(3), 327–339.

Harding, S. (2006). *Taking on ADHD*. YoungMinds, (80), 21.

Higgins, I. and McDougall, T. (2006). Nursing children and adolescents who are aggressive or violent: a psychological approach. In: McDougall, T. (ed). *Child and Adolescent Mental Health Nursing*. London: Blackwell.

Hill, P. and Taylor, E. (2001). Current topic: an auditable protocol for treating attention deficit/hyperactivity disorder. *Archives of Disease in Childhood*, (84), 404–409.

Hinshaw, S. (1994). *Attention Deficits and Hyperactivity in Children*. California: Sage.

Hinton, C. E. and Wolpert, M. (1998) Why is ADHD such a compelling story? *Clinical Child Psychology and Psychiatry*, 3(2), 315–317.

Jones, J. (2004). *The Post-Registration Education and Training Needs of Nurses Working with Children and Young People with Mental Health Problems in the UK: A Research Study Conducted by the Mental Health Programme, Royal College of Nursing Institute, in Collaboration with the RCN Children and Young People's Mental Health Forum*. London: RCN Institute.

Jones, J. and Baldwin, L. (2004). Tiers before bedtime: a survey shows post-registration CAMHS education is missing the mark. *Mental Health Practice*, 7(6), 14–17.

Joseph, B. (1998). Thinking about a playroom. *Journal of Child Psychotherapy*, (24), 359–366.

Keen, D. (2005). ADHD and the paediatrician: a guide to management. *Current Paediatrics*, 15(2), 133–142.

Keen, T. and Keen, J. (2003). Developing collaborative assessment. In: Barker, P. (Ed). *Psychiatric and Mental Health Nursing: the Craft of Caring*. London: Arnold.

Kelly, C. and Rounsley, C. (2004). Introducing a school-based monitoring system for children taking methylphenidate. *Royal College of Nursing: Nursing Minds*, (Autumn 2004), 6–7.

Koskelainen, M., Sourander, A. and Kaljonen, A. (2000). The Strengths and Difficulties Questionnaire among Finnish school-aged children and adolescents. *European Child and Adolescent Psychiatry*, 9(4), 277–284.

Lahey, B., McBurnett, K. and Piacentini, J. (1987). Agreement of parent and teacher rating scales with comprehensive clinical assessment of attention deficit disorder with hyperactivity. *Journal of Psychopathology and Behavioral Assessment*, 9(4), 429–439.

Laver-Bradbury, C. (2003). The role of the nurse: helping children with ADHD and their families. *Child and Adolescent Mental Health in Primary Care*, 1(3), 77–81.

Law, J. and Garnett, Z. (2004) Speech and language therapy: its potential role in CAMHS. *Child and Adolescent Mental Health*, 9(2), 50–55.

Leighton, S. (2006). Nursing children and young people with emotional disorders. In: McDougall, T. (ed). *Child and Adolescent Mental Health Nursing*. London: Blackwell.

Lewer, L. (2006). Nursing children and young people with eating disorders. In: McDougall, T. (ed). *Child and Adolescent Mental Health Nursing*. London: Blackwell.

Ludwikowski, K. and DeValk, M. (1998). Attention deficit/hyperactivity disorder: a neurodevelopmental approach. *Journal of Child and Adolescent Psychiatric Nursing*, 11(1), 17–29.

McDougall, T. (2006). *Child and Adolescent Mental Health Nursing*. London: Blackwell.

McGoldrick, M. and Gerson, R. (1985). *Genograms in Family Assessment*. New York: Norton.

McMorrow, R. (2006). Nursing children and young people in a multicultural society: an acculturation model. In: McDougall, T. (ed). *Child and Adolescent Mental Health Nursing*. London: Blackwell.

Miller, W. and Rollnick, S. (2002). *Motivational Interviewing: Preparing People for Change* (2nd Edition). New York: Guilford Press.

Ministry of Health. (2001). *New Zealand Guidelines for the Assessment and Treatment of Attention Deficit Hyperactivity Disorder*. Wellington: Ministry of Health.

Mitchell, P. (2006). Adolescent forensic mental health nursing. In: McDougall, T. (ed). *Child and Adolescent Mental Health Nursing*. London: Blackwell.

Moncher, F. and Josephson, A. (2004). Religious and spiritual assessment of the family. *Child and Adolescent Psychiatric Clinics of North America*, (13), 49–70.

National Institute for Health and Clinical Excellence. (2008). *Attention Deficit Hyperactivity Disorder: Diagnosis and Management of ADHD in Children, Young People and Adults*. London: NCCMH.

Osman, K. and Parker, J. (2003). ADHD: how are specialist nurses doing? *Child and Adolescent Mental Health in Primary Care*, 1(3), 82–84.

Parke, R. (2000). Beyond white and middle class: cultural variations in families, assessments, processes and policies. *Journal of Family Psychology*, (14), 331–333.

Partridge, I., Richardson, G., Casswell, G and Jones, N. (2003). Multi-disciplinary team-working. In: Richardson, G. and Partridge, I. (Eds). *Child and Adolescent Mental Health Services, An Operational Handbook*. London: Gaskell.

Porter, L. (1988). The what, why and how of hyperkinesis. *Journal of Advanced Nursing*, (13), 229–236.

Power, T. (1994). The school psychologist as manager of programming for ADHD. *School Psychology Review*, 23(2), 279–291.

Prochaska, J. and DiClemente, C. (1982). Transtheoretical therapy: toward a more integrative model of change. *Psychotherapy: Theory, Research and Practice*, (19), 276–288.

Reder, P. and Fredman, G. (1996). The relationship to help: interacting beliefs about the treatment process. *Clinical Child Psychology and Psychiatry*, (1), 457–467.

Richardson-Todd, B. (2003). Setting up a nurse-run young people's drop in clinic. *Nursing Standard*, 17(47), 38–41.

Ronning, J., Handegaard, B., Sourander, A. and Morch, W. (2003). The Strengths and Difficulties Self Report Questionnaire as a screening instrument in Norwegian community samples. *European Child and Adolescent Psychiatry*, 13(2), 73–82.

Ryan, N. (2006). Nursing children and young people with ADHD. In: McDougall, T. (Ed). *Child and Adolescent Mental Health Nursing*. London: Blackwell.

Ryan, N. (2007a). Non-medical prescribing in a child and adolescent mental health service. *Mental Health Practice*, 11(1), 40–44.

Ryan, N. (2007b). Nurse prescribing in child and adolescent mental health services. *Mental Health Practice*, 10(10), 35–37.

Safer, D. (2000). Commentary. *Journal of American Academy of Child and Adolescent Psychiatry*, (39), 989–992.

Safren, S., Otto, M., Sprich, S., Winett, C., Wilens, T. and Biederman, J. (2005). Cognitive-behavioral therapy for ADHD in medication treated adults with continued symptoms. *Behaviour Research and Therapy*, 43(7), 831–842.

Salmon, G., Cleave, H. and Samuel, C. (2006). Development of multi-agency referral pathways for attention deficit hyperactivity disorder, developmental coordination disorder and autistic spectrum disorders: reflections on the process and suggestions for new ways of working. *Clinical Child Psychology and Psychiatry*, 11(1), 63–81.

Scahill, L., Lynch, K. and Ort, S. (1995). Tourette syndrome: update and review. *Journal of School Nursing*, (11), 26–32.

Scahill, L. and Ort, S. (1995). Selection and use of clinical rating instruments in child psychiatric nursing. *Journal of Child and Adolescent Psychiatric Nursing*, 8(3), 33–34.

Schacher, R. and Tannock, R. (2002). Syndromes of hyperactivity and attention deficit. In: Rutter, M. and Taylor, E. (Eds). *Child and Adolescent Psychiatry* (4th Edition). Oxford: Blackwell Publishing.

Stevenson, C. (2003). The context of assessment: families. In: Barker, P. (Ed). *Psychiatric and Mental Health Nursing: the Craft of Caring*. London: Arnold.

Tan, J. and Jones, D. (2001). Children's consent. *Current Opinion in Psychiatry*, (14), 303–307.

Taylor, E., Dopfner, M., Sergeant, J., Asherson, P., Banaschewski, T., Rothenberger, A., Buitelaar, J., Coghill, D., Danckaerts, M., Sonuga-Barke, E., Steinhausen, H. and Zuddas, A. (2004). European clinical guidelines for hyperkinetic disorder: first upgrade. *European Child and Adolescent Psychiatry*, 13(1), 1–30.

Wagner, S. (2008). *Motivation to Change Parenting in Mothers of Children with and without ADHD: Associations with Demographic and Psychological Characteristics*. Unpublished thesis, West Virginia University, Morgantown, West Virginia.

Welsh Assembly Government. (2005). *National Service Framework for Children, Young People and Maternity Services.* Cardiff: WAG.

Wilkin, P. (2003) The craft of psychiatric-mental health nursing practice. In: Barker, P. (Ed). *Psychiatric and Mental Health Nursing: the Craft of Caring.* London: Arnold.

Wilson, P. (1991). Psychotherapy with adolescents. In: Holmes, J. (Ed). *Textbook of Psychotherapy in Psychiatric Practice.* New York: Churchill Livingstone.

Wright, P., Turner, C. and Clay, D. (2006). *The Participation of Children and Young People in Developing Social Care.* London: SCIE.

Young, S. and Bramham, J. (2007). *ADHD in Adults: a Psychological Guide to Practice.* London: Wiley and Sons.

Chapter 4 What are the costs of ADHD?

ADDISS. (2006). *ADHD is Real: ADDISS Families Survey.* London: ADDISS Resource Centre.

Anastopoulous, A., Guevremont, D., Shelton, T. and DuPaul, G. (1992). Parenting stress among families of children with attention deficit hyperactivity disorder. *Journal of Abnormal Child Psychology,* 20(5), 503–520.

Anastopolous, A., Shelton, T., DuPaul, G. and Guevremont, D. (1993). Parent training for attention deficit hyperactivity disorder: its impact on parent functioning. *Journal of Abnormal Child Psychology,* (21), 581–596.

Barkley, R., Fischer, M., Smallish, L. and Fletcher, K. (2004). Young adult follow-up of hyperactive children: antisocial activities and drug use. *Journal of Child Psychology and Psychiatry,* 45(2), 195–211.

Biederman, J. (2003). Pharmacotherapy for attention deficit hyperactivity disorder decreases the risk for substance misuse: findings from a longitudinal follow-up of youths with and without ADHD. *Journal of Clinical Psychiatry,* 64(11), 3–8.

Biederman, J., Newcorn, J. and Sprich, S. (1991). Comorbidity of attention deficit hyperactivity disorder with conduct, depressive, anxiety and other disorders. *American Journal of Psychiatry,* (148), 564–577.

Bijur, P., Stewart-Brown, S. and Butler, N. (1986). Child behaviour and accidental injury in 11,966 preschoolchildren. *American Journal of Diseases of Childhood,* (140), 487–492.

Blachman, D. and Hinshaw, S. (2002). Patterns of friendship among girls with and without attention deficit/hyperactivity disorder. *Journal of Abnormal Child Psychology,* (30), 625–640.

Black, D., Arndt, S., and Hale, N. (2004). Use of the MINI International Neuropsychiatric Interview (MINI) as a screening tool in prisons: results of a preliminary study. *Journal of American Academy of Psychiatry and Law,* (32), 158–162.

Brown, R. and Pacini, J. (1989). Perceived family functioning, marital status, and depression in parents of boys with attention deficit disorder. *Journal of Learning Disabilities,* (22), 581–587.

Brown, T. and McMullen, W. (2001). Attention deficit disorders and sleep/arousal disturbance. *Annals of the New York Academy of Sciences,* (931), 271–286.

Bukstein, O., Brent, D. and Kaminer, Y. (1989). Comorbidity of substance abuse and other psychiatric disorders in adolescents. *American Journal of Psychiatry,* (146), 1131–1141.

Cantwell, R., Berwin, J., Glazebrook, C., Dalkin, T., Fox, R., Medley. I., and Harrison, G. (1999). Substance misuse: prevalence of substance misuse in first episode psychosis. *British Journal of Psychiatry*, (174), 150–153.

Charman, T., Carroll, F. and Sturge, C. (2001). Theory of mind, executive function and social competence in boys with ADHD. *Emotional and Behavioural Difficulties*, 6(1), 31–49.

Cramond, B. (1994). Attention deficit disorder and creativity: what is the connection? *Journal of Creative Behaviour*, (28), 193–209.

Crome, I. (2004). Psychiatric comorbidity. In: Crome, I., Ghodse, H., Gilvarry, E. and McArdle, P. (Eds). *Young People and Substance Misuse*. London: Gaskell.

Cunningham, C., Benness, B. and Siegel, L. (1988). Family functioning, time allocation and parental depression in the families of normal and ADHD children. *Journal of Clinical and Child Psychology*, 17(1), 69–77.

Dean, D. (2005). ADHD and its impact on family life. *Mental Health Practice*, 8(9), 22–23.

Department for Education and Skills. (2006). *School Nurse Practice Development Resource Pack: Specialist Community Public Health Nurse*. London: HMSO.

Department of Health. (2004a). *National Service Framework for Children, Young People and Maternity Services: Standard 9 – Mental Health and Psychological Wellbeing*. London: HMSO.

Department of Health. (2004b). *Choosing Health: Making Healthier Choices Easier*. London: HMSO.

DiScala, C., Lescohier, I., Barthel, M. and Li, G. (1998). Injuries to children with attention deficit hyperactivity disorder. *Pediatrics*, (102), 1415–1421.

DuPaul, G., McGoey, K., Eckert, T. and Vanbrakle, J. (2001). Preschool children with attention deficit hyperactivity disorder: impairments in behavioural, social and school functioning. *Journal of the American Academy of Child and Adolescent Psychiatry*, 40(5), 508–515.

Edwards, G., Barkley, R., Laneri, M., Fletcher, K. and Metevia, L. (2001). Parent–adolescent conflict in teenagers with ADHD and ODD. *Journal of Abnormal Child Psychology*, (29), 557–572.

Efron, D., Jarman, F., and Barker, M. (1998). Child and parent perceptions of stimulant medication treatment in attention deficit hyperactivity disorder. *Journal of Paediatrics and Child Health*, 34(3), 288–292.

Fergusson, D., Woodward, L. and Horwood, L. (2000). Risk factors and life processes associated with the onset of suicidal behaviour during adolescence and early adulthood. *Psychological Medicine*, 30(1), 23–29.

Fischer, M., Barkley, R., Fletcher, K. and Smallish, L. (1993). The adolescent outcome of hyperactive children: predictors of psychiatric, academic, social and emotional adjustment. *Journal of the American Academy of Child and Adolescent Psychiatry*, (32), 324–332.

Flicek, M. (1992). Social status of boys with both academic problems and attention deficit hyperactivity disorder. *Journal of Abnormal Child Psychology*, 20(4), 353–366.

Fryers, T. (2007). *Children at Risk: Childhood Determinants of Adult Psychiatric Disorder*. Helsinki: Stakes.

Gerring, J., Brady, K. and Cher A. (1998). Premorbid prevalence of ADHD and development of secondary ADHD after closed head injury. *Journal of American Academy of Child and Adolescent Psychiatry*, (37), 647–654.

Green, R., Biederman, J., Faraone, S. Monuteaux, M., Mick, E. and DuPre, E. (2001).

Social impairment in girls with ADHD: patterns, gender comparisons and correlates. *Journal of the American Academy of Child and Adolescent Psychiatry*, (40), 704–710.

Green, H., McGinnity, A., Meltzer, H., Ford, T. and Goodman, R. (2005). *Mental Health of Children and Young People in Great Britain*. London: ONS.

Greene, R., Biederman, J., Faraone, S., Ouellette, C., Penn, C. and Griffin, M. (1996). Toward a new psychometric definition of social disability in children with attention deficit hyperactivity disorder. *Journal of American Academy of Child and Adolescent Psychiatry*, (35), 571–578.

Guevara, J. and Mandell, D. (2003). Costs associated with attention deficit hyperactivity disorder: overview and future projections. *Expert Review on Pharmacoeconomics and Outcomes Research*, (3), 201–210.

Hall, C., Peterson, A., Webster, R., Bolen, L. and Brown, M. (1999). Perception of non-verbal social cues by regular education, ADHD, and ADHD/LD students. *Psychology in the Schools*, 36(6), 505–514.

Harpin, V. (2005). The effect of ADHD on the life of an individual, their family, and community from preschool to adult life. *Archives of Disease in Childhood*, 90(1), 2–7.

Haynes, N. (1990). Influence of self concept on school adjustment among middle school students. *Journal of Social Psychology*, (130), 199–207.

Henker, B. and Whalen, C. (1999). The child with attention deficit/hyperactivity disorder. In: Quay, H. and Hagen, A. (Eds). *Handbook of Disruptive Behavior Disorders*. New York: Plenum.

Hinshaw, S. (1991). Stimulant medication in the treatment of aggression in children with attentional deficits. *Journal of Clinical Child Psychology*, (12), 301–312.

International Narcotics Control Board. (2003). *Psychotropic Substances: Statistics for 2003, Assessments of Medical and Scientific Requirements for Substances in Schedule II, III and IV*. Retrieved 16 March 2005 from *www.incb.org/e/ind_ar*.

Johnston, C. and Mash, E. (2001). Families of children with attention deficit/hyperactivity disorder: review and recommendations for future research. *Clinical Child and Family Psychology Review*, (4), 183–207.

Kidd, P. (2000). Attention deficit/hyperactivity disorder in children: rationale for its integrative management. *Alternative Medicine Review*, 5(5), 402–428.

King, C., Guaziuddin, N. and McGovern, L. (1996). Predictors of comorbid alcohol and substance misuse in depressed adolescents. *Journal of the American Academy of Child and Adolescent Psychiatry*, (35), 743–751.

King, S., Griffin, S., Hodges, Z. (2006). *A Systematic Review and Economic Model of the Effectiveness and Cost-effectiveness of Methylphenidate, Dexamphetamine and Atomoxetine for the Treatment of Attention Deficit Hyperactivity Disorder in Children and Adolescents*. Health Technology Assessment 10. Tunbridge Wells: Gray Publishing.

Kreuger, M. and Kendall, J. (2001). Descriptions of self: an exploratory study of adolescents with ADHD. *Journal of Child and Adolescent Psychiatric Nursing*, 14(2), 61–72.

Kutner, D. (1999). Blurred brilliance: what AD/HD looks like in gifted adults. *Advanced Development Journal*, (8), 87–112.

Landgraf, J., Rich, M. and Rappaport, L. (2002). Measuring quality of life in children with attention deficit hyperactivity disorders and their families: development and evaluation of a new tool. *Archives of Pediatric and Adolescent Medicine*, (156), 384–391.

Lecendreux, M., Konofal, E., Bouvard, M., Falissard, B., Mouren-Simeoni, M. (2000). Sleep and alertness in children with ADHD. *Journal of Child Psychology and Psychiatry and Allied Disciplines*, (41), 803–812.

Mannuzza, S. and Klein, R. (2000). Long-term prognosis in attention deficit/hyperactivity disorder. *Child and Adolescent Psychiatric Clinics of North America.* (9), 711–726.

Mannuzza, S., Klein, R. and Bessler, A. (1998). Adult psychiatric status of hyperactive boys grown up. *American Journal of Psychiatry*, (155), 493–498.

Mash, E. and Johnston, C. (1983). Parental perceptions of child behaviour problems, parenting self-esteem and mother's reported stress in younger and older hyperactive and normal children. *Journal of Consulting Clinical Psychology*, (51), 86–99.

Maughan, B., Brock, A. and Ladva, G. (2004). Chapter 12: mental health. In: Office for National Statistics. (Ed). *The Health of Children and Young People.* London: ONS.

Melrose, M. and Brodie, I. (2000). Vulnerable Young People and their Vulnerability to Drug Misuse. London: Drugscope.

Merton, R. (1968). *Social Theory and Social Structure.* New York: Free Press.

Molina, B. and Pelham, W. (2003). Childhood predictors of substance misuse in a longitudinal study of children with ADHD. *Journal of Abnormal Psychology*, 112(3), 497–507.

Murphy, K. and Barkley, R. (1996). Parents of children with attention deficit hyperactivity disorder: psychological and attentional impairment. *American Journal of Orthopsychiatry*, (66), 93–102.

Muthukrishna, N. (2007). Inclusion and exclusion in school: experiences of children labelled 'ADHD' in South Africa. In: Lloyd, D., Stead, J. and Cohen, D. (Eds). *Critical New Perspectives on ADHD.* London: Routledge.

National Institute for Health and Clinical Excellence. (2008). *Attention Deficit Hyperactivity Disorder: Diagnosis and Management of ADHD in Children, Young People and Adults.* London: NCCMH.

NHS Information Centre. (2006). *Prescription Cost Analysis (England 2006).* London: Prescribing Support Unit.

Nixon, E. (2001). The social competence of children with attention deficit hyperactivity disorder: a review of the literature. *Child Psychology and Psychiatry Review*, 6(4), 172–180.

Owens, J. (2005). The ADHD and sleep conundrum: a review. *Journal of Developmental Behavioral Pediatrics*, 26(4), 312–322.

Philo, G. (1993). *Mass Media Representation of Mental Health/Illness: Report for the Health Education Board for Scotland.* Glasgow: Glasgow University.

Rasmussen, K., Almvik, R. and Levander, S. (2001). Attention deficit disorder, reading disability and personality disorders in a prison population. *Journal of American Academy of Psychiatry and Law*, (29), 186–193.

Repper, J. and Perkins, R. (2001). Mental health nursing and social inclusion. *Mental Health Practice*, 4(5), 29–32.

Rosen, B. and Peterson, L. (1990). Gender differences in children's outdoor play injuries: a review and an integration. *Clinical Psychology Review*, (10), 187–205.

Rosenberg, M., Schooler, C. and Schoenbach, C. (1989). Self-esteem and adolescent problems: modeling reciprocal effects. *American Sociological Review*, (54), 1004–1018.

Rosler, M., Retz, W., Retz-Junginger, P., Hengesch, G., Schneider, M., Supprian, T., Schwitzgebel, P., Pinhard, K., Dovi-Aku, N., Wender, P. and Thome, J. (2004). Prevalence of attention deficit/hyperactivity disorder (ADHD) and comorbid disorders in young male prison inmates. *European Archives of Psychiatry and Clinical Neuroscience*, (254), 365–371.

Rutter, M. (1990). Psychosocial resilience and protective mechanisms. In: Rolf, J., Garmezy, N., Masten, A., Cicchetti, D., Nuchterlein, K. and Weintraub, S. (Eds). *Risk and Protective Factors in the Development of Psychopathology.* Cambridge: Cambridge University Press.

Satterfield, J., Swanson, J., Schell, A. and Lee, F. (1994). Prediction of antisocial behavior in attention-deficit hyperactivity disorder in boys from aggression/defiance scores. *Journal of American Academy of Child and Adolescent Psychiatry*, (26), 56–64.

Schacher, R. and Tannock, R. (2002). Syndromes of hyperactivity and attention deficit. In: Rutter, M. and Taylor, E. (Eds). *Child and Adolescent Psychiatry* (4th Edition). Oxford: Blackwell Publishing.

Schlander, M. (2007). Impact of attention deficit hyperactivity disorder (ADHD) on prescription drug spending for children and adolescents: increasing relevance of health economic evidence. *Child and Adolescent Psychiatry and Mental Health*, (1), 1–13.

Scott, S., Knapp, M., Henderson, J. and Maughan, B. (2001). Financial cost of social exclusion: follow-up study of anti-social children into adulthood. *British Medical Journal*, (323), 1–5.

Selikowitz, M. (2006). *ADHD: The Facts.* New York: Oxford University Press.

Shattell, M., Bartlett, R. and Rowe, T. (2008). 'I have always felt different': the experience of attention-deficit/hyperactivity disorder. *Journal of Pediatric Nursing*, 23(1), 49–57.

Stein, M. (1999). Unravelling sleep problems in treated and untreated children with ADHD. *Journal of Child and Adolescent Psychopharmacology*, 9(3), 157–168.

Swenson, A., Birnbaum, H., Hamadi, R., Greenberg, P., Cremieux, P. and Secnik, K. (2004). Incidence and costs of accidents among attention deficit/hyperactivity disorder patients. *Journal of Adolescent Health*, (35), 346–356.

Swenson, A., Birnbaum, H., Secnik, K., Marynchenko, M., Greenberg, P. and Claxton, A. (2003). Attention deficit/hyperactivity disorder: increased costs for patients and their families. *Journal of American Academy of Child and Adolescent Psychiatry*, 42(12), 1415–1423.

Taylor, E., Sandberg, S., Thorley, G. and Giles, S. (1991). The epidemiology of childhood hyperactivity. *Maudsley Monographs*, Number 33. London: Institute of Psychiatry.

Vermeiren, R. (2003). Psychopathology and delinquency in adolescents: a descriptive and developmental perspective. *Clinical Psychology Review*, (23), 277–318.

Webb, T. and Latimer, D. (1993). ADHD and children who are gifted. *Exceptional Children*, (60), 60–64.

Wexler, H. (1996). ADHD substance abuse and crime. *Attention*, 2(3), 27–32.

Wilens, T., Biederman, J. and Millstein, R. (1999). Risk of substance use disorders in youths with child and adolescent onset bipolar disorder. *Journal of American Academy of Child and Adolescent Psychiatry*, (38), 680–685.

Young, S. and Bramham, J. (2007). *ADHD in Adults: A Psychological Guide to Practice.* London: Wiley and Sons.

Young, S., Heptinstall, E., Sonuga-Barke, E., Chadwick, O. and Taylor, E. (2005). The adolescent outcome of hyperactive girls: self report of psychosocial status. *Journal of Child Psychology and Psychiatry*, 46(3), 255–262.

Young, S., Mikulich, S. and Goodwin, M. (1995). Treated delinquent boys: substance misuse onset pattern relationship to conduct and mood disorders. *Drug and Alcohol Dependence*, (37), 149–162.

Chapter 5 Major mental health problems and ADHD

American Psychiatric Association. (1994). *Diagnostic and Statistical Manual of Mental Disorders* (4th Edition). Washington: APA.

August, G. and Garfinkel, B. (1990). Comorbidity of ADHD and reading disability among clinic-referred children. *Journal of Abnormal Child Psychology*, 18(1), 10.1007/BF00919454.

Atwood, T. (1998). *Asperger's Syndrome: a Guide for Parents and Professionals*. London: Jessica Kingsley.

Banaschewski, T., Hollis, J., Oosterlaan, J., Roeyers, H., Rubia, K., Willcutt, E. and Taylor, E. (2005). Towards an understanding of unique and shared pathways in the psychopathophysiology of ADHD. *Developmental Science*, 8(2), 132–140.

Barkley, R., DuPaul, G., McMurray, M. (1990). Comprehensive evaluation of attention deficit disorder with and without hyperactivity as defined by research criteria. *Journal of Consulting and Clinical Psychology*, (58), 775–789.

Baron-Cohen, S., Tager-Flusberg, H. and Cohen, D. (1993). *Understanding Other Minds: Perspectives from Autism*. Oxford: Oxford University Press.

Biederman, J., Mick, E., and Bostic, J. (1998). The naturalistic course of pharmacologic treatment of children with manic-like symptoms: a systematic chart review. *Journal of Clinical Psychiatry*, (59), 628–637.

Biederman, J., Newcorn, J. and Sprich, S. (1991). Comorbidity of attention deficit hyperactivity disorder with conduct, depressive, anxiety and other disorders. *American Journal of Psychiatry*, (148), 564–577.

Butler, S., Arrendondo, D. and McCloskey, V. (1995). Affective comorbidity in children and adolescents with attention deficit hyperactivity disorder. *Annals of Clinical Psychiatry*, 7(2) 51–55.

Chadwick, O., Taylor, E. and Bernard, S. (1998). *The Prevention of Behaviour Disorders in Children with Severe Learning Disability. Final Report to the NHS Executive*. London: Institute of Psychiatry.

Clark, T., Feehan, C., Tinline, C. and Vostanis, P. (1999). Autistic symptoms in children with attention deficit hyperactivity disorder. *European Child and Adolescent Psychiatry*, (8), 50–55.

Crome, I. and Gilvarry, E. (2005). Young People and substance misuse. In: Williams, R. and Kerfoot, M. (eds). *Child and Adolescent Mental Health Services: Strategy, Planning, Delivery and Evaluation*. Oxford: Oxford University Press.

Dalsgaard, S., BoMortensen, P., Frydenberg, M. and Thomsen, P. (2002). Conduct problems, gender and adult psychiatric outcomes of children with attention-deficit hyperactivity disorder. *British Journal of Psychiatry*, (181), 416–421.

Dunn, D., Austin, J. and Harezlak, J. (2003). ADHD and epilepsy in childhood. *Developmental Medicine and Child Neurology*, (45), 50–54.

Emerson, M. (2003). Prevalence of psychiatric disorders in children and adolescents with and without intellectual disability. *Journal of Intellectual Disability Research*. (47), 51–58.

Farrington, D. (2007). Childhood risk factors and risk-focused prevention. In: McGuire, M., Morgan, R. and Reiner, R. (Eds). *The Oxford Handbook of Criminology* (4th Edition). Oxford: Oxford University Press.

Fitzgerald, M. and Corvin, A. (2001). Diagnosis and differential diagnosis of Asperger Syndrome. *Advances in Psychiatric Treatment*, (7), 310–318.

Fonagy, P., Target, M., Cottrell, D., Phillips, J. and Kurtz, Z. (2002). *What Works for*

Whom? A Critical Review of Treatments for Children and Adolescents. London: Guilford Press.

Fox, R. and Wade, E. (1998). Attention deficit hyperactivity disorders among adults with severe and profound mental retardation. *Research in Developmental Disabilities*, (19), 275–280.

Furman, L. (2005). What is attention deficit hyperactivity disorder? *Journal of Child Neurology*, 20(12), 994–1002.

Geller, B. and Luby, J. (1997). Child and adolescent bipolar disorder: a review of the past 10 years. *Journal of the American Academy of Child and Adolescent Psychiatry*, 36(9), 1168–1176.

Geller, B., Williams, M., Zimerman, B. and Frazier, J. (1996), *Washington University in St. Louis Kiddie Schedule for Affective Disorders and Schizophrenia (WASH-U-KSADS)*. St Louis: Washington University.

Geller, B., Zimerman, B. and Williams, M. (2002). DSM-IV mania symptoms in a prepubertal and early adolescent bipolar disorder phenotype compared to attention deficit hyperactive and normal controls. *Journal of Child and Adolescent Psychopharmacology*, (12), 11–26.

Gillberg, C. (2003). Deficits in attention, motor control and perception: a brief review. *Archives of Disease in Childhood*, (88), 904–910.

Gillberg, C. and Billstedt, E. (2000). Autism and Asperger syndrome: coexistence with other clinical disorders. *Acta Psychiatrica Scandinavica*, 102(5), 321–330.

Gillberg, C., Gillberg, I., Rasmussen, P., Kadesjö, B., Söderström, H., Rästam, M., Johnson, M., Rothenberger, A., Niklasson, L. (2004). Co-existing disorders in ADHD – implications for diagnosis and intervention. *European Child and Adolescent Psychiatry*, (13), supplement 1, 180–192.

Gillis, J., Gilger, J., Pennington, B. and DeFries, J. (1992). Attention deficit disorder in reading disabled twins: evidence for a genetic etiology. *Journal of Abnormal Child Psychology*, (20), 303–314.

Green, H., McGinnity, A., Meltzer, H., Ford, T. and Goodman, R. (2005). *Mental Health of Children and Young People in Great Britain*. London: ONS.

Hardy, S. and Bouras, N. (2002). The presentation and assessment of mental health problems in people with learning disabilities. *Learning Disability Practice*, 5(3), 33–38.

Hesdorffer, D., Ludvigsson, P., Olafsson, E., Gudmundsson, G., Kjartansson, O. and Hauser, A. (2004). ADHD as a risk factor for incident unprovoked seizures and epilepsy in children. *Archives of General Psychiatry*, 61(7), 731–736.

Hindley, P. and Kroll, L. (1998). Theoretical and epidemiological aspects of attention deficit and overactivity in deaf children. *Journal of Deaf Studies and Deaf Education*, (3), 64–72.

Hinshaw, S. (2002). Preadolescent girls with attention deficit/hyperactivity disorder. 1: background characteristics, comorbidity, cognitive and social functioning, and parenting practices. *Journal of Consulting and Clinical Psychology*, (70), 1086–1098.

Hinshaw. S. (1994). *Attention Deficits and Hyperactivity in Children*. Sage: California.

Hurtig, T., Ebeling, H. Taanila, A., Miettunen, J., Smalley, S., McGough, J., Loo, S., Jarvelin, M-R. and Moilanen, I. (2007). ADHD and comorbid disorders in relation to family environment and symptom severity. *Journal of European Child and Adolescent Psychiatry*, (16), 362–369.

Hyun-Rhee, S., Willcutt, E., Hartman, C., Pennington, B. and DeFries, J. (2006). Test of alternative hypotheses explaining the comorbidity between attention deficit/hyperactivity disorder and conduct disorder. *Journal of Abnormal Child Psychology*, (36), 29–40.

Jensen, P., Martin, D. and Cantwell, D. (1997). Comorbidity in ADHD: implications for research, practice and DSM-V. *Journal of the American Academy of Child and Adolescent Psychiatry*. (36), 1065–1079.

Kaplan, B., Dewey, D., Crawford, S. and Wilson, B. (2001). The term 'comorbidity' is of questionable value in reference to developmental disorders: data and theory. *Journal of Learning Disabilities*, (34), 555–565.

Khune, M., Schacher, R. and Tannock, R. (1997). Impact of comorbid oppositional or conduct problems on ADHD. *Journal of the American Academy of Child and Adolescent Psychiatry*. (36), 1715–1725.

Levitas, A. *et al.* (2001). The mental state examination in patients with mental retardation and developmental disabilities. *Mental Health Aspects of Developmental Disabilities*, 4(2), 2–16.

Loeber, R., Russo, M., Stouthamer-Loeber, M. and Lahey, B. (1994). Internalizing problems and their relation to the development of disruptive behaviors in adolescence. *Journal of Research on Adolescence*, (4), 615–637.

Losse, A., Henderson, S., Elliman, D., Hall, D., Knight, E. and Jongmans, M. (1991). Clumsiness in children – do they grow out of it? A 10-year follow-up study. *Developmental Medicine and Child Neurology*, (33), 55–68.

Love, A. and Thompson, M. (1988). Language disorders and attention deficit disorders in young children referred for psychiatric services: analysis of prevalence and a conceptual synthesis. *American Journal of Orthopsychiatry*, (58), 52–64.

McDougall, T. (2006). Nursing children and young people with learning disabilities and mental health problems. In: McDougall, T. (Ed). *Child and Adolescent Mental Health Nursing*. London: Blackwell.

McGee, R., Williams, S. and Feehan, M. (1992). Attention deficit disorder and age of onset of problem behaviours. *Journal of Abnormal Child Psychology*, (20), 487–502.

Mannuzza, S., Klein, R., Bessler, A., Malloy P. and Lapadula, M. (1998). Adult psychiatric status of hyperactive boys grown up. *American Journal of Psychiatry*, 155(4), 493–498.

Marzocchi, G., Oosterlaan, J., Zuddas, A., Cavolina, P., Geurts, H., Redigolo, D., Vio, C. and Sergeant, J. (2008). Contrasting deficits on executive functions between ADHD and reading-disabled children. *Journal of Child Psychology and Psychiatry and Allied Disciplines*, 49(5), 543–562.

MTA Cooperative Group. (1999). A 14-month randomised clinical trial of treatment strategies for attention-deficit hyperactivity disorder. *Archives of General Psychiatry*, (56), 1073–1086.

National Collaborating Centre for Mental Health. (2008) *Attention Deficit Hyperactivity Disorder: Diagnosis and Management of ADHD in Children, Young People and Adults*. London: NCCMH.

National Collaborating Centre for Mental Health. (2005). *Depression in Children and Young People: Identification and Management in Primary, Community and Secondary Care*. London: NCCMH.

National Institute for Health and Clinical Excellence. (2006). *Methylphenidate, Atomoxetine and Dexamfetamine for Attention Deficit Hyperactivity Disorder (ADHD) in Children and Adolescents: Review of Technology Appraisal 13*. London: NICE.

National Institute for Clinical Excellence. (2004). *Anxiety: Management of Generalised Anxiety Disorder and Panic Disorder (With or Without Agoraphobia) in Adults in*

Primary, Secondary and Community Care (Draft for Second Consultation). London: National Institute for Clinical Excellence.

Nolan, M. and Carr, A. (2000). Attention deficit hyperactivity disorder. In: Carr, A. (Ed). *What Works with Children and Adolescents? A Critical Review of Psychological Interventions with Children, Adolescents and their Families*. London: Routledge.

O'Connor, T. and Rutter, M. (2000). Attachment disorder behavior following early severe deprivation: extension and longitudinal follow-up. English and Romanian Adoptees Study Team. *Journal of the American Academy of Child and Adolescent Psychiatry*. (39), 703–712.

Post, R., Chang, K., Findling, R., Geller, B., Kowatch, R., Kutcher, S., and Leverich, G. (2004). Prepubertal bipolar I disorder and bipolar disorder NOS are separable from ADHD. *Journal of Clinical Psychiatry*, 65(7), 898–902.

Quine, L. (1993). Teaching parents of children with severe handicaps to manage sleep disturbance by using behavioural methods. In Harris, J. (ed). *Innovations in Training For Those Working With People Who Have Severe Learning Difficulties*. Kidderminster: BIMH.

Quine, L. (1992). Severity of sleep problems in children with severe learning disabilities: description and correlates. *Journal of Community and Applied Social Psychology*, (2), 247–268.

Quine, L. (1991). Sleep problems in children with mental handicap. *Journal of Mental Deficiency Research*, (35), 269–290.

Quist, J., Barr, C., Schacher, R., Roberts, W., Malone, M., Tannock, R., Basile, V., Beitchman, J. and Kennedy, J. (2003). The serotonin 5-HT1B receptor gene and attention deficit hyperactivity disorder. *Molecular Psychiatry*, (8), 98–102.

Rasmussen, P. and Gillberg, C. (2000). Natural outcome of ADHD with developmental coordination disorder at age 22 years: a controlled longitudinal community-based study. *Journal of the American Academy of Child and Adolescent Psychiatry*, (39), 1424–1431.

Reierson, A., Constantino, J., Volk, H. and Todd, R. (2007). Autistic traits in a population-based ADHD twin sample. *Journal of Child Psychology and Psychiatry*, 48(5), 464–472.

Rothenberger, A. and Banaschewski, T. (2004). In: Gillberg, C., Harrington, R. and Steinhausen, H. (Eds). *A Clinician's Handbook of Child and Adolescent Psychiatry*. Cambridge. Cambridge University Press.

Salmon, G., Cleave, H. and Samuel, C. (2006). Development of multi-agency referral pathways for attention deficit hyperactivity disorder, developmental coordination disorder and autistic spectrum disorders: reflections on the process and suggestions for new ways of working. *Clinical Child Psychology and Psychiatry*, 11(1), 63–81.

Spencer, T. (2001). *Depressive Disorders and ADHD: Program and Abstracts of the 154th Annual Meeting of the American Psychiatric Association*. 5–10 May 2001. New Orleans. Louisiana. Industry Symposium 46C.

Szatmari, P., Offord, D. and Boyle, M. (1989). Correlates, associated impairments and patterns of service utilization of children with attention deficit hyperactivity disorders: findings from the Ontario child health study. *Journal of Child Psychology and Psychiatry*, (30), 205–217.

Taylor, E. (1994). Syndromes of attention deficit and overactivity. In: Rutter, M., Taylor, E. and Hersov, L. (Eds). *Child and Adolescent Psychiatry: Modern Approaches* (3rd Edition). London. Blackwell.

Taylor, E., Chadwick, O., Heptinstall, E., and Danckaerts, M. (1996). Hyperactivity and conduct problems as risk factors for adolescent development. *Journal of American Academy of Child and Adolescent Psychiatry*, (35), 1213–1226.

Taylor, E., Doepfner, M., Sergeant, J., Asherson, P., Banaschewski, T., Buitelaar, J., Coghill, D., Danckaerts, M., Rothenberger, A., Sonuga-Barke, E., Steinhausen, H. and Zuddas, A. (2004). European clinical guidelines for hyperkinetic disorder – first upgrade. *Journal of European Child and Adolescent Psychiatry*, (13), Supplement 1, 1–30.

Taylor, E., Sandberg, E., Thorley, G., and Giles, S. (1991). The epidemiology of childhood hyperactivity. *Maudsley Monographs.* (33). Oxford. Oxford University Press.

Thapar, A., Harrington, R. and McGuffin, P. (2001). Examining the comorbidity of ADHD related behaviours and conduct problems using a twin study design. *British Journal of Psychiatry*, (179), 224–229.

Van Lier, P., van der Ende, J., Koot, H. and Verhulst, F. (2007). Which better predicts conduct problems? The relationship of trajectories of conduct problems with ODD and ADHD symptoms from childhood into adolescence. *Journal of Child Psychology and Psychiatry*, 48(6), 601–608.

Willoughby, M. (2003). Developmental course of ADHD symptomatology during the transition from childhood to adolescence: a review with recommendations. *Journal of Child Psychology and Psychiatry*, 44(1), 88–106.

World Health Organisation. (1993). *The ICD-10 Classification of Mental and Behavioural Disorders: Clinical Descriptions and Diagnostic Guidelines.* Geneva: WHO.

Chapter 6 What do children, young people and families tell us about living with ADHD?

Banaschewski, T., Coghill, D., Santosh, P., Zuddas, A., Asherson, P., Buitelaar, J., Danckaerts, M., Doepfner, M., Faraone, S., Rothenberger, A., Sergeant, J., Steinhausen, H., Sonuga-Barke, E. and Taylor, E. (2006) Long-acting medications for the hyperkinetic disorders: a systematic review and European treatment guideline. *European Child and Adolescent Psychiatry*, 15(8), 476–495.

Barber, S., Grubbs, L. and Cottrell, B. (2005) Self-perception in children with attention deficit/hyperactivity disorder. *Journal of Pediatric Nursing*, 20(4) 232–245.

Baxley, G., Turner, P. and Greenwold, W. (1978). Hyperactive children's knowledge and attitudes concerning drug treatment. *Journal of Pediatric Psychology*, 3(4), 172–176.

Bennett, D., Power, T., Rostain, A. and Carr, D. (1996). Parent acceptability and feasibility of ADHD interventions: assessment, correlates and predictive validity. *Journal of Pediatric Psychology*, 21(5), 643–657.

Blunt-Bugental, D. (2003). The child in a world apart: the experiences of children who appear to be socially unresponsive. In: Bunt-Bugental, D. (Ed). *Thriving in the Face of Childhood Adversity.* New York: Psychology Press.

Brody, G., Stoneman, Z. and Gauger, K. (1996). Parent–child relationships, family problem-solving behavior and sibling relationship quality: the moderating role of sibling temperaments. *Child Development*, (67), 1289–1300.

Bull, C. and Whelan, T. (2006). Parental schemata in the management of children with attention deficit-hyperactivity disorder. *Qualitative Health Research*, 16 (5), 664–678.

Bussing, R. and Gary F. (2001). Practice guidelines and parental ADHD treatment evaluations: friends or foes? *Harvard Review of Psychiatry*, (9), 223–233.

Bussing, R., Gary, F., Mills, T. and Wilson-Garvan, C. (2003). Parental explanatory models of ADHD: gender and cultural variations. *Social Psychiatry and Psychiatric Epidemiology*, (38), 563–575.

Coghill, D. (2003). Current issues in child and adolescent psychopharmacology: part 1: attention deficit hyperactivity and affective disorders. *Advances in Psychiatric Treatment*, (9), 86–94.

Colley, M. (2005). The parent's perspective. *Archives of Disease in Childhood*, 90(1), doi:10.1136/adc.2004.058016.

Concannon, P. and Tang, Y. (2005). Management of attention deficit hyperactivity disorder: a parental perspective. *Journal of Paediatrics and Child Health*, 41, 625–630.

Cohen, N. and Thompson, L. (1982). Perceptions and attitudes of hyperactive children and their mothers regarding treatment with methylphenidate. *Canadian Journal of Psychiatry*, (27), 40–42.

Cooper, P. and Shea, T. (2000). ADHD from the inside: an empirical study of young people's perceptions of the experience of ADHD. In: Cooper, P. and Bilton, K. (Eds). *ADHD: Research, Practice and Opinion*. London: Whurr.

Cronin, A. (2004). Mothering a child with hidden impairments. *American Journal of Occupational Therapy*, (58), 83–92.

Department for Education and Skills. (2006). *Working Together to Safeguard Children: a Guide to Interagency Working to Safeguard and Promote the Welfare of Children*. London: HMSO.

Department for Education and Skills. (2003). *Every Child Matters*. London: HMSO.

Douglas, A. (1999) *ADHD: a Mother's Story* Available: *http://www.lanc.uk.com/ADHD_article.pdf* [2008, March 30].

Efron, D., Jarman, F., and Barker, M. (1998). Child and parent perceptions of stimulant medication treatment in attention deficit hyperactivity disorder. *Journal of Paediatrics and Child Health*, 34(3), 288–292.

Faraone, S., Biederman, J. and Chen, W. (1995). Genetic heterogeneity in attention deficit hyperactivity disorder (ADHD): gender, psychiatric comorbidity, and maternal ADHD. *Journal of Abnormal Psychology*, (104), 334–345.

Faux, S. (1993). Siblings of children with chronic physical and cognitive disabilities. *Journal of Pediatric Nursing*, (8), 305–317.

Foreward, S., Brown, T. and McGrath, P. (1996). Mother's attitudes and behavior towards medicating children's pain. *Pain*, 67(2), 469–474.

Frame, K., Kelly, L. and Bayley, E. (2003). Increasing perceptions of self-worth in preadolescents diagnosed with ADHD. *Journal of Nursing Scholarship*, 35(3), 225–229.

Gerdes, A., Hoza, B., Pelham, W., Swanson, J., Conners, C. and Hinshaw, S. (2003). Attention deficit/hyperactivity disordered boys' relationships with their mothers and fathers: child, mother and father perceptions. *Development and Psychopathology*, (15), 363–382.

Gordon, K., Dooley, J., Camfield, P., Camfield, C. and MacSween, J. (2001). Treatment of febrile seizures: the influence of treatment efficacy and side effect profile on value to parents. *Pediatrics*, (108), 1080–1088.

Hansen, D. and Hansen, E. (2006). Caught in a balancing act: parents' dilemmas regarding their ADHD child's treatment with stimulant medication. *Qualitative Health Research*, (16), 1267–1287.

Harborne, A., Wolpert, M. and Clare, L. (2004). Making sense of ADHD: a battle for understanding parents' views of their children being diagnosed with ADHD. *Clinical Child Psychology and Psychiatry*, 9(3), 327–339.

Harpin, V. (2005). The effect of ADHD on the life of an individual, their family, and community from preschool to adult life. *Archives of Disease in Childhood*, 90(1), 2–7.

Hazell, P., McDowell, M. and Walton, J. (1996). Management of children prescribed psychostimulant medication for attention deficit hyperactivity disorder in the Hunter region of NSW. *Medical Journal of Australia*, (165), 477–480.

Hinshaw, S. (2005). The stigmatization of mental illness in children and parents: developmental issues, family concerns and research needs. *Journal of Child Psychology and Psychiatry*, (46), 714–734.

Hinton, C. and Wolpert, M. (1998). Why is ADHD such a compelling story? *Clinical Child Psychology and Psychiatry*, 3(2), 315–317.

Hoza, B., Owens, J., Pelham, W., Swanson, J., Conners, C. and Hinshaw, S. (2000). Parental cognitions as predictors of child treatment response in attention deficit/ hyperactivity disorder. *Journal of Abnormal Psychology*, (28), 569–583.

Hurt, E., Hoza, B. and Pelham, W. (2007). Parenting, family loneliness and peer functioning in boys with attention deficit/hyperactivity disorder. *Journal of Abnormal Child Psychology*, (35), 543–555.

Jackson, J. (2003). *Multicoloured Mayhem: Parenting the Many Shades of Adolescents and Children with Autism, Asperger Syndrome and AD/HD*. London: Jessica Kingsley.

Jones, K., Welsh, R., Glassmire, D. and Tavegia, B. (2006). Psychological functioning in siblings of children with attention deficit hyperactivity disorder. *Journal of Child and Family Studies*, 15(6), 753–759.

Kendall, J. (1999). Sibling accounts of attention deficit hyperactivity disorder (ADHD). *Family Process*, (38), 117–136.

Kendall, J. (1998). Outlasting disruption: the process of reinvestment in families with ADHD children. *Qualitative Health Research*, (8), 839–857.

Kendall, J. (1997) The use of qualitative methods in the study of wellness in children with attention deficit hyperactivity disorder. *Journal of Child and Adolescent Psychiatric Nursing*, 10(4), 27–38.

Kendall, J., Hatton, D., Beckett, A. and Leo, M. (2003). Children's accounts of attention deficit hyperactivity disorder. *Advanced Nursing Science*, 26(2), 114–130.

Kendall, J., Leo, M., Perrin, N. and Hatton, D. (2005). Modeling ADHD child and family relationships. *Western Journal of Nursing Research*, 27(500), doi: 10.1177/ 0193945905275513.

Kendall, J. and Shelton, K. (2003). A typology of management styles in families with children with ADHD. *Journal of Family Nursing*, (9), 257.

Klasen, H. and Goodman, R. (2000). Parents and GPs at cross purposes over hyperactivity: a qualitative study of possible barriers to treatment. *British Journal of General Practice*, (50), 199–202.

Krueger, M. and Kendall, J. (2001). Descriptions of self: an exploratory study of adolescents with ADHD. *Journal of Child and Adolescent Psychiatric Nursing*, 14(2), 61–72.

Litner, B. (2003). Teens with ADHD: the challenge of high school. *Child and Youth Care Forum*, 32(3), 137–158.

Liu, C., Robin, A., Brenner, S. and Eastman, J. (1991). Social acceptability of methylphenidate and behavior modification for treating attention deficit hyperactivity disorder. *Pediatrics*, (88), 560–565.

Ludwikowski, K. and DeValk, M. (1998). Attention deficit/hyperactivity disorder: a neurodevelopmental approach. *Journal of Child and Adolescent Psychiatric Nursing*, 11(1), 17–29.

McElearney, C., Fitzpatrick, C., Farrell, N., King, M. and Lynch, B. (2005). Stimulant medication in ADHD: what do children and their parents say? *Irish Journal of Psychological Medicine*, 22(1), 5–9.

McHale, S., Crouter, A., McGuire, S. and Updegraff, K. (1995). Congruence between mothers' and fathers' differential treatment of siblings: links with family relations and children's wellbeing. *Child Development*, (66), 116–128.

McNeal, R., Roberts, M. and Barone, V. (2004). Mother's and children's perceptions of medication for children with attention deficit hyperactivity disorder. *Child Psychiatry and Human Development*, 30(3), 173–187.

Meaux, J., Hester, C., Smith, B. and Shoptaw, A. (2006). Stimulant medications: a trade-off?: the lived experiences of adolescents with ADHD. *Journal for Specialists in Pediatric Nursing*, 11(4), 214–226.

Muthukrishna, N. (2007). Inclusion and exclusion in school: experiences of children labelled 'ADHD' in South Africa. In: Lloyd, D., Stead, J. and Cohen, D. (Eds). *Critical New Perspectives on ADHD*. London: Routledge.

National Institute for Health and Clinical Excellence. (2008). *Attention Deficit Hyperactivity Disorder: Diagnosis and Management of ADHD in Children, Young People and Adults*. London: NCCMH.

Paton, M. (2002). *Qualitative Research and Evaluation Methods* (3rd Edition). California: Sage.

Peterson-Sweeney, K., McMullen, A., Yoos, L. and Kitzman, H. (2003). Parental perceptions of their child's asthma: management and medication use. *Journal of Pediatric Health Care*, 17(3), 118–125.

Petersson, C., Petersson, K. and Hakansson, A. (2003). General parental education in Sweden: participants and non participants. *Scandinavian Journal of Primary Health Care*, 21(1), 43–46.

Pryjmachuk, S. (1999). Learning how to live with a child with ADHD was a long and arduous process. *Evidence-Based Nursing*, (2), 60.

Rolland, J. (1994). *Families, Illness and Disability: an Integrated Treatment Model*. New York: Basic Books.

Rostain, A., Power, T. and Atkins, M. (1993). Assessing parents' willingness to pursue treatment for children with attention deficit hyperactivity disorder. *Journal of the American Academy of Child and Adolescent Psychiatry*, (32), 175–181.

Schmidt-Neven, R., Anderson, V. and Godber, T. (2000). *Attention Deficit Disorder: an Illness for our Time*. Melbourne: Full Circle.

Seligman, M. and Darling, R. (1997). *Ordinary Families, Special Children* (2nd Edition). New York: Guilford Press.

Shattell, M., Bartlett, R. and Rowe, T. (2008). 'I have always felt different': the experience of attention-deficit/hyperactivity disorder. *Journal of Pediatric Nursing*, 23(1), 49–57.

Singh, I. (2004). Doing their jobs: mothering with Ritalin in a culture of mother-blame. *Social Science and Medicine*, (59), 1193–1205.

Singh, I. (2003). Boys will be boys: fathers' perspectives on ADHD symptoms, diagnosis and drug treatment. *Harvard Review of Psychiatry*, 11(6), 308–316.

Singh, I. (2002). Bad boys, good mothers and the 'miracle' of Ritalin. *Science in Context*, 15(4), 577–603.

Sobol, M., Ashbourne, D., Earn, B. and Cunningham, C. (1989). Parents' attributions for achieving compliance from attention deficit disordered children. *Journal of Abnormal Child Psychology*, (17), 359–369.

Stocker, C., Dunn, J. and Plomin, R. (1989). Sibling relationships: links with child temperament, maternal behavior and family structure. *Child Development*, (60), 715–727.

Stoneman, Z. and Brody, G. (1993). Sibling temperaments, conflict, warmth and role asymmetry. *Child Development*, (64), 1786–1800.

Tallmadge, J. and Barkley, R. (1983). The interactions of hyperactive and normal boys with their fathers and mothers. *Journal of Abnormal Child Psychology*, 11(4), 565–577.

Taylor, E., Dopfner, M., Sergeant, J., Asherson, P., Banaschewski, T., Rothenberger, A., Buitelaar, J., Coghill, D., Danckaerts, M., Sonuga-Barke, E., Steinhausen, H. and Zuddas, A. (2004). European clinical guidelines for hyperkinetic disorder: first upgrade. *European Child and Adolescent Psychiatry*, 13(1), 1–30.

Tollefson, N. and Chen, J. (1988). Consequences of teachers' attributions for students' failure. *Teaching and Teacher Education*, (4), 259–265.

Winsler, A. (1998). Parent–child interaction and private speech in boys with ADHD. *Applied Developmental Science*, (2), 17–39.

Young, S. and Bramham, J. (2007). *ADHD in Adults: a Psychological Guide to Practice*. London: Wiley and Sons.

Chapter 7 Treatment and management strategies

Abikoff, H. (1991). Cognitive training in ADHD children: less to it than meets the eye. *Journal of Learning Disabilities*, (24), 205–209.

ADDISS. (2006). *ADHD is Real: ADDISS Families Survey*. London: ADDISS Resource Centre.

American Academy of Child and Adolescent Psychiatry. (2007a). Practice parameters for the assessment and treatment of children and adolescents with oppositional defiant disorder. *Journal of the American Academy of Child and Adolescent Psychiatry*, 46(1), 126–141.

American Academy of Child and Adolescent Psychiatry. (2007b). Practice parameters for the assessment and treatment of children and adolescents with attention deficit/hyperactivity disorder. *Journal of the American Academy of Child and Adolescent Psychiatry*, 46(7), 894–921.

American Academy of Child and Adolescent Psychiatry. (1997). Practice parameters for the assessment and treatment of children and adolescents with conduct disorders. *Journal of the American Academy of Child and Adolescent Psychiatry*, Retrieved May 2008, from *www.aacap.org/page.ww?section=Practice+Parametersandname= Practice+Parameters*.

Anastopolous, A., DuPaul, G. and Barkley, R. (1991). Stimulant medication and parent training therapies for attention deficit hyperactivity disorder. *Journal of Learning Disabilities*, (24), 210–218.

Anastopolous, A., Shelton, T., DuPaul, G. and Guevremont, D. (1993). Parent training for attention deficit hyperactivity disorder: its impact on parent functioning. *Journal of Abnormal Child Psychology*, (21), 581–596.

Baguley, I. and Baguley, C. (1999). Psychosocial interventions in the treatment of psychosis. *Mental Health Care*, 2(9), 314–316.

Banaschewski, T., Coghill, D., Santosh, P., Zuddas, A., Asherson, P., Buitelaar, J., Danckaerts, M., Doepfner, M., Faraone, S., Rothenberger, A., Sergeant, J., Steinhausen, H., Sonuga-Barke, E. and Taylor, E. (2006) Long-acting medications for the hyperkinetic disorders: a systematic review and European treatment guideline. *European Child and Adolescent Psychiatry*, 15(8), 476–495.

Bennett, D., Power, T., Rostain, A. and Carr, D. (1996). Parental acceptability and feasibility of ADHD interventions: assessment, correlates and predictive validity. *Journal of Pediatric Psychology*, 21(5), 643–657.

Bernier, J. and Siegel, D. (1994). Attention deficit hyperactivity disorder: a family and ecological systems perspective. *Families in Society*, (75), 142–151.

Biederman, J. and Faraone, S. (2005). Attention deficit hyperactivity disorder. *Lancet*, (366), 237–248.

Biederman, J., Faraone, S., Monuteaux, M., Plunkett, E., Gifford, J. and Spencer, T. (2003). Growth deficits and attention deficit hyperactivity disorder revisited: impact of gender, development and treatment. *Pediatrics*, 111(5), 1010–1016.

Biederman, J. and Spencer, T. (2000). Non-stimulant treatments for ADHD. *European Child and Adolescent Psychiatry*, 9(1), 151–159.

Bjornstad, G. and Montgomery, P. (2005). Family therapy for attention deficit disorder or attention deficit/hyperactivity disorder in children and adolescents. *Cochrane Database of Systematic Reviews*, (2). The Cochrane Collaboration.

Bor, W., Sanders, M. and Markie-Dadds, C. (2002). The effects of the Triple P Positive Parenting Program on pre-school children with co-occurring disruptive behavior and attentional/hyperactive difficulties. *Journal of Abnormal Child Psychology*, 30(6), 571–587.

Bull, C. and Whelan, T. (2006) Parental schemata in the management of children with attention deficit-hyperactivity disorder. *Qualitative Health Research*, 16(5), 664–678.

Camp. B. and Bash, M. (1981). *Think Aloud: Increasing Cognitive and Social Skills – a Problem-Solving Program for Children: Primary Level*. Illinois: Research Press.

Cantor, D. (2000). The role of group therapy in promoting identity development in ADHD adolescents. *Journal of Psychotherapy in Independent Practice*, 1(2), DOI: 10.1300/J288v01n02_07.

Carlson, C., Pelham, W., Milich, R. and Dixon, J. (1992). Single and combined effects of methylphenidate and behavior therapy on the classroom performance of children with attention deficit hyperactivity disorder. *Journal of Abnormal Child Psychology*, (20), 213–232.

Carr, A. (2000a). *Family Therapy: Concepts, Process and Practice*. Chichester: John Wiley and Sons.

Carr, A. (2000b). Evidence-based practice in family therapy and systemic consultation 1: child focused problems, *Journal of Family Therapy*, (22), 29–60.

Coghill, D. (2003). Current issues in child and adolescent psychopharmacology: part 1: attention deficit hyperactivity and affective disorders. *Advances in Psychiatric Treatment*, (9), 86–94.

Concannon, P. and Tang, Y. (2005). Management of attention deficit hyperactivity disorder: a parental perspective. *Journal of Paediatrics and Child Health*, 41, 625–630.

Coulter, M. and Dean, M. (2007). Homeopathy for attention deficit hyperactivity disorder or hyperkinetic disorder. *Cochrane Database of Systematic Reviews*, (4). Cochrane Library.

Cousins, L. and Weiss, G. (1993). Parent training and social skills training for children with attention deficit hyperactivity disorder: how can they be combined for greater effectiveness? *Canadian Journal of Psychiatry*, (39), 449–457.

Crystal, D., Ostrander, R., Chen, R. and August, G. (2001). Multimethod assessment of psychopathology among DSM-IV subtypes of children with attention deficit/hyperactivity disorder: self, parent and teacher reports. *Journal of Abnormal Child Psychology*, 29(3), 189–205.

Department of Health. (2008). *Medicines Management: Everybody's Business*. London: HMSO.

Department of Health. (2007). *Commissioning a Brighter Future: Improving Access to Psychological Therapies*. London: HMSO.

Department of Health. (2006). *From Values to Actions: the Chief Nursing Officer's Review of Mental Health Nursing*. London: HMSO.

Department of Health (2004b). *Choosing Health: Making Healthier Choices Easier*. London: HMSO.

Department of Health. (2004a). *The National Service Framework for Children, Young People and Maternity Services: Standard 9 – Mental Health and Psychological Wellbeing of Children and Young People*. London: HMSO.

DuPaul, G. and Eckert, T. (1997). Interventions for students with attention deficit/hyperactivity disorder: one size does not fit all. *School Psychology Review*, 26(3), 369–382.

DuPaul, G., Guevremont, D. and Barkley, R. (1992). Behavioral treatment of attention deficit hyperactivity disorder in the classroom. *Behavior Modification*, (16), 204–225.

Dwivedi, K. (1993). *Group Work with Children and Adolescents: a Handbook*. London: Jessica Kingsley.

Findling, R. and Dogin, J. (1998). Psychopharmacology of ADHD: children and adolescents. *Journal of Clinical Psychiatry*, 59(7), 42–49.

Fonagy, P, Target, M, Cottrell, D, Phillips, J. and Kurtz, Z. (2002). *What Works for Whom?: a Critical Review of Treatments for Children and Adolescents*. London: Guilford Press.

Ford, T., Fowler, T., Langley, K., Whittinger, N. and Thapar, A. (2007). Five years on: public sector service use related to mental health in young people with ADHD or hyperkinetic disorder five years after diagnosis. *Journal of Child and Adolescent Mental Health*, doi 10.1111/j.1475–3588.2007.00466.x.

Fryers, T. (2007). *Children at Risk: Childhood Determinants of Adult Psychiatric Disorder*. Helsinki: Stakes.

Goldman, L., Genel, M. and Bezman, R. (1998). Diagnosis and treatment of attention-deficit/hyperactivity disorder in children and adolescents. *Journal of the American Medical Association*, (279), 1100–1107.

Gordon, T. (1975). *PET: Parent Effectiveness Training*. New York: Plume.

Green, H., McGinnity, A., Meltzer, H., Ford, T. and Goodman, R. (2005). *Mental Health of Children and Young People in Great Britain*. London: ONS.

Greenhill, L., Halperin, J. and Abikoff, H. (1999). Stimulant medications. *Journal of the American Academy of Child and Adolescent Psychiatry*, (38), 503–512.

Hall, K., Irwin, M., Bowman, K., Frankenberger, W. and Jewett, D. (2005). Illicit use of prescribed stimulant medication among college students. *Journal of American College Health*, 53(4), 164–174.

Harrison, L., Manocha, R. and Rubia, K. (2004). Sahaja yoga meditation as a family treatment programme for children with attention deficit hyperactivity disorder. *Clinical Child Psychology and Psychiatry*, 9(4), 479–497.

Hill, P. and Taylor, E. (2001). An auditable protocol for treating attention deficit hyperactivity disorder. *Archives of Diseases in Childhood*, (84), 404–409.

Hinshaw, S. (1994). *Attention Deficit and Hyperactivity in Children: Developmental Clinical Psychology and Psychiatry*. London: Sage.

Hoath, F. and Sanders, C. (2002). A feasibility study of enhanced Triple P positive parenting program for parents of children with attention deficit hyperactivity disorder. *Behaviour Change*, 19(4), 191–206.

Indiana Prevention Resource Center. (1998). *Factline on Non-medical Use of Ritalin*. Bloomington: Indiana University.

Jackson, B. and Farrugia, D. (1997). Diagnosis and treatment of adults with attention deficit hyperactivity disorder. *Journal of Counselling and Development*, (75), 312–319.

Jensen, P., Arnold, E., Swanson, J., Vitiello, B., Abikoff, H., Greenhill, L., Hechtman, L., Hinshaw, S., Pelham, W., Wells, K., Conners, K., Elliott, G., Epstein, J., Hoza, B., March, J., Brooke, M., Newcorn, J., Severe, J., Wigal, T., Gibbons, R. and Hur, K. (2007). 3-year follow-up of the NIMH MTA study. *Child and Adolescent Psychiatry*, 46(8), 989–1002.

Jensen, P., Martin, D. and Cantwell, D. (1997). Comorbidity in ADHD: implications for research, practice and DSM-V. *Journal of the American Academy of Child and Adolescent Psychiatry*. (36), 1065–1079.

Johnson, J. and Clark, A. (2001). Prescribing of unlicensed medicines or licensed medicines for unlicensed applications in child and adolescent psychiatry. *Psychiatric Bulletin*, (25), 465–466.

Jones, K., Welsh, R., Glassmire, D. and Tavegia, B. (2006). Psychological functioning in siblings of children with attention deficit hyperactivity disorder. *Journal of Child and Family Studies*, 15(6), 753–759.

Kendall, P. and Braswell, L. (1982). *Cognitive Behavioural Therapy for Impulsive Children*. New York: Guilford Press.

Kendall, P. and Finch, A. (1978). A cognitive-behavioural treatment for impulsivity: a group comparison study. *Journal of Consulting and Clinical Psychology*, (46), 110–118.

Kendall, P., Panichelli-Mindel, S. and Gerow, M. (1995). Cognitive behavioral therapies with children and adolescents. In: van Bilsen, H., Kendall, P. and Slavenburg, J. (Eds). *Behavioral Approaches for Children and Adolescents: Challenges for the Next Century*. New York: Plenum Press.

Kidd, P. (2000). Attention deficit/hyperactivity disorder in children: rationale for its integrative management. *Alternative Medicine Review*, 5(5), 402–428.

Klein, R., Lander, B., Mattes, J. and Klein, D. (1988). Methylphenidate and growth in hyperactive children: a controlled withdrawal study. *Archives of General Psychiatry*, (45), 1127–1130.

Kramer, J., Loney, J. and Ponto, L. (2000). Predictors of adult height and weight in boys treated with methylphenidate for childhood behavior problems. *Journal of the American Academy of Child and Adolescent Psychiatry*. (39), 517–524.

Kratochvil, C., Heiligenstein, J., Dittmann, R., Spencer, T., Biederman, J., Wernicke, J., Newcorn, J., Casat, C., Milton, D. and Michelson, D. (2002). Atomoxetine and methylphenidate treatment in children with ADHD: a prospective, randomised, open label trial. *Journal of the American Academy of Child and Adolescent Psychiatry*. 41(7), 776–784.

Leon, L. (2001). *Time to Listen: the Mental Health Needs of Young People*. London: ChildRight.

Lim, L., Faught, P., Chalasani, N. and Molleston, J. (2006). Severe liver injury after initiating therapy with atomoxetine in two children. *Journal of Pediatrics*, 148(6), 831–834.

Linden, M., Habib, T. and Radojevic, V. (1996). A controlled study of the effects of EEG biofeedback on cognition and behavior of children with attention deficit disorder and learning disabilities. *Applied Psychophysiology and Biofeedback*, 21(1), 35–49.

Liu, C., Robin, A., Brenner, S. and Eastman, J. (1991). Social acceptability of methylphenidate and behavior modification for treating attention deficit hyperactivity disorder. *Pediatrics*, (88), 560–565.

Long, N. (1997). Parent education/training in the USA: current status and future trends. *Clinical Child Psychology and Psychiatry*, 2(4), 501–515.

Long, N., Rickert, V. and Ashcraft, E. (1993). Bibliotherapy as an adjunct to stimulant medication in the treatment of attention-deficit hyperactivity disorder. *Journal of Pediatric Health Care*, (7), 82–88.

Marcus, S., Wan, G., Kemner, J. and Olfson, M. (2005). Continuity of methylphenidate treatment for attention deficit/hyperactivity disorder. *Archives of Pediatric and Adolescent Medicine*, (159), 572–578.

Martins, S., Tramontina, S., Polanczyk, G., Eizirik, M., Swanson, J. and Rohde, L. (2004). Weekend holidays during methylphenidate use in ADHD children: a randomised clinical trial. *Journal of Child and Adolescent Psychopharmacology*, 14(2), 195–206.

Meaux, J., Hester, C., Smith, B. and Shoptaw, A. (2006). Stimulant medications: a trade-off?: the lived experiences of adolescents with ADHD. *Journal for Specialists in Pediatric Nursing*, 11(4), 214–226.

Meichembaum, D. and Goodman, J. (1971) Training impulsive children to talk to themselves, a means of developing self-control. *Journal of Abnormal Psychology*, 70, 117–126.

Mental Health Foundation. (2001). *Turned Upside Down: Developing Community-Based Crisis Services for 16–25-Year-Olds Experiencing a Mental Health Crisis*. London: Mental Health Foundation.

Michelson, D., Adler, L., Spencer, T., Reimherr, F., West, S., Allen, A., Kelsey, D., Wernicke, J., Dietrich, A. and Milton, D. (2003). Atomoxetine in adults with ADHD: two randomised, placebo-controlled studies. *Biological Psychiatry*, (53), 112–120.

Michelson, D., Faries, D., and Wernicke, J. (2001). Atomoxetine in the treatment of children and adolescents with attention deficit/hyperactivity disorder: a randomised, placebo-controlled, dose-response study. *Pediatrics*, 108(5), 83.

Mitchell, P. (2006). Adolescent forensic mental health nursing. In: McDougall, T. (Ed). *Child and Adolescent Mental Health Nursing*. London: Blackwell.

MTA Cooperative Group. (1999). A 14-month randomised clinical trial of treatment strategies for attention-deficit hyperactivity disorder. *Archives of General Psychiatry*, (56), 1073–1086.

National Institute for Health and Clinical Excellence. (2008). *Attention Deficit Hyperactivity Disorder: Diagnosis and Management of ADHD in Children, Young People and Adults*. London: NCCMH.

National Institute for Clinical Excellence. (2006a). *Methylphenidate, Atomoxetine and*

Dexamfetamine for the Treatment of Attention Deficit Hyperactivity Disorder in Children and Adolescents. Technology Assessment 98. London: NICE.

National Institute for Clinical Excellence. (2006b). *Parent Training/Education Programmes in the Management of Children with Conduct Disorders*. Technology Assessment 102. London: NICE.

Nissen, S. (2006). ADHD drugs and cardiovascular risk. *New England Journal of Medicine*, (354), 1445–1448.

Pelham, W. and Waschbusch, D. (1999). Behavioral intervention in attention deficit/ hyperactivity disorder. In: Quay, H. and Hogan, A. (Eds). *Handbook of Disruptive Disorders*. New York: Plenum Press.

Pelham, W., Wheeler, T. and Chronis, A. (1998). Empirically supported psychosocial treatments for attention deficit hyperactivity disorder. *Journal of Clinical Child Psychology*, (27), 190–205.

Pentecost, D. (2000). *Parenting the ADD Child: Can't Do? Won't Do?: Practical Strategies for Managing Behaviour Problems in Children with ADD and ADHD*. London: Jessica Kingsley.

Perring, C. (1997). Medicating children: the case of Ritalin. *Bioethics*, (11), 228–240.

Pisterman, S., Firestone, P., McGrath, P., Goodman, J., Webster, L., Mallory, R. and Goffin, B. (1992). The role of parent training in treatment of preschoolers with ADHD. *American Journal of Orthopsychiatry*, (62), 397–408.

Poduska, J. (2000). Parents' perceptions of their first graders' need for mental health and educational services. *Journal of the American Academy of Child and Adolescent Psychiatry*, (39), 584–591.

Purdie, N., Hattie, J., and Carroll, A. (2002). A review of research on interventions for attention deficit hyperactivity disorder: what works best? *Review of Educational Research*, (72), 61–99.

Rapport, M. and Moffitt, C. (2002). Attention deficit/hyperactivity disorder and methylphenidate: a review of height/weight, cardiovascular, and somatic complaint side effects. *Clinical Psychology Review*, (22), 1107–1131.

Reid, J., Webster-Stratton, C. and Hammond, M. (2003). Follow-up of children who received the incredible years' intervention for oppositional-defiant disorder: maintenance and prediction of 2-year outcome. *Behavior Therapy*, 34(4), 471–491.

Rice, D. and Richmond, C. (1997). Attention deficit hyperactivity disorder and the family. In: Bailey, J. and Rice, D. (Eds). *Attention Deficit/Hyperactivity Disorder: Medical, Psychological and Educational Perspectives*. Sydney: Australian Association of Special Education.

Roberts, I. and McDougall, T. (2006). Clinical governance for specialist child and adolescent mental health nurses. In: McDougall, T. (Ed). *Child and Adolescent Mental Health Nursing*. London: Routledge.

Rosack, J. (2005). Lilly agrees to add warning on Strattera labelling. *Psychiatric News*, 40(20), 1.

Royal College of Paediatrics and Child Health. (2000). *The Use of Unlicensed Medicines or Licensed Medicines for Unlicensed Applications in Paediatric Practice: Policy Statement*. London: Royal College of Paediatrics and Child Health.

Ryan, N. (2007). Non medical prescribing in a child and adolescent mental health service. *Mental Health Practice*, 11(1), 40–44.

Ryan, N. (2006). Nursing children and young people with ADHD. In: McDougall, T. (Ed). *Child and Adolescent Mental Health Nursing*. London: Routledge.

Safer, D., Zito, J., and Fine, E. (1996). Incresaed methylphenidate usage for attention deficit disorder in the 1990s. *Pediatrics*, (98). 10–84–1088.

Safren, S., Otto, M., and Sprich, S. (2005). Cognitive behavioral therapy for ADHD in medication-treated adults with continued symptoms. *Behavior Research and Therapy*, (43), 831–842.

Sanders, M., Markie-Dadds, C. and Turner, K. (2003). Theoretical, scientific and clinical foundations of the Triple P Positive Parenting Programme: a population approach to the promotion of parenting competence. *Parenting Practice and Research Monograph No. 1*. Parenting and Family Support Centre: University of Queensland.

Sanders, M., Mazzucchelli, T. and Studman, L. (2004). Stepping Stones Triple P – an evidence-based positive parenting program for families with a child who has a disability: its theoretical basis and development. *Journal of Intellectual and Developmental Disability*, (29), 1–19.

Santosh, P. and Taylor, E. (2000). Stimulant drugs. *European Child and Adolescent Psychiatry*, 9(1), 127–143.

Santosh, P., Taylor, E., Swanson, J., Wigal, T. (2005). Refining the diagnoses of inattention and overactivity syndromes: a reanalysis of the multimodal treatment study of attention deficit hyperactivity disorder (ADHD) based on ICD-10 criteria for hyperkinetic disorder. *Clinical Neuroscience Research*, (5), 307–314.

Satterfield, J., Cantwell, D. and Saul, R. (1973). Response to stimulant drug treatment in hyperactive children: prediction from EEG and neurological findings. *Journal of Autism and Childhood Schizophrenia*, (3), 35–48.

Schachar, R., Tannock, R. and Cunningham, C. (1997). Behavioral, situational and temporal effects of treatment of ADHD with methylphenidate. *Journal of the American Academy of Child and Adolescent Psychiatry*, (36), 754–763.

Shattell, M., Bartlett, R. and Rowe, T. (2008). 'I have always felt different': the experience of attention-deficit/hyperactivity disorder. *Journal of Pediatric Nursing*, 23(1), 49–57.

Singh, I. (2005). Will the 'real boy' please behave: dosing dilemmas for parents of boys with ADHD. *American Journal of Bioethics*, 5(3), 34–47.

Skuse, D. (2003). *Child Psychology and Psychiatry: an Introduction*. Abingdon: Medicine Publishing Company.

Smyth, B. and Gowers, S. (2005). Principles of treatment, service delivery and psychopharmacology. In: Gowers, S. (Ed). *Seminars in Child and Adolescent Psychiatry* (2nd Edition). London: Gaskell.

Sonuga-Barke, E., Daley, D. and Thompson, M. (2001). Parent-based therapies for preschool attention/hyperactivity disorder: a randomised controlled trial with a community sample. *Journal of the American Academy of Child and Adolescent Psychiatry*, (40), 402–408.

Spencer, T., Beiderman, J. and Harding, M. (1996). Growth deficits in ADHD children revisited: evidence for disorder-associated growth delays? *Journal of the American Academy of Child and Adolescent Psychiatry*, (35), 1460–1469.

Spencer, T., Biederman, J. and Wilens, T. (1998). Growth deficits in children with attention deficit hyperactivity disorder. *Pediatrics*, (102), 501–506.

Spencer, T., and Heiligenstein, J. (2001). An open-label, dose-ranging study of atomoxetine in children with attention deficit hyperactivity disorder. *Journal of Child and Adolescent Psychopharmacology*, (11), 251–265.

Stead, J., Lloyd, G. and Cohen, D. (2007). Widening our view of ADHD. In: Lloyd, G., Stead, J. and Cohen, D. (Eds). *Critical New Perspectives on ADHD*. Oxford: Routledge.

Steer, C. (2005). Managing attention deficit/hyperactivity disorder: unmet needs and future directions. *Archives of Disease in Childhood*, 90(1), doi: 10.1136/adc2004.059352.

Stein, M. (1999). Unravelling sleep problems in treated and untreated children with ADHD. *Journal of Child and Adolescent Psychopharmacology*, 9(3), 157–168.

Stevens, S. (2005). Attention deficit/hyperactivity disorder: working the system for better diagnosis and treatment. *Journal of Pediatric Nursing*, (20), 47–51.

Swanson, J., Lerner, M. and Williams, M. (1995). More frequent diagnosis of ADHD. *New England Journal of Medicine*, (333), 944.

Swanson, J., Sergeant, J., Taylor, E., Sonuga-Barke, E., Jensen, P. and Cantwell, D. (1998a). Attention deficit hyperactivity disorder and hyperkinetic disorder. *Lancet*, (351), 429–433.

Tatano-Beck, C. (1999). Maternal depression and child behaviour problems: a meta-analysis. *Journal of Advanced Nursing*, 29(3), 623–629.

Taylor, E., Dopfner, M., Sergeant, J., Asherson, P., Banaschewski, T., Rothenberger, A., Buitelaar, J., Coghill, D., Danckaerts, M., Sonuga-Barke, E., Steinhausen, H. and Zuddas, A. (2004). European clinical guidelines for hyperkinetic disorder: first upgrade. *European Child and Adolescent Psychiatry*, 13(1), 1–30.

Thompson, M. and Laver-Bradbury, C. (1999a). *On the Go: the Hyperactive Child: a Video for Parents and Professionals*. Southampton: University of Southampton Media Services.

Thompson, M. and Laver-Bradbury, C. (1999b). *Always on the Go: the Hyperactive Child: a Video for Teachers*. Southampton: University of Southampton Media Services.

Till, U. (2007). The values of recovery within mental health nursing. *Mental Health Practice*, 11(3), 3–7.

Utting, D., Monteiro, H. and Ghate, D. (2006). *Interventions for Children at Risk of Developing Antisocial Personality Disorder: Report to the Department of Health and Prime Minister's Strategy Unit*, London: Policy Research Bureau.

Vlam, S. (2006). Attention deficit/hyperactivity disorder: diagnostic assessment methods used by advanced practice registered nurses. *Pediatric Nursing*, (32), 18–24.

Volkow, N., Wang, G. and Fowler, J. (1998). Dopamine transporter occupancies in the human brain induced by therapeutic doses of oral methylphenidate. *American Journal of Psychiatry*, (155), 1325–1331.

Webster-Stratton, C. (2000). *The Incredible Years: Parent, Teachers and Children Training Series*. Washington: Haworth Press.

Webster-Stratton, C. (1998). Preventing conduct problems in Head Start children: strengthening parental competencies. *Journal of Consulting and Clinical Psychology*, (66), 715–730.

Webster-Stratton, C. (1981), Videotape modelling: a method of parent education. *Journal of Clinical Child Psychology*, (10), 93–98.

Weeks, A., Laver-Bradbury, C. and Thompson, M. (1999). *Manual for Professionals Working with Hyperactive Children*. Southampton: Southampton Community Health Services Trust.

Whalen, C. and Henker, B. (1991). Therapies for hyperactive children: comparisons, combinations and compromises. *Journal of Consulting and Clinical Psychology*, (59), 126–137.

Wolraich, M., Greenhill, L., Pelham, W., Swanson, J., Wilen, T., Palumbo, D., Atkins, M. and McBurnett, K. (2001). Randomised controlled trials of methylphenidate once a day in children with attention deficit hyperactivity disorder. *Pediatrics*, (108), 833–892.

Wood, A. and Hughes, S. (2005). Psychosocial approaches and psychotherapies. In: Gowers, S. (Ed). *Seminars in Child and Adolescent Psychiatry* (2nd Edition). London: Gaskell.

Woolley, I. (2006). Treatment interventions for children and young people with mental health problems. In: McDougall, T. (Ed). *Child and Adolescent Mental Health Nursing*. London: Routledge.

Zimmerman, T., Jacobson, R., MacIntyre, Y. and Watson, C. (1996). Solution-focused parenting groups: an empirical study. *Journal of Family Therapy*, 19. 159–172.

Chapter 8 Service provision and care pathways

ADDISS. (2006). *ADHD is Real: ADDISS Families Survey*. London: ADDISS Resource Centre.

American Academy of Child and Adolescent Psychiatry. (2002). Practice parameter for the use of stimulant medications in the treatment of children, adolescents and adults. *Journal of the American Academy of Child and Adolescent Psychiatry*, (41), 26–49.

American Academy of Pediatrics. (2000). Clinical practice guidelines: diagnosis and evaluation of the child with attention deficit hyperactivity disorder. *Pediatrics*, (105), 1158–70.

Asherson, P. (2005). Clinical assessment and treatment of attention deficit hyperactivity disorder in adults. *Expert Review of Neurotherapeutics*, 5(4), 525–539.

Audit Commission. (1999). *Children in Mind: Child and Adolescent Mental Health Services*. London: Audit Commission.

Barton, J., Aitken, K., Butler, S., Harbour, R., Johnstone, R., Eunson, P., Nairn, M., Nasir, J., Norton, B., Puckering, C., Robb, C., Steer, C., and Stone, D. (2001). *Attention Deficit and Hyperactivity Disorder in Children and Young People: a National Clinical Guideline*. Scotland: Scottish Intercollegiate Guidelines Network.

Beresford, B. (2004). On the road to nowhere? Young disabled people and transition. *Child: Health Care and Development*, 30(6), 581–587.

Cohen, D. (2007). How does the decision to medicate children arise in cases of 'ADHD'? In: Lloyd, D., Stead, J. and Cohen, D. (Eds). *Critical New Perspectives on ADHD*. London: Routledge.

Conners, C. (1997). *Conners' Rating Scales Revised Technical Manual*. New York. Multi Health Systems.

Department of Health and Department for Education and Skills. (2001). *The Connexions Framework for Assessment, Planning, Implementation and Review: Guidance for Personal Advisors*. London: HMSO.

Dulcan, M., Dunne, J., Ayres, W., Arnold, V., Benson, R., Bernett, W., Bulkstein, O., Kinlan, J., Leonard, H., Licamele, W., and McClellan, J. (1997). Practice parameters for the assessment and treatment of children and adolescents and adults with attention deficit hyperactivity disorder. *Journal of the American Academy of Child and Adolescent Psychiatry*, (36), 85–121.

Goodman, R. (1997). The strengths and difficulties questionnaire: a research note. *Journal of Child Psychology and Psychiatry*, (38), 581–586.

Health Advisory Service. (1995). *Together We Stand: the Commissioning, Role and Management of Child and Adolescent Mental Health Services*. London: HMSO.

Hill, P. and Taylor, E. (2001). Current topic: an auditable protocol for treating attention deficit/hyperactivity disorder. *Archives of Disease in Childhood*, (84), 404–409.

Hoagwood, K., Kelleher, K., Feil, M. and Comer, D. (2000). Treatment services for children with ADHD: a national perspective. *Journal of the American Academy of Child and Adolescent Psychiatry*, 39(2), 198–206.

Horstmann, K. and Steer, J. (2007). Transition into a secondary school for children with a diagnosis of attention deficit hyperactivity disorder or autistic spectrum disorder: a pilot group. *Clinical Psychology Forum*, (176), August 2007.

Keen, D., Olurin-Lynch, L. and Venables, K. (1997). Getting it all together: developing a forum for a multi-agency approach to assessing and treating ADHD. *Educational and Child Psychology*, (14), 82–90.

Kendall, T., Pilling, S., Whittington, C., Pettinari, C. and Burbeck, R. (2005). Clinical guidelines in mental health II: a guide to making NICE guidelines. *Psychiatric Bulletin*, 29(1), 3–8.

Klasen, H. and Goodman, R. (2002). Parents and GPs at cross-purposes over hyperactivity: a qualitative study of possible barriers to treatment. *British Journal of General Practice*, (50), 199–202.

Litner, B. (2003). Teens with ADHD: the challenge of high school. *Child and Youth Care Forum*, 32(3), 137–158.

McDougall, T. and Crocker, A. (2001). Referral pathways through a specialist child mental health service: the role of the specialist practitioner. *Mental Health Practice*, 5(1), 15–20.

Mann, T. (1996). *Clinical Guidelines: Using Clinical Guidelines to Improve Patient Care within the NHS*. London: Department of Health NHS Executive.

National Institute for Health and Clinical Excellence. (2008). *Attention Deficit Hyperactivity Disorder: Diagnosis and Management of ADHD in Children, Young People and Adults*. London: NCCMH.

National Institute for Clinical Excellence. (2001). *Guidance on the Use of Methylphenidate*. London: NICE.

NHS Quality Improvement Scotland. (2007). *ADHD: Services over Scotland: Report of the Service-Profiling Exercise 2007*. Edinburgh: NHS Scotland.

Nutt, D., Fone, K., Asherson, P., Bramble, D., Hill, P., Matthews, K., Morris, K., Santosh, P., Sonuga-Barke, E., Taylor, E., Weiss, M., and Young, S. (2007). Evidence-based guidelines for management of attention deficit hyperactivity disorder in adolescents in transition to adult services and in adults: recommendations from the British Association for Psychopharmacology. *Journal of Psychopharmacology*, 21(1), 10–41.

Pryjmachuk, S. (1999). Learning how to live with a child with ADHD was a long and arduous process. *Evidence-Based Nursing*, (2), 60.

Ryan, N. (2007a). Nurse prescribing in child and adolescent mental health services. *Mental Health Practice*, 10(10), 35–37.

Ryan, N. (2007b). Non-medical prescribing in a child and adolescent mental health service. *Mental Health Practice*, 11(1), 40–44.

Salmon, G., Cleave, H. and Samuel, C. (2006). Development of multi-agency referral pathways for attention deficit hyperactivity disorder, developmental coordination disorder and autistic spectrum disorders: reflections on the process and suggestions for new ways of working. *Clinical Child Psychology and Psychiatry*, 11(1), 63–81.

Salmon, J. (2005). Hyperactive children. In: Williams, R. and Kerfoot, M. (Eds).

Child and Adolescent Mental Health Services: Strategy, Planning, Delivery and Evaluation. Oxford: Oxford University Press.

Sayal, K., Taylor, E., Beecham, J. and Byrne, P. (2002). Pathways to care in children at risk of attention deficit hyperactivity disorder. *British Journal of Psychiatry*, (181), 43–48.

Scottish Intercollegiate Guidelines Network. (2001). *Attention Deficit and Hyperkinetic Disorders in Children and Young People.* SIGN Publication Number 52. SIGN. Edinburgh.

Skuse, D. (2003). *Child Psychology and Psychiatry: an Introduction.* Abingdon: Medicine Publishing Company.

Steer, C. (2005). Managing attention deficit/hyperactivity disorder: unmet needs and future directions. *Archives of Disease in Childhood*, 90(1), doi: 10.1136/adc2004.059352.

Taylor, E., Dopfner, M., Sergeant, J., Asherson, P., Banaschewski, T., Rothenberger, A., Buitelaar, J., Coghill, D., Danckaerts, M., Sonuga-Barke, E., Steinhausen, H. and Zuddas, A. (2004). European clinical guidelines for hyperkinetic disorder: first upgrade. *European Child and Adolescent Psychiatry*, 13(1), 1–30.

Thapar, A. and Thapar, A. (2002). Is primary care ready to take on attention deficit hyperactivity disorder. *BMC Family Practice*, (3), 7.

Ward, L., Mallett, R., Heslop, P. and Simons, K. (2003). Planning for health at transition. *Learning Disability Practice*, 6(3), 24–27.

While, A., Forbes, A., and Fullman, R. (2004). Good practices that address continuity during transition from child to adult care: syntheses of the evidence. *Child: Health Care and Development*, 30(5), 439–452.

Willoughby, M. (2003). Developmental course of ADHD symptomatology during the transition from childhood to adolescence: a review with recommendations. *Journal of Child Psychology and Psychiatry*, 44(1), 88–106.

Wolpert, M. and Fredman, G. (1994). Remodelling the referral pathway to mental health services for children. *Association for Child Psychology and Psychiatry Review Newsletter*, 1(3), 98–103.

Chapter 9 School-based interventions for ADHD

Abikoff, H. and Gittelman, R. (1985). The normalizing effects of methylphenidate on the classroom behaviour of ADDH children: *Journal of Abnormal Child Psychology*, (13), 33–44.

Abramowitz, A., O'Leary, S. and Rosen, L. (1987). Reducing off-task behavior in the classroom: a comparison of encouragement and reprimands. *Journal of Abnormal Psychology*, 15(2), 153–163.

Agency for Health Care Policy and Research. (1999). *Diagnosis of Attention Deficit/ Hyperactivity Disorder: Summary. Technical Review: Number 3.* Rockville, MD.

American Academy of Child and Adolescent Psychiatry. (2007). Practice parameter for the assessment and treatment of children and adolescents with attention deficit/hyperactivity disorder. *Journal of the American Academy of Child and Adolescent Psychiatry*, (46), 894–921.

Antrop, I., Roeyers, H. and Van Oost, P. (2000). Stimulation seeking and hyperactivity in children with ADHD. *Journal of Child Psychology and Psychiatry*, (41), 225–232.

Bandura, A. (1977). *Social Learning Theory.* New Jersey: Prentice Hall.

Barbaresi, W., Katusic, S. and Colligan, R. (2007). Long-term school outcomes for children with attention deficit/hyperactivity disorder: a population-based perspective. *Journal of Developmental and Behavioral Pediatrics*, (28), 265–273.

Barber, B. and Olsen, J. (2003). Assessing the transitions to middle and high school. *Journal of Adolescent Research*, 19(1), 3–30.

Barkley, R. (1997a). Behavioral inhibitions, sustained attention and executive functions: constructing a unifying theory of ADHD. *Psychiatric Bulletin*, 121(1), 65–94.

Barkley, R. (1997b). *ADHD and the Nature of Self-Control*. New York Press.

Barkley, R. and Cunningham, C. (1978). Do stimulant drugs improve the performance of hyperkinetic children? *Clinical Pediatrics*, (17), 85–92.

Biederman, J., Newcorn, J. and Sprich, S. (1991). Comorbidity of attention deficit hyperactivity disorder with conduct, depressive, anxiety and other disorders. *American Journal of Psychiatry*, (148), 564–577.

Bitsakou, P., Psychchogiou, L., Thompson, M., and Sonuga-Barke, E. (2008). Inhibitory deficits in attention deficit hyperactivity disorder are independent of basic processing efficiency and IQ. *Journal of Neural Transmission*, 115(2), 261–268.

Brown, G. (2003). Assessment of attention deficit hyperactivity disorder. *Nursing Times*, 99(25), 34–36.

Bussing, R., Gary, F., Mills, T. and Wilson-Garvan, C. (2003). Parental explanatory models of ADHD: gender and cultural variations. *Social Psychiatry and Psychiatric Epidemiology*, (38), 563–575.

Cantor, D. (2000). The role of group therapy in promoting identity development in ADHD adolescents. *Journal of Psychotherapy in Independent Practice*, 1(2), DOI: 10.1300/J288v01n02_07.

Clark, T., Feehan, C., Tinline, C. and Vostanis, P. (1999). Autistic symptoms in children with attention deficit hyperactivity disorder. *European Child and Adolescent Psychiatry*, (8), 50–55.

Compas, B., Benson, M. and Boyer, M. (2002). Problem-solving and problem-solving therapies. In: Rutter, M., Taylor, E. and Hersov, L. (Eds). *Child and Adolescent Psychiatry* (4th Edition). Oxford: Blackwell Publishing.

Conners, C. and MHS Staff. (2000). *Conners' Continuous Performance Test II*: Computer Program for Windows Technical Guide and Software Manual. New York: Multi-Health Systems.

Conners C., Sitarenios G., Parker J. and Epstein J. (1998). Revision and restandardization of the Connors' Teacher Rating Scale (CTRS-R): factor structure, reliability, and criterion validity. *Journal of Abnormal Child Psychology*, 26 (4), 279–291.

Connors, C. (1989). *Connors Teacher Rating Scales Manual*. New York. Multi-Health Systems.

Davis, J. and Watson, N. (2000). Disabled children's rights in everyday life: problematizing notions of competency and promoting self-empowerment. *International Journal of Children's Rights*, (8), 211–228.

Department for Children, Schools and Families. (2008). *The Children's Plan*. London: HMSO.

Department for Education and Skills and Department of Health. (2006). *Looking for a School Nurse*. London: HMSO.

Department for Education and Skills and Department of Health. (2005). *Managing Medicines in Schools and Early-Years Settings*. London: HMSO.

Department of Health. (2004). *National Service Framework for Children, Young People and Maternity Services*. London: HMSO.

Department for Education and Skills. (2003). *Every Child Matters*. London: HMSO.

Department for Education and Skills. (2001). *Promoting Children's Mental Health within Early-Years and Schools Settings*. London: HMSO.

Douglas, V., Barr, R., O'Neill, M. (1986). Short-term effects of methylphenidate on the cognitive, learning and academic performance of children with attention deficit disorder in the laboratory and the classroom. *Journal of Child Psychology and Psychiatry*, (27), 191–211.

Drabman, Spitalnik, R., and O'Leary, K. (1973). *Journal of Abnormal Psychology*, (82), 20–16.

DuPaul, G. and Eckert, T. (1997a). Interventions for students with attention deficit/hyperactivity disorder: one size does not fit all. *School Psychology Review*, 26(3), 369–382.

DuPaul, G. and Eckert, T. (1997b). The effects of school-based interventions for attention deficit hyperactivity disorder: a meta-analysis. *School Psychology Review*, 26(1), 5–27.

Ervin, R., DuPaul, G., Kern, L. and Friman, P. (1998). Classroom-based functional and adjunctive assessments: proactive approaches to intervention selection for adolescents with attention deficit hyperactivity disorder. *Journal of Applied Behavior Analysis*, (31), 65–78.

Fonagy, P, Target, M, Cottrell, D, Phillips, J. and Kurtz, Z. (2002). *What Works for Whom?: a Critical Review of Treatments for Children and Adolescents*. London: Guilford Press.

Ford, T., Goodman, R. and Meltzer, H. (2004). The relative importance of child, family, school and neighbourhood correlates of childhood psychiatric disorder. *Social Psychiatry and Psychiatric Epidemiology*, (39), 487–496.

Frame, K., Kelly, L. and Bayley, E. (2003). Increasing perceptions of self-worth in pre-adolescents diagnosed with ADHD. *Journal of Nursing Scholarship*, 35(3), 225–229.

Frankel, F., Myatt, R., Cantwell, D. and Feinberg, D. (1997). Parent-assisted transfer of social skills training: effects on children with and without attention deficit hyperactivity disorder. *Journal of the American Academy of Child and Adolescent Psychiatry*, (36), 1056–64.

Frazier, T., Youngstrom, E. and Glutting, J. (2007). ADHD and achievement: meta-analysis of the child, adolescent and adult literatures and a concomitant study with college students. *Journal of Learning Disabilities*, (40), 49–65.

Furman, L. (2005). What is attention deficit hyperactivity disorder? *Journal of Child Neurology*, 20(12), 994–1002.

Galton, M., Gray, J. and Ruddock, J. (1999). *The Impact of School Transitions and Transfers on Pupil Progress and Attainment*. London: Department for Education and Skills.

Gaub, M. and Carlson, C. (1997). Behavioral characteristics of DSM-IV ADHD subtypes in a school-based population, Journal of Abnormal Child Psychology 25(2), 103–111.

Gelfand, D. and Hartmann, D. (1984). *Child Behavior Analysis and Therapy*. New York: Pergamon Press.

Gol, D. and Jarus, T. (2005). Effect of a social skills training group on everyday activities of children with attention deficit hyperactivity disorder. *Developmental Medicine and Child Neurology*, (47), 539–545.

Goodman, R. (1997). The extended version of the Strengths and Difficulties Questionnaire as a guide to child psychiatric caseness and consequent burden. *Journal of Child Psychology and Psychiatry and Allied Disciplines*, (40), 791–799.

Gowers, S., Thomas, S. and Deeley, S. (2004). Can primary schools contribute effect-ively to tier 1 child mental health services? *Clinical Child Psychology and Psychiatry*, (9), 419–425.

Green, C. and Chee, K. (2001). *Understanding ADHD* (3rd Edition). Sydney: Doubleday Press.

Green, H., McGinnity, A., Meltzer, H., Ford, T. and Goodman, R. (2005). *Mental Health of Children and Young People in Great Britain*. London: ONS.

Hartsough, C. and Lambert, N. (1985). Medical factors in hyperactive and normal children: prenatal, development and health history findings. *American Journal of Orthopsychiatry*, (55), 190–210.

Hill, P. (2005). Attention deficit hyperactivity disorder. *Archives of Disease in Childhood*, 90(1), doi: 10.1136/adc.2004.058842.

Hinshaw, S. (2002). Pre-adolescent girls with attention deficit hyperactivity dis-order (1): background characteristics, comorbidity, cognitive and social function-ing and parenting practices. *Journal of Consulting and Clinical Psychology*, (70), 1086–1098.

Hjorne, E. (2007). Pedagogy in the 'ADHD classroom'. In: Lloyd, D., Stead, J. and Cohen, D. (Eds). *Critical New Perspectives on ADHD*. London: Routledge.

Horstmann, K. and Steer, J. (2007). Transition into a secondary school for children with a diagnosis of attention deficit hyperactivity disorder or autistic spectrum disorder: a pilot group. *Clinical Psychology Forum*, (176), August 2007.

Jensen, P., Martin, D. and Cantwell, D. (1997). Comorbidity in ADHD: implications for research, practice and DSM-V. *Journal of the American Academy of Child and Adolescent Psychiatry*. (36), 1065–1079.

Jerome, L., Gordon, M., and Hustler, P. (1994). Comparison of American and Canadian teachers' knowledge and attitudes towards attention deficit hyperactivity disorder (ADHD). *Canadian Journal of Psychiatry*, (39), 563–566.

Kagan, J. (1965). Reflection-impulsivity and reading ability in primary grade child-ren. *Child Development*, 36(3), 609–628.

Kendall, J. (1999). Sibling accounts of attention deficit hyperactivity disorder (ADHD). *Family Process*, (38), 117–136.

Kidd, P. (2000). Attention deficit/hyperactivity disorder in children: rationale for its integrative management. *Alternative Medicine Review*, 5(5), 402–428.

Klingberg, T., Forssberg, H. and Westerberg, H. (2002). Training of working memory in children with ADHD. *Journal of Clinical and Experimental Neuropsychology*, 24(6), 781–791.

Leighton, S. (2006). Nursing and school-based mental health services. In: McDougall, T. (Ed). *Child and Adolescent Mental Health Nursing*. London: Routledge.

Leroux, J. and Levitt-Perlman, M. (2000). The gifted child with attention deficit dis-order: an identification and intervention challenge, *Roeper Review*, (22), 171–176.

Levine, M. (1997). *Frames of Mind*. Cambridge, MA: Educators Publishers.

McArdle, P. (2005). Disorders of conduct. In: Gowers, S. (Ed). *Seminars in Child and Adolescent Psychiatry* (2nd Edition). London: Gaskell.

McDougall, T. and Davren, M. (2006). The bigger picture: CAMHS, nursing and the strategic context. In: McDougall, T. (Ed). *Child and Adolescent Mental Health Nursing*. London: Routledge.

McGee, R., Prior, M. and Williams, S. (2002). The long-term significance of teacher-rated hyperactivity and reading ability in childhood: findings from two longi-tudinal studies. *Journal of Child Psychology and Psychiatry*, (43), 1004–1017.

Mental Health Foundation. (2003). *Effective Joint Working between Child and Adolescent Mental Health Services (CAMHS) and Schools*. London: HMSO.

Merrell, C. and Tymms, P. (2004). *Screening and Classroom Interventions for Inattentive, Hyperactive and Impulsive Young Children: a Longitudinal Study*. Paper presented at the Annual General Meeting of the American Educational Research Association. San Diego. 2004.

Merrell, C. and Tymms, P. (2001). Inattention, hyperactivity and impulsiveness: their impact on academic achievement and progress. *British Journal of Educational Psychology*, (71), 43–56.

Mitchell, G., Baptiste, L. and Potel, D. (2004). Developing links between school nursing and CAMHS. *Nursing Times*, 100(5), 36–39.

Morris, J. (1999). *Hurtling into a Void*. Brighton: Pavilion Publishing.

Mulligan, S. (2001). Classroom strategies used by teachers of students with attention deficit hyperactivity disorder. *Physical and Occupational Therapy in Paediatrics*, 20(4), 25–44.

National Institute for Health and Clinical Excellence. (2008a). *Social and Emotional Wellbeing in Primary Education*. (NICE Public Health Guidance 12). London: NICE.

National Institute for Health and Clinical Excellence. (2008b). *Attention Deficit Hyperactivity Disorder: Diagnosis and Management of ADHD in Children, Young People and Adults*. London: NCCMH.

Offler, E. (2000). Bullying: everybody's problem. *Paediatric Nursing*, 12(9), 22–26.

O'Regan, F. (2006). *How to Teach and Manage Children with ADHD*. London: LDA.

Pavlov, I. (1955). *Selected Works*. Moscow: Foreign Languages Publishing House.

Pelham, W., Gnagy, E., Greenslade, K., and Milich, R. (1992). Teacher ratings of DSM-III-R symptoms for the disruptive behaviour disorders. *Journal of the American Academy of Child and Adolescent Psychiatry*, (31), 210–218.

Pfiffner, L., Barkley, R. and DuPaul, G. (2006). Treatment of ADHD in School Settings: In: Barkley, R. and Murphy, K. (Eds). *Attention Deficit Hyperactivity Disorder: a Clinical Workbook* (3rd Edition). New York: Guilford Press.

Pitcher, T., Piek, J. and Hay, D. (1987). Fine and gross motor ability in males with ADHD. *Developmental Medicine and Child Neurology*, (45), 525–535.

Poduska, J. (2000). Parents' perceptions of their first graders' need for mental health and educational services. *Journal of the American Academy of Child and Adolescent Psychiatry*, (39), 584–591.

Porter, L. (1988). The what, why and how of hyperkinesis. *Journal of Advanced Nursing*, (13), 229–236.

Rapport, M., Denney, C., DuPaul, G. and Gardner, M. (1994). Attention deficit disorder and methylphenidate: normalisation rates, clinical effectiveness and response prediction in 76 children. *Journal of the American Academy of Child and Adolescent Psychiatry*, (33), 882–893.

Reid, G. (2007). Managing attention difficulties in the classroom. In: Lloyd, D., Stead, J. and Cohen, D. (Eds). *Critical New Perspectives on ADHD*. London: Routledge.

Rhodes, J. and Ajmal, Y. (1995). *Solution-Focused Thinking in Schools*. London: BT Press.

Rigby, K. (2002). *New Perspectives on Bullying*. London: Jessica Kingsley.

Rones, M. and Hoagwood, K. (2000). School-based mental health services: a research review. *Clinical Child and Family Psychology Review*, 3(4), 223–241.

Rucklidge, J. and Tannock, R. (2001). Psychiatric, psychosocial and cognitive functioning of female adolescents with ADHD. *Journal of American Academy of Child and Adolescent Psychiatry*, (40), 530–540.

Sandberg, S. (2002). Psychosocial contributions. In: Sandberg, S. (Ed). *Hyperactivity and Attention Disorder of Childhood* (2nd Edition). Cambridge: Cambridge University Press.

Sayal, K., Hornsey, H. and Warren, S. (2006a). Identification of children at risk of attention deficit/hyperactivity disorder: a school-based intervention. *Social Psychiatry and Psychiatric Epidemiology*, (47), 744–750.

Sayal, K., Goodman, R. and Ford, T. (2006b). Barriers to the identification of children with attention deficit/hyperactivity disorder. *Journal of Child Psychology and Psychiatry*, (47), 744–750.

Sergeant, J., Geurts, H. and Oosterlaan, J. (2002). How specific is a deficit of executive functioning for attention deficit hyperactivity disorder? *Behavioural Brain Research*, 130(1), 3–28.

Skinner, B. (1974). *About Behaviourism*. London: Cape.

Sloan, M., Jensen, P. and Kettle, L. (1999). Assessing the services for children with ADHD: gaps and opportunities. *Journal of Attention Disorders*, (3), 13–29.

Snider, V., Busch, T. and Arrowood, L. (2003). Teacher knowledge of stimulant medication and ADHD. *Remedial and Special Education*, 24(1), 46–56.

Swanson, J., (2001). Clinical relevance of the primary findings of the MTA: success rates based on severity of ADHD and ODD symptoms at the end of treatment. *Journal of the American Academy of Child and Adolescent Psychiatry*, 40(2), 168–179.

Swanson, H., Mink, J. and Bocian, K. (1999). Cognitive processing deficits in poor readers with symptoms of reading disabilities and ADHD: more alike than different? *Journal of Educational Psychology*, 91(2), 321–333.

Tannock, R. (1999). ADHD: Advances in cognitive neurobiological and genetic research. *Journal of Child Psychology and Psychiatry*, 39(1), 65.

Taylor, E., Chadwick, O., Heptinstall, E. and Danckaerts, M. (1996). Hyperactive and conduct problems as risk factors for adolescent development. *Journal of the American Academy of Child and Adolescent Psychiatry*, (35), 1213–1226.

Thomas, G. (2004). What do we mean by EBD? In: Clough, P., Garner, P., Pardeck, J., and Yeun, F. (Eds). *Handbook of Emotional and Behavioural Difficulties*. London: Sage Publications.

Tripp, G. and Alsop, B. (2001). Sensitivity to reward delay in children with attention deficit hyperactivity disorder. *Journal of Child Psychology and Psychiatry and Allied Disciplines*, (42), 691–698.

Turpin, A. and Titheridge, A. (2001). Groupwork in schools: supporting children with behavioural difficulties. *Young Minds Magazine*, (50), 21–24.

Van der Krol, R., Oosterbaan, H., Weller, S. and Koning, A. (1998). Attention deficit hyperactivity disorder. In: Graham, P. (Ed) *Cognitive Behaviour Therapy for Children and Families*. London: Cambridge.

Weber, K., Frankenberger, W. and Heilman, K. (1992). The effects of Ritalin on the academic achievement of children diagnosed with attention deficit hyperactivity disorder. *Developmental Disabilities Bulletin*, (20), 49–68.

West, J., Taylor, M., Houghton, S. and Hudyma, S. (2005). A comparison of teachers' and parents' knowledge and beliefs about attention deficit hyperactivity disorder. *School Psychology International*, 26(2), 192–208.

World Health Organisation. (1997). *Child Mental Health and Psychosocial Development: Technical Report Series 613*. Geneva: WHO.

Weare, K. (1999). *Promoting Mental, Emotional and Social Health: a Whole-School Approach*. London: Routledge.

Wells, K., Pelham, W. and Kotkin, R. (2000). Psychosocial treatment strategies in the MTA study: rationale, methods and critical issues in design and implementation. *Journal of Abnormal Child Psychology*, (28), 483–505.

Whalen, C., Henker, B. and Collins, B. (1979). A social ecology of hyperactive boys: medication effects in structured classroom environments. *Journal of Applied Behavior Analysis*, (12), 65–81.

Wood, A. and Hughes, S. (2005). Psychosocial approaches and psychotherapies. In: Gowers, S. (Ed). *Seminars in Child and Adolescent Psychiatry* (2nd Edition). London: Gaskell.

Woolley, I. (2006). Treatment interventions for children and young people with mental health problems. In: McDougall, T. (Ed). *Child and Adolescent Mental Health Nursing*. London: Routledge.

Young, S. and Bramham, J. (2007). *ADHD in Adults: a Psychological Guide to Practice*. London: Wiley and Sons.

Zentall, S. (1993). Research on the educational implications of attention deficit hyperactivity disorder. *Exceptional Children*, (60), 143–153.

Chapter 10 Adults with ADHD

Adler, L. and Chua, H. (2002). Management of ADHD in adults. *Journal of Clinical Psychiatry*, 63(12), 29–35.

Asherson, P. (2005). Clinical assessment and treatment of attention deficit hyperactivity disorder in adults. *Expert Review of Neurotherapeutics*, 5(4), 525–539.

Barkley, R. (1997). Advancing age, declining ADHD. *American Journal of Psychiatry*, 154(9), 1323–1325.

Barkley, R., Murphy, K. and Kwasnik, D. (1996). Psychological adjustment and adaptive impairments in young adults with ADHD. *Journal of Attention Disorders*, 1(1), 41–54.

Barkley, R. Murphy, K. and Fischer, M. (2007). *ADHD in Adults: What the Science Says*. New York: Guildford Publications.

Biederman, J., Mick, E. and Faraone, S. (2000). Age-dependent decline of symptoms of attention deficit hyperactivity disorder: impact of remission, definition and symptom type. *American Journal of Psychiatry*, (157), 816–818.

Boonstra, A., Oosterlaan, J., Sergeant, J. and Buitelaar, J. (2005). Executive functioning in adult ADHD: a meta-analytic review. *Psychological Medicine*, (35), 1097–1108.

Brown, T. (1996). *Brown Attention Deficit Disorder Scales*. Texas: Psychological Corporation, Harcourt Brace and Company.

Conners, C., Erhardt, D., Epstein, J., Parker, J., Sitarenios, G. and Sparrow, E. (1999). Self-ratings of ADHD symptoms in adults 1: factor structure and normative data. *Journal of Attention Disorders*, 3(3), 141–151.

Conners, C., Erhardt, D. and Sparrow, E. (1998). *The Conners Adult ADHD Rating Scale (CAARS)*. Toronto: Multi-Health Systems Inc.

Copeland, E. (1991). *Medications for Attention Disorders (ADHD/ADD) and Related Medical Problems (Tourette's Syndrome, Sleep Apnea, Seizure Disorders)*. Atlanta: SPI Press.

Dalsgaard, S., Mortensen, P., and Frydenberg, M. (2002). Conduct problems, gender and the adult psychiatric outcome of children with attention deficit hyperactivity disorder. *British Journal of Psychiatry*, (181), 416–421.

Eakin, L., Minde, L., Hetchman, E., Ochs, E., Krane, E., Bouffard, B., Greenfield, B., and Looper, K. (2004). The marital and family functioning of adults with ADHD and their spouses. *Journal of Attention Disorders*, 8(1), 1–9.

Elliot, H. (2002). Attention deficit hyperactivity disorder in adults: a guide for the primary care physician. *Southern Medical Journal*, 95(7), 736–742.

Faraone, S. and Biederman, J. (2005). What is the prevalence of adult ADHD?: results of a population screen of 966 adults. *Journal of Attention Disorders*, 9, 384–391.

Faraone, S., Biederman, J., Mennin, D., Wozniak, J. and Spencer, T. (1997). Attention deficit hyperactivity with bipolar disorder: a familial subtype? *Journal of the American Academy of Child and Adolescent Psychiatry*, 36(10), 1378–1390.

Faraone, S., Biederman, J. and Mick, E. (2006). The age-dependent decline of attention deficit hyperactivity disorder: a meta-analysis of follow-up studies. *Psychological Medicine*, 36, 159–165.

Fergusson, D. and Boden, J. (2007). Cannabis use and adult ADHD symptoms. *Drug and Alcohol Dependence*, (95), 90–96.

Fryers, T. (2007). *Children at Risk: Childhood Determinants of Adult Psychiatric Disorder*. Helsinki: Stakes.

Gunter, T., Arndt, S., Wenman, G., Allen, J., Loveless, P., Sieleni, B. and Black, D. (2008). Frequency of mental and addictive disorders among 320 men and women entering the Iowa prison system: use of the MINI-Plus. *Journal of the American Academy of Psychiatry and the Law*, (36), 27–34.

Hallowell, E. and Ratey, J. (1994). *Driven to Distraction: Recognizing and Coping with Attention Deficit Disorder from Childhood to Adulthood*. New York: Pantheon Press.

Harpin, V. (2005). The effect of ADHD on the life of an individual, their family, and community from preschool to adult life. *Archives of Disease in Childhood*, 90(1), 2–7.

Ingram, S., Hechtman, L. and Morgenstern, G. (1999). Outcome issues in ADHD: adolescent and adult long-term outcomes. *Mental Retardation and Developmental Disabilities Research Reviews*, 5(3), 243–250.

Keen, D., Bramble, D. and Olurin-Lynch, J. (2000). Attention deficit hyperactivity disorder: how much do we see? *Child Psychology and Psychiatry Review*, (5), 164–168.

Kessler, R., Adler, L., Ames, M. (2005a). The prevalence and effects of adult attention deficit hyperactivity disorder on work performance in a nationally representative sample of workers. *Journal of Occupational and Environmental Medicine*, (47), 565–572.

Kessler, R., Adler, L., Ames, M., Demler, O., Faraone, S., Hiripi, E., Howes, M., Jin, R., Secnik, K., Spencer, T., Ustun, B., and Walters, E. (2005b). The World Health Organisation adult ADHD self report scale (ASRS): a short screening scale for use in the general population. *Psychological Medicine*, (35), 245–256.

McDougall, T. (2007). Target practice: are children's services up to scratch? *Mental Health Practice*, 10(6), 11–14.

McGough, J. and Barkley, R. (2004). Diagnostic controversies in adult attention deficit hyperactivity disorder. *American Journal of Psychiatry*, (161), 1948–1956.

Millstein, R., Wilens, T., Biederman, J. and Spencer, T. (1997). Presenting ADHD symptoms and subtypes in clinically referred adults with ADHD. *Journal of Attention Disorders*, 2(3), 159–166.

Murray, C. and Johnston, C. (2006). Parenting in mothers with and without attention deficit/hyperactivity disorder. *Journal of Abnormal Psychology*, 115(1), 52–61.

Murphy, K. and Adler, L. (2004). Assessing attention deficit/hyperactivity disorder in adults: focus on rating scales. *Journal of Clinical Psychiatry*, 65(3), 7.

National Institute for Health and Clinical Excellence. (2008). *Attention Deficit Hyperactivity Disorder: Diagnosis and Management of ADHD in Children, Young People and Adults*. London: NCCMH.

NHS Quality Improvement Scotland. (2007). *ADHD: Services over Scotland: Report of the Service Profiling Exercise 2007*. Edinburgh: NHS Scotland.

Nutt, D., Fone, K., Asherson, P., Bramble, D., Hill, P., Matthews, K., Morris, K., Santosh, P., Sonuga-Barke, E., Taylor, E., Weiss, M., and Young, S. (2007). Evidence-based guidelines for management of attention deficit hyperactivity disorder in adolescents in transition to adult services and in adults: recommendations from the British Association for Psychopharmacology. *Journal of Psychopharmacology*, 21(1), 10–41.

Ramsay, R. and Rostain, A. (2003). A cognitive therapy approach for adult attention deficit/hyperactivity disorder. *Journal of Cognitive Psychotherapy: an International Quarterly*, (17), 319–333.

Rapport, L., Friedman, S., Tzelepis, A. and Van Voorhis, A. (2002). Experienced emotion and affect recognition in adult attention deficit hyperactivity disorder. *Neuropsychology*, 16(1), 102–110.

Rosler, M., Retz, W., Retz-Junginger, P., Hengesch, G., Schneider, M., Supprian, T., Schwitzgebel, P., Pinhard, K., Dovi-Akue, N., Wender, P. and Thome, P. (2004). Prevalence of attention-deficit/hyperactivity disorder (ADHD) and comorbid disorders in young male prison inmates. *European Archives of Psychiatry and Clinical Neurosciences*, (254), 365–371.

Rostain, A. and Ramsay, R. (2006). A combined treatment approach for adults with ADHD – results of an open study of 43 patients. *Journal of Attention Disorders*, 10(2), 150–159.

Rutter, M. (1989). Isle of Wight revisited: twenty-five years of child psychiatric epidemiology. *Journal of the American Academy of Child and Adolescent Psychiatry*, 28(5), 633–653.

Safren, S., Otto, M., Sprich, S., Winett, C., Wilens, T., and Biederman, J. (2005a). Cognitive behavioral therapy for ADHD in medication-treated adults with continued symptoms. *Behaviour Research and Therapy*, 43(7), 831–842.

Safren, S., Sprich, S. and Chulvick, M. (2005b). Psychosocial treatments for adults with attention deficit hyperactivity disorder. *Psychiatric Clinics of North America*, 27(2), 349–360.

Sayal, K. (2008). Attention deficit hyperactivity disorder. In: Jackson, C., Hill, K. and Lavis, P. (Eds). *Child and Adolescent Mental Health Today: a Handbook*. London: Pavilion.

Sonuga-Barke, E., Daley, D. and Thompson, M. (2005). Does maternal ADHD reduce the effectiveness of parent training for pre-school children's ADHD? *Journal of American Academy of Child and Adolescent Psychiatry*, (41), 696–702.

Spencer, T., Biederman, J. and Wilens, T. (1998). Adults with attention deficit hyperactivity disorder: a controversial diagnosis. *Journal of Clinical Psychiatry*, (59 supplement 7), 59–68.

Taylor, E., Chadwick, O., Heptinstall, E., and Danckaerts, M. (1996). Hyperactivity and conduct problems as risk factors for adolescent development. *Journal of American Academy of Child and Adolescent Psychiatry*, (35), 1213–1226.

Ward, M., Wender, P., and Reimherr, F. (1993). The Wender Utah Rating Scale: an aid in the retrospective diagnosis of attention deficit hyperactivity disorder. *American Journal of Psychiatry*, (150), 885–890.

Weiss, G. and Hechtman, L. (1993). *Hyperactive Children Grown Up* (2nd Edition). New York: Guilford.

Weiss, M. and Murray, C. (2003). Assessment and management of attention deficit hyperactivity disorder in adults. *Canadian Medical Association Journal*, (168), 717–722.

Wender, P. (2000). *Attention Deficit Hyperactivity Disorder in Children and Adults*. New York: Oxford University Press.

Wender, P., Reimherr, F. and Wood, D. (1981). Attention deficit disorder ('minimal brain dysfunction') in adults. *Archives of General Psychiatry*, (38), 449–456.

Wexler, H. (1996). ADHD substance abuse and crime. *Attention*, 2(3), 27–32.

Wilens, T., Biederman, J., Spencer, T. and Prince, J. (1995). Pharmacotherapy of adult attention deficit hyperactivity disorder: a review. *Journal of Clinical Psychopharmacology*, 15(4), 270–279.

Wilens, T., Gignac, M., Swezey, A., Monuteaux, M. and Biederman, J. (2006). Characteristics of adolescents and young adults with ADHD who divert or misuse their prescribed medications. *Journal of the Academy of Child and Adolescent Psychiatry*, 45(4), 408–414.

Wilens, T., Spencer, T. and Biederman, J. (2002). A review of the pharmacotherapy of adults with attention deficit/hyperactivity disorder. *Journal of Attention Disorders*, 5(4), 189–202.

Wood, D., Reimherr, F., Wender, P. and Johnson, G. (1976). Diagnosis and treatment of minimal brain dysfunction in adults: a preliminary report. *Archives of General Psychiatry*, (33), 1453–1460.

Woods, S., Lovejoy, D., and Ball, J. (2002). Neuropsychological characteristics of adults with ADHD: a comprehensive review of initial studies. *The Clinical Neuropsychologist*, (16), 12–34.

Young, S., Toone, B. and Tyson, C. (2003a). Comorbidity and psychosocial profile of adults with attention deficit hyperactivity disorder. *Personality and Individual Differences*, (35), 743–755.

Young, S., Gudjonsson, G., Ball, S. and Lam, J. (2003b). Attention deficit hyperactivity disorder (ADHD) in personality-disordered offenders and the association with disruptive behavioural problems. *Journal of Forensic Psychiatry and Psychology*, 14 (3), 491–505.

Young, S. and Bramham, J. (2007). *ADHD in adults: a psychological guide to practice*. London: Wiley and Sons.

Young, S., Bramham, J., Gray, K. and Rose, E. (2008). The experience of receiving a diagnosis and treatment of ADHD in adulthood: a qualitative study of clinically referred patients using interpretative phenomenological analysis. *Journal of Attention Disorders*, 11(4), 493–503.

Chapter 11 Nurse prescribing and ADHD

Armstrong, M. (2006). Self-harm, young people and nursing. In: McDougall, T. (Ed). *Child and Adolescent Mental Health Nursing*. London: Blackwell.

Ashmore, R. and Carver, N. (2001). Concerns over the influences that pharmaceutical representatives have as nurses. *Mental Health Practice*, 5(2), 18–19.

Avery, A. and Pringle, M. (2005). Extended prescribing by UK nurses and pharmacists. *British Medical Journal*, (331), 1154–1155.

Bailey, K. (2003). Pharmacological treatments for ADHD and the novel agent atomoxetine. *Journal of Psychosocial Nursing*, 41(8), 12–17.

Bailey, K. (1999). Framework for prescriptive practice. In: Shea, C. and Pelletier, L. *et al.* (Eds). *Advanced Practice Nursing in Psychiatric and Mental Health Care*. St Louis: Mosby.

Barlow, M., Magorrain, K., Jones, M. and Edwards, K. (2008). Nurse prescribing in an Alzheimer's disease service: a reflective account. *Mental Health Practice*, 11(7), 32–35.

Bradley, E. and Nolan, P. (2005). Non-medical prescribing and mental health nursing: prominent issues. *Mental Health Practice*, 8(5), 16–20.

Brimblecombe, N., Parr, A. and Gray, R. (2005). Medication and mental health nurses: developing new ways of working. *Mental Health Practice*, 8(5), 12–14.

British National Formulary. (2008). *BNF for Children*. London: BNF Publications.

Coghill, D. (2003). Current issues in child and adolescent psychopharmacology. Part 1: attention deficit hyperactivity and affective disorders. *Advances in Psychiatric Treatment*, (9), 86–94.

Conners, C. (1989a). *Conners Adolescent Self Report Rating Scale Manual*. New York: Multi-Health System.

Conners, C. (1989b). *Conners Parent Rating Scale Manual*. New York: Multi-Health System.

Conners, C. (1989c). *Conners Teacher Rating Scale Manual*. New York: Multi-Health System.

Department of Health. (2008). *Medicines Management: Everybody's Business*. London: HMSO.

Department of Health. (2007). *New Ways of Working for Everyone: Developing and Sustaining a Capable and Flexible Workforce*. London: HMSO.

Department of Health. (2006). *Improving Patients' Access to Medicines: a Guide to Implementing Nurse and Pharmacist Independent Prescribing in the NHS in England*. London: HMSO.

Department of Health. (2004a). *The NHS Knowledge and Skills Framework (NHS KSF) and the Development Review Process*. London: HMSO.

Department of Health. (2004b). *National Service Framework for Children, Young People and Maternity Services. Medicines for Children and Young People*. London: HMSO.

Department of Health. (2003). *Supplementary Prescribing by Nurses and Pharmacists within the NHS in England: a Guide for Implementation*. London: HMSO.

Department of Health. (2001). *Medicines and Older People: National Service Framework*. London: HMSO.

Department of Health. (1999). *Review of Prescribing, Supply and Administration of Medicines* (Crown Report). London. HMSO.

Department of Health. (1989). *Report for the Advisory Group on Nurse Prescribing*. (Crown Report). London. HMSO.

Department of Health. (1986). *Nursing: a Focus for Care. Report of the Community Nursing Review*. (The Cumberledge Report). London: DHSS.

Greenhill, L. (1995). Pharmacologic treatment of attention deficit hyperactivity disorder. *Psychiatric Clinics of North America*, (15), 1–28.

Gunn, J. (1990). Nurses and prescriptive authority. *Specialty Nursing Forum*, (2), 1–6.

Hemingway, S. (2003). Mental health nursing and the pharmaceutical industry. *Mental Health Practice*, 7(2), 22–23.

Heyman, I. and Santosh, P. (2002). Pharmacological and other physical treatments. In: Rutter, M. and Taylor, E. (Eds). *Child and Adolescent Psychiatry* (4th Edition). Oxford: Blackwell Publishing.

Hill, P. and Taylor, E. (2001). An auditable protocol for treating attention deficit/hyperactivity disorder. *Archives of Disease in Childhood*, (84), 404–409.

Horton, R. (2002). Nurse prescribing in the UK: right but also wrong. *Lancet*, 359(9321), 1875–1876.

Jones, A., Doyle, V., Pyke, S. and Harborne, G. (2005). New roles for nurses and psychiatrists in the management of long-term conditions. *Mental Health Practice*, 9(3), 16–20.

Jones, A. and Harbone, G. (2005). Supplementary prescribing in hospital settings. *Mental Health Practice*, 9(1), 38–40.

Jones, S. and Bhadrinath, B. (1998). GPs' views on prioritisation of child and adolescent mental health problems. *Psychiatric Bulletin*, (22), 484–486.

Keogh, B. and Doyle, L. (2008). Psychopharmacological adverse effects. *Mental Health Practice*, 11(6), 28–30.

Kersenich, C. (2000). The garden of good and evil: pharmaceutical companies and the prescriptive practices of PNPs. *Journal of Paediatric Care*, 14(6), 324–326.

Lipley, N. (2000). Rich pickings. *Nursing Standard*, 14(36), 12–13.

Ludwikowski, K. and DeValk, M. (1998). Attention deficit/hyperactivity disorder: a neurodevelopmental approach. *Journal of Child and Adolescent Psychiatric Nursing*, 11(1), 17–29.

McDougall, T. and Ryan, N. (2008). Nurse prescribing in the UK: invited commentary. *Journal of Child and Adolescent Psychiatric Nursing* (accepted for publication).

Morrison-Griffiths, S. (2002). Pre-registration nurse education in pharmacology: is it adequate for the roles that nurses are expected to fulfil? *Nurse Education Today*, (22), 447–456.

MTA Cooperative Group. (1999). A 14-month randomised clinical trial of treatment strategies for attention-deficit hyperactivity disorder. *Archives of General Psychiatry*, (56), 1073–1086.

National Institute for Health and Clinical Excellence. (2008). *Attention Deficit Hyperactivity Disorder: Diagnosis and Management of ADHD in Children, Young People and Adults*. London: NCCMH.

National Institute for Clinical Excellence. (2006). *Methylphenidate, Atomoxetine and Dexamphetamine for Attention Deficit Hyperactivity Disorder (ADHD) in Children and Adolescents*: Review of Technology Appraisal 13. London: NICE.

National Institute for Clinical Excellence. (2005a). *Bipolar Disorder: the Management of Bipolar Disorder in Adults and Adolescents in Primary and Secondary Care*. London: NICE.

National Institute for Health and Clinical Excellence. (2005b). *Depression in Children and Young People: Identification and Management in Primary, Community and Secondary Care*. Clinical Guideline 28. London: NICE.

National Institute for Health and Clinical Excellence. (2005c). *Obsessive Compulsive Disorder: Core Interventions in the Treatment of Obsessive Compulsive Disorder and Body Dysmorphic Disorder*. Clinical Guideline 31. London: NICE.

National Patient Safety Agency. (2002). *Building a Safer NHS for Patients*. London: NPSA.

National Prescribing Centre. (1999) Signposts for prescribing nurses – general principles of good prescribing. *Nurse Prescribing Bulletin*, 1, 1, 1–4.

Nursing and Midwifery Council. (2008). *The Standards of Conduct, Performance and Ethics for Nurses and Midwives*. London: NMC.

Nursing and Midwifery Council. (2007). *Standards for Medicines Management*. London: NMC.

Nursing and Midwifery Council. (2006a). *Standards for Proficiency for Nurse and Midwife Prescribers: Protecting the Public Through Professional Standards*. London: NMC.

Nursing and Midwifery Council. (2006b). *Prescribing Practice: Clinical Management Plans*. London: NMC News.

Nolan, P. and Badger, F. (2000). Mental health nurse prescribing: added chore or golden opportunity? *Mental Health Practice*, 4(1), 12–15.

Nolan, P., Bradley, E. and Carr, N. (2004a). Nurse prescribing and the enhancement of mental health services. *Nurse Prescriber*, (1), 207.

Nolan, P., Carr, N. and Doran, M. (2004b). Nurse prescribing: the experiences of psychiatric nurses in the United States. *Nursing Standard*, 18(26), 33–38.

Nolan, P., Carr, N. and Harold, L. (2001). Mental health nurse prescribing: the US experience. *Mental Health Practice*, 4(8), 4–7.

O'Dowd, A. (2007). The power to prescribe. *Nursing Times*, 103(3), 16–18.

Rains, A. and Scahill, L. (2006). Psychopharmacology notes. Nonstimulant medications for the treatment of ADHD. *Journal of Child and Adolescent Psychiatric Nursing*, 19(1), 44–47.

Ryan, N. (2007). Non-medical prescribing in a child and adolescent mental health service. *Mental Health Practice*, 11(1), 40–44.

Ryan, N. (2006). Nursing children and young people with attention deficit hyperactivity disorder (ADHD) In: McDougall, T. (Ed). *Child and Adolescent Mental Health Nursing*. London: Blackwell.

Scahill, L., Carroll, D. and Burke, K. (2004). Psychopharmacology notes: Methylphenidate: mechanism of action and clinical update. *Journal of Child and Adolescent Psychiatric Nursing*. 17, (2), 85–86.

Shuttle, B. (2004). Non-medical prescribing in a multidisciplinary team context. In: Courtenay, M. and Griffiths, M. (Eds). *Independent and Supplementary Prescribing: an Essential Guide*. Cambridge: Greenwich Medical Media.

Sutcliffe, A. (1999). Prescribing medicines for children. *British Medical Journal*, (319), 70–71.

Swanson, J., Wigal, S. and Greenhill, L. (1998). Analog classroom assessment of Adderall in children with ADHD. *Journal of the American Academy of Child and Adolescent Psychiatry*, (37), 519–526.

Taylor, E., Doepfner, M., Sergeant, J., Asherson, P., Banaschewski, T., Buitelaar, J., Coghill, D., Danckaerts, M., Rothenberger, A., Sonuga-Barke, E., Steinhausen, H. and Zuddas, A. (2004). European clinical guidelines for hyperkinetic disorder – first upgrade. *Journal of European Child and Adolescent Psychiatry*, (13), Supplement 1, 1–30.

Terry, J. (2003). Brief intervention: a pilot initiative in a child and adolescent mental health service. *Mental Health Practice*, 6(5), 18–20.

Till, U. (2007). The values of recovery within mental health nursing. *Mental Health Practice*, 11(3), 3–7.

Turner, T. (2007). Non-medical prescribing in community health settings. *Mental Health Practice*, 11(4), 29–32.

Chapter 12 Good practice and the legal framework

ADDISS. (2006). *ADHD is Real: ADDISS Families Survey*. London: ADDISS Resource Centre.

Department for Children, Schools and Families. (2008). *The Children's Plan*. London: HMSO.

Department for Education and Skills. (2006). *Working Together to Safeguard Children: a Guide to Interagency Working to Safeguard and Promote the Welfare of Children*. London: HMSO.

Department for Education and Skills. (2003). *Every Child Matters*. London: HMSO.

Department of Health. (2004). *National Service Framework for Children, Young People and Maternity Services*. London: HMSO.

Department of Health. (2002). *Listening, Hearing and Responding: Department of Health Action Plan Summary*. London: HMSO.

Department of Health. (2001). *Consent – What You Have a Right to Expect: a Guide for Children and Young People*. London: HMSO.

Department of Health. (2000). *The NHS Plan*. London: HMSO.

Foreman, D. (2006). Attention deficit hyperactivity disorder: legal and ethical aspects. *Archives of Diseases in Childhood*, (91), 192–194.

Gowers, S., Harrington, R. and Whitton, A. (1998). *Health of the Nation Outcome Scales for Children and Adolescents (HoNOSCA)*. London: Royal College of Psychiatrists Research Unit.

Gowers, S., Levine, W., Bailey-Rogers, S., Shore, A., and Burhouse, E. (2002). Use of a routine, self report outcome measure (HoNOSCA-SR) in two adolescent mental health services. *British Journal of Psychiatry*, (180), 266–269.

Jones, D. (2003). *Communicating with Vulnerable Children*. London: Gaskell.

Laws, S. (1999). Involving children and young people in the monitoring and evaluation of mental health services. *Healthy Minds*, (6), 3–5.

Nursing and Midwifery Council. (2008). *The Standards of Conduct, Performance and Ethics for Nurses and Midwives*. London: NMC.

Office of the Children's Commissioner. (2007). *Pushed into the Shadows: Young People's Experience of Adult Mental Health Facilities*. London: OCC.

Pugh, K, McHugh, A. and McKinstrie, F. (2006). *Two Steps Forward, One Step Back? 16–25-Year-Olds on their Journey to Adulthood*. London: YoungMinds.

Street, C. and Herts, B. (2005). *Putting Participation into Practice: a Guide for Practitioners Working in Services to Promote the Mental Health and Wellbeing of Children and Young People*. London: YoungMinds.

Tan, J. and Jones, D. (2001). Children's consent. *Current Opinion in Psychiatry*, (14), 303–307.

United Nations, (1989). Convention on the Rights of the Child. [World Wide Web] Available: *http://www.unicef.org/crc/* [2008, March 24].

Vasiliou-Theodore, C. and Penketh, K. (2008). Listen up!: young people's participation in service design and delivery. In: Jackson, C., Hill, K. and Lavis, P. (Eds). *Child and Adolescent Mental Health Today: a Handbook*. London: Pavilion.

Index

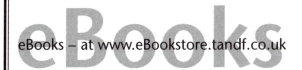

3